T0195195

Piecing Together the Puzzle of Adherence in Sleep Medicine

Editor

JESSIE P. BAKKER

SLEEP MEDICINE CLINICS

www.sleep.theclinics.com

Consulting Editor
TEOFILO LEE-CHIONG Jr

March 2021 • Volume 16 • Number 1

ELSEVIER

1600 John F. Kennedy Boulevard • Suite 1800 • Philadelphia, Pennsylvania, 19103-2899

http://www.theclinics.com

SLEEP MEDICINE CLINICS Volume 16, Number 1
March 2021, ISSN 1556-407X, ISBN-13: 978-0-323-76148-2

Editor: Joanna Collett
Developmental Editor: Donald Mumford

Sleep Medicine Clinics (ISSN 1556-407X) is published quarterly by Elsevier Inc., 360 Park Avenue South, New York, NY 10010-1710. Months of issue are March, June, September and December. Business and Editorial Offices: 1600 John F. Kennedy Blvd., Ste. 1800, Philadelphia, PA 19103-2899. Customer Service Office: 3251 Riverport Lane, Maryland Heights, MO 63043. Periodicals postage paid at New York, NY and additional mailing offices. Subscription prices are $225.00 per year (US individuals), $100.00 (US and Canadian students), $625.00 (US institutions), $272.00 (Canadian individuals), $252.00 (international individuals), $135.00 (International students), $656.00 (Canadian and International institutions). Foreign air speed delivery is included in all *Clinics* subscription prices. All prices are subject to change without notice. **POSTMASTER:** Send change of address to *Sleep Medicine Clinics*, Elsevier Health Sciences Division, Subscription Customer Service, 3251 Riverport Lane, Maryland Heights, MO 63043. Customer Service: **Tel: 1-800-654-2452 (U.S. and Canada); 314-447-8871 (outside U.S. and Canada). Fax: 314-447-8029. E-mail: journalscustomerservice-usa@elsevier.com (for print support); journalsonline-support-usa@elsevier.com (for online support)**.

Reprints. For copies of 100 or more of articles in this publication, please contact the Commercial Reprints Department, Elsevier Inc., 360 Park Avenue South, New York, NY 10010-1710. Tel.: 212-633-3874; Fax: 212-633-3820; E-mail: reprints@elsevier.com.

Sleep Medicine Clinics is covered in *MEDLINE/PubMed (Index Medicus)*.

SLEEP MEDICINE CLINICS

SERIES OF RELATED INTEREST

Clinics in Chest Medicine
Available at: https://www.chestmed.theclinics.com/

THE CLINICS ARE AVAILABLE ONLINE!
Access your subscription at:
www.theclinics.com

Contributors

EDITOR

JESSIE P. BAKKER, MS, PhD
Lecturer in Medicine, Division of Sleep
Medicine, Harvard Medical School, Associate
Epidemiologist, Division of Sleep and
Circadian Disorders, Brigham and Women's
Hospital, Boston, Massachusetts, USA;
Associate Director of Clinical Affairs, Sleep and
Respiratory Care, Philips, Monroeville,
Pennsylvania, USA

AUTHORS

PETER A. CISTULLI, MD PhD
Sleep Research Group, Charles Perkins
Centre, University of Sydney, Department of
Respiratory and Sleep Medicine, Royal North
Shore Hospital, Sydney, New South Wales,
Australia

SOMMER AGNEW, MSc
School of Psychological Sciences and Health,
University of Strathclyde, Glasgow, United
Kingdom

BIMAJE AKPA, MD
Assistant Professor of Medicine, Division of
Pulmonary, Allergy, Critical Care and Sleep
Medicine, University of Minnesota,
Minneapolis, Minnesota, USA

DELWYN J. BARTLETT, PhD
Clinical Associate Professor, Sleep and
Circadian Research Group, Woolcock Institute
of Medical Research, The University of Sydney,
Sydney Medical School, Sydney, New South
Wales, Australia

**RAKESH BHATTACHARJEE, MD,
DABP(SM), FRCPC, CBSM, DBSM, RPSGT**
Associate Professor of Clinical Pediatrics,
Division of Respiratory Medicine, Department
of Pediatrics, University of California, San

Diego, Rady Children's Hospital, San Diego,
California, USA

CYNTHIA L. BIANCO, MS
Clinical Research Coordinator, Department of
Psychiatry Research, Dartmouth-Hitchcock,
Concord, New Hampshire, USA

MARTHA E. BILLINGS, MD, MSc
Associate Professor of Medicine, Division of
Pulmonary, Critical Care and Sleep Medicine,
University of Washington School of Medicine,
UW Medicine Sleep Center at Harborview
Medical Center, Seattle, Washington, USA

AMY BLASE, CCRA
ResMed Corporation, San Diego, California,
USA

LUIS F. BUENAVER, PhD
Assistant Professor of Psychiatry and
Neurology, Director, Johns Hopkins Behavioral
Sleep Medicine Program, Johns Hopkins
University School of Medicine, Baltimore,
Maryland, USA

**CHING LI CHAI-COETZER, MBBS, FRACP,
PhD**
Associate Professor, Respiratory and Sleep
Consultant and Senior Post-Doctoral Research
Fellow, Adelaide Institute for Sleep Health,

College of Medicine and Public Health, Flinders University and Southern Adelaide Local Health Network, SA Health, Bedford Park, South Australia, Australia

MEGAN R. CRAWFORD, PhD
School of Psychological Sciences and Health, University of Strathclyde, Glasgow, United Kingdom

EARL CHARLES CREW, PhD
Behavioral Health Program, Mental Health Care Line, Michael E. DeBakey VA Medical Center, Psychology Division, Menninger Department of Psychiatry and Behavioral Sciences, Baylor College of Medicine, Houston, Texas, USA

ANGELA L. D'ROZARIO, PhD
School of Psychology, Faculty of Science, Brain and Mind Centre and Charles Perkins Centre, Sleep and Circadian Research Group, Woolcock Institute of Medical Research, The University of Sydney, Sydney Medical School, Sydney, New South Wales, Australia

OYKU DALCI, DDS PhD
Department of Orthodontics and Paediatric Dentistry, University of Sydney, Department of Orthodontics, Sydney Dental Hospital, Surry Hills, New South Wales, Australia

BRADLEY A. EDWARDS, PhD
Associate Professor, Department of Physiology, School of Biomedical Sciences and Biomedicine Discovery Institute, Turner Institute for Brain and Mental Health, Monash University, Melbourne, Victoria, Australia

LEANNE FLEMING, PhD
School of Psychological Sciences and Health, University of Strathclyde, Glasgow, United Kingdom

KAREN L. FORTUNA, PhD, LICSW
Assistant Professor, Department of Psychiatry, Dartmouth College, Concord, New Hampshire, USA

YAEL GALGUT, PGDip (ProfPsych)
Sleep and Circadian Research Group, Woolcock Institute of Medical Research, The University of Sydney, Sydney, New South Wales, Australia

NICOLE GRIVELL, B Nurs (Hons)
PhD Candidate, Adelaide Institute for Sleep Health, College of Medicine and Public Health, Flinders University, Bedford Park, South Australia, Australia

AILIE HAMILTON, MSc
School of Psychological Sciences and Health, University of Strathclyde, Glasgow, United Kingdom

SIMON A. JOOSTEN, MBBS, BMedSc, PhD
Monash Lung and Sleep, Monash Medical Centre, Monash Partners – Epworth, Clayton, Victoria, Australia; School of Clinical Sciences, Monash University, Melbourne, Victoria, Australia

BRENDAN T. KEENAN, MS
Co-director, Biostatistics Core, Division of Sleep Medicine, Department of Medicine, University of Pennsylvania, Translational Research Laboratories, Philadelphia, Pennsylvania, USA

ROO KILLICK, MBBS, FRACP, PhD
Honorary Affiliate, Woolcock Institute of Medical Research, The University of Sydney, Sydney, New South Wales, Australia

SAMUEL T. KUNA, MD
Professor of Medicine, University of Pennsylvania Perelman School of Medicine, Center for Sleep and Circadian Neurobiology, Chief, Sleep Medicine, Sleep Medicine Section, Corporal Michael J. Crescenz VA Medical Center, Philadelphia, Pennsylvania, USA

SIMON D. KYLE, PhD
Sleep and Circadian Neuroscience Institute, Nuffield Department of Clinical Neurosciences, University of Oxford, Oxford, United Kingdom

SHANE A. LANDRY, PhD
Department of Physiology, School of Biomedical Sciences and Biomedical Discovery Institute, Turner Institute for Brain and Mental Health, Monash University, Melbourne, Victoria, Australia

NATHANIEL S. MARSHALL, PhD
Honorary Affiliate, Woolcock Institute of Medical Research, Associate Professor,

Faculty of Medicine and Health, The University of Sydney, Sydney, New South Wales, Australia

STEPHANIE McCRORY, MSc
School of Psychological Sciences and Health, University of Strathclyde, Glasgow, United Kingdom

BABAK MOKHLESI, MD, MSc
Professor of Medicine, Section of Pulmonary and Critical Care, Director, Sleep Disorders Center, Director, Sleep Medicine Fellowship, The University of Chicago, Chicago, Illinois, USA

AMANDA L. MYERS, BS
Master of Public Health Candidate, Department of Public Health, Rivier University, Nashua, New Hampshire, USA

MAREK NIKOLIC, MSc
School of Psychological Sciences and Health, University of Strathclyde, Glasgow, United Kingdom

AARON OH, MBBS, FRACP
Respiratory and Sleep Consultant, Adelaide Institute for Sleep Health, College of Medicine and Public Health, Flinders University, Bedford Park, South Australia, Australia

SANJAY R. PATEL, MD, MS
Center for Sleep and Cardiovascular Outcomes Research, University of Pittsburgh, Pittsburgh, Pennsylvania, USA

SACHIN R. PENDHARKAR, MD, MSc
Associate Professor, Departments of Medicine and Community Health Sciences, Cumming School of Medicine, University of Calgary, Calgary, Alberta, Canada

NARESH M. PUNJABI, MD, PhD
Chief, Division of Pulmonary, Critical Care, and Sleep Medicine, University of Miami Miller School of Medicine, Miami, Florida, USA

BRUNO SACONI, MS, RN
Predoctoral Student, University of Pennsylvania School of Nursing, Philadelphia, Pennsylvania, USA

AMY M. SAWYER, PhD, RN
Associate Professor of Sleep and Health Behavior, Department of Biobehavioral Health Science, University of Pennsylvania School of Nursing, Corporal Michael J. Crescenz VA Medical Center, University of Pennsylvania Perelman School of Medicine, Center for Sleep and Circadian Neurobiology, Philadelphia, Pennsylvania, USA

RICHARD J. SCHWAB, MD
Chief, Division of Sleep Medicine, Professor, Department of Medicine, University of Pennsylvania, University of Pennsylvania Medical Center, Philadelphia, Pennsylvania, USA

STEPHEN SMAGULA, PhD
Assistant Professor, Department of Psychiatry, University of Pittsburgh School of Medicine, Pittsburgh, Pennsylvania, USA

KATE SUTHERLAND, PhD
Sleep Research Group, Charles Perkins Centre, University of Sydney, Department of Respiratory and Sleep Medicine, Royal North Shore Hospital, Sydney, New South Wales, Australia

ANNIE VALLIÈRES, PhD
École de psychologie, Pavillon Félix-Antoine-Savard, Université Laval, Québec, Québec, Canada

DOUGLAS M. WALLACE, MD
Associate Professor of Clinical Neurology, Department of Neurology, Sleep Medicine Division, University of Miami Miller School of Medicine, Miami VA Healthcare System, Neurology Service, Bruce W. Carter Department of Veterans Affairs Medical Center, Miami, Florida, USA

ALEXA J. WATACH, PhD, RN
Postdoctoral Research Fellow, University of Pennsylvania Perelman School of Medicine, Center for Sleep and Circadian Neurobiology, University of Pennsylvania School of Nursing, Philadelphia, Pennsylvania, USA

JEREMY WEARN, MD
Assistant Professor, Sleep Medicine and Internal Medicine, Oregon Health & Science University, Portland VAMC, Portland, Oregon, USA

NATASHA J. WILLIAMS, EdD, MPH
Department of Population Health, Division of Health and Behavior, Center for Healthful Behavior Change, New York University Grossman School of Medicine, New York, New York, USA

WILLIAM K. WOHLGEMUTH, PhD
Psychology Service, Bruce W. Carter Department of VA Medical Center, Miami VA Healthcare System, Sleep Disorders Center, Neurology Service, Bruce W. Carter Department of Veterans Affairs Medical Center, Miami, Florida, USA

AI-MING WONG, MBBS, BMedSc, PhD
Monash Lung and Sleep, Monash Medical Centre, Clayton, Victoria, Australia; School of Clinical Sciences, Monash University, Melbourne, Victoria, Australia

Contents

limited information on the characteristics and pattern of positive airway pressure (PAP) adherence in patients with OHS compared with eucapnic patients with obstructive sleep apnea (OSA). This article discusses in detail the impact of PAP therapy on outcomes in patients with OHS, compares adherence between continuous PAP and noninvasive ventilation in OHS, and compares PAP adherence in patients with OHS to patients with moderate to severe OSA enrolled in clinical trials designed to improve CPAP adherence.

The high burden of obstructive sleep apnea (OSA), combined with inadequate supply of sleep specialists and constraints on polysomnography resources, has prompted interest in alternative models of care to improve access and treatment effectiveness. In appropriately selected patients, ambulatory clinical pathways and use of nonphysicians or primary care providers to manage OSA can improve timely access and costs without compromising adherence or other clinical outcomes. Although initial studies show promising results, there are several potential barriers that must be considered before broad implementation, and further implementation research and economic evaluation studies are required.

This article reviews the evidence to date examining whether adherence to positive airway pressure (PAP) therapy is affected by any device modifications to pressure delivery. To date there is no robust evidence from systematic reviews and meta-analyses indicating that any modification to standard fixed-pressure PAP makes a clinically significant difference to patient adherence to therapy. The main modifications are reviewed in this article and whether improving pressure could drive adherence, in turn improving patient outcomes, is discussed.

The ability to remotely monitor positive airway pressure therapy adherence and efficacy provides a unique opportunity for the field of sleep medicine to quickly and efficiently improve patient adherence. Smaller randomized studies and larger-scale retrospective evaluations show that telemedicine interventions leveraging these data can increase average usage and efficiency of care. However, more evidence on the impact of these programs on longer-term adherence and improving patient-reported outcomes is needed. Combining data from remote monitoring with clinical information in electronic health records may prove to be invaluable to the future of clinical sleep medicine practice and research.

Preface

Piecing Together the Puzzle of Adherence in Sleep Medicine

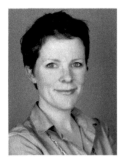

Jessie P. Bakker, MS, PhD
Editor

This issue of *Sleep Medicine Clinics* focuses primarily on our current understanding and future directions regarding adherence to therapy for sleep disorders, as described by experts in the field. The title, "Piecing Together the Puzzle of Adherence," nods to how much we have learned to date while acknowledging that adherence remains a complex and puzzling behavioral phenomenon.

Much of our understanding of adherence to sleep therapies has arisen from studies of positive airway pressure (PAP) treatment of sleep-disordered breathing, and as such, eight reviews in this issue are devoted to various PAP topics. Successful application of PAP was first reported in a seminal 1981 publication,[1] and although widespread thought at the time was that PAP would represent a useful research tool rather than a first-line therapy,[2] research regarding self-reported use of PAP at home appeared just three years later[3] and has remained a major focus of study since. Early home use of PAP required medical-grade silicone rubber to seal the mask that was made for each patient from a facial mold,[4] and thus, the rate of adhesive consumption provided the first surrogate measure of objective adherence. This metric soon gave way to meter readings beginning in the late 1980s,[5] and eventually it became possible to identify "mask on" time linked to clock time, providing a temporal understanding of usage patterns. Data transmission progressed similarly, moving from pen-and-paper readings, to secure digital and universal serial bus memory cards, and more recently, to wireless transmission with cloud-based remote access. These advancements have allowed adherence research to flourish alongside the expanding use of PAP in various settings.

Looking beyond PAP, Sutherland and colleagues present a review of adherence to oral appliances, which can now be monitored objectively using temperature microsensors. Agnew and colleagues present a systematic review of the cognitive behavioral therapy for insomnia literature and provide five key recommendations regarding the measurement and reporting of adherence to behavioral therapy in future studies. New and emerging therapies for sleep-disordered breathing, including hypoglossal nerve stimulation, expiratory resistance valves, suction devices, and pharmaceuticals, present their own adherence-related challenges, as reviewed by Joosten and colleagues. Together, these articles emphasize that as various modalities for treating complex and often overlapping sleep disorders become more established, methods for supporting adherence will continue to be needed.

As the 40th anniversary of PAP approaches this year, it is timely to reflect on the fact that in this short period of time, PAP technology has advanced to the point of providing what is arguably the most prolific method of monitoring detailed, objective therapy adherence in real-world settings.[6,7] The recent expansion of digital

Sleep Med Clin 16 (2021) xiii–xiv
https://doi.org/10.1016/j.jsmc.2020.12.002

medicine, however, has led to substantial technological advancements in digital monitoring tools across other therapeutic areas.[8,9] Until recently, monitoring adherence to pharmaceutical treatments has been limited to assaying biomarkers, which is impractical in most settings, or surrogate measurements, such as refill rates, pill counts, and Bluetooth-enabled pill bottles, which record the times at which the device is used, but not whether the drug was actually taken.[10] It is now possible to measure objective adherence to pharmaceuticals with devices such as digital pills, which are capsules containing a digital radiofrequency emitter alongside the medication,[11] or smart inhalers, which allow for audio analysis of inhalation, breath-hold, and exhalation.[12] Thus, despite sleep medicine being one of the more advanced fields of adherence research, there is much we can learn from investigators focused on other diseases. As such, this issue concludes with a review by Bianco and colleagues of smartphone app interventions designed to assist people with mental illness take their medications as prescribed, as a perspective on adherence research from outside of the sleep field. I wish to thank all authors sincerely for their valuable contributions to this issue.

DISCLOSURE

Dr Bakker is a full-time employee of Philips, which is a company that focuses on sleep and respiratory care. Dr Bakker also has a part-time appointment at Brigham and Women's Hospital. Dr Bakker's interests were reviewed and are managed by Brigham and Women's Hospital and Partners HealthCare in accordance with their conflict-of-interest policies.

Jessie P. Bakker, MS, PhD
Division of Sleep and Circadian Disorders
Brigham and Women's Hospital
221 Longwood Avenue
Boston, MA 02115, USA

E-mail address:
jpbakker@bwh.harvard.edu

REFERENCES

1. Sullivan CE, Issa FG, Berthon-Jones M, et al. Reversal of obstructive sleep apnoea by continuous positive airway pressure applied through the nares. Lancet 1981;1(8225):862–5.
2. Sullivan CE. Nasal positive airway pressure and sleep apnea. Reflections on an experimental method that became a therapy. Am J Respir Crit Care Med 2018;198(5):581–7.
3. McEvoy RD, Thornton AT. Treatment of obstructive sleep apnea syndrome with nasal continuous positive airway pressure. Sleep 1984;7(4):313–25.
4. Grunstein RR. Nasal continuous positive airway pressure treatment for obstructive sleep apnoea. Thorax 1995;50(10):1106–13.
5. Krieger J, Kurtz D. Objective measurement of compliance with nasal CPAP treatment for obstructive sleep apnoea syndrome. Eur Respir J 1988; 1(5):436–8.
6. Patel SR, Bakker JP, Stitt CJ, et al. Age and sex disparities in adherence to CPAP. Chest 2020, in press.
7. Cistulli PA, Armitstead J, Pepin JL, et al. Short-term CPAP adherence in obstructive sleep apnea: a big data analysis using real world data. Sleep Med 2019;59:114–6.
8. Godfrey A, Vandendriessche B, Bakker JP, et al. Fit-for-purpose biometric monitoring technologies: leveraging the laboratory biomarker experience. Clin Transl Sci 2020.
9. Manta C, Patrick-Lake B, Goldsack JC. Digital measures that matter to patients: a framework to guide the selection and development of digital measures of health. Digit Biomark 2020;4(3):69–77.
10. Mehta SJ, Asch DA, Troxel AB, et al. Comparison of pharmacy claims and electronic pill bottles for measurement of medication adherence among myocardial infarction patients. Med Care 2019;57(2):e9–14.
11. Martani A, Genevieve LD, Poppe C, et al. Digital pills: a scoping review of the empirical literature and analysis of the ethical aspects. BMC Med Ethics 2020;21(1):3.
12. Sulaiman I, Seheult J, MacHale E, et al. Irregular and ineffective: a quantitative observational study of the time and technique of inhaler use. J Allergy Clin Immunol Pract 2016;4(5):900–9 e902.

What is a Clinically Meaningful Target for Positive Airway Pressure Adherence?

Aaron Oh, MBBS, FRACP[a], Nicole Grivell, B Nurs (Hons)[b],
Ching Li Chai-Coetzer, MBBS, FRACP, PhD[b,c,*]

KEYWORDS

• PAP • Adherence • Positive airway pressure • Obstructive sleep apnea • Compliance

KEY POINTS

- Good positive airway pressure (PAP) adherence often is defined as usage greater than or equal to 4 hours/night, or greater than or equal to 4 hours/night and greater than or equal to 70% of nights; however, the rationale for this is unclear.
- Research evidence has shown that the optimum duration of PAP usage per night is variable, depending on the patient outcome of interest.
- Studies suggest that target PAP usage in patients with moderate–severe obstructive sleep apnea (OSA) to improve daytime sleepiness is greater than or equal to 4 hours/night to 5 hours/night; quality of life is greater than or equal to 4 hours/night to 7 hours/night; neurocognitive outcomes is greater than or equal to 6 hours/night; depression is greater than or equal to 3.5 hours/night to 5 hours/night; and hypertension (in particular, resistant hypertension) is greater than or equal to 4 hours/night to 5.5 hours/night.
- Recent large-scale, randomized controlled trials have failed to show a benefit in cardiovascular disease (CVD) outcomes and mortality with PAP, thus treatment of OSA with PAP to reduce CVD and mortality risk in otherwise asymptomatic patients cannot currently be recommended.

INTRODUCTION

Positive airway pressure (PAP) is the first-line treatment of symptomatic, moderate–severe obstructive sleep apnea (OSA),[1,2] a prevalent disorder characterized by recurrent upper airway obstruction during sleep. PAP provides positive air pressure that splints the upper airway, prevents airway collapse during sleep, and corrects intermittent hypoxia. Despite being highly effective for the treatment of OSA, PAP intolerance and poor usage remain common problems.[3–5]

Good PAP adherence commonly is defined as use greater than or equal to 4 hours/night, or greater than or equal to 4 hours/night on 70% of nights in a consecutive 30-day period, as used by the US Center for Medicare & Medicaid Services.[6] The origins of and rationale for these definitions, however, are unclear. Evidence suggests that target PAP usage varies, depending on the clinical outcome of interest. This article reviews the current literature to answer the question, What can be considered a clinically meaningful target for PAP adherence?

[a] College of Medicine and Public Health, Flinders University, Sturt Road, Bedford Park, South Australia 5042, Australia; [b] Adelaide Institute for Sleep Health, College of Medicine and Public Health, Flinders University, Mark Oliphant Building, 5 Laffer Drive, Bedford Park, South Australia 5042, Australia; [c] Respiratory and Sleep Service, Southern Adelaide Local Health Network, SA Health, Flinders Drive, Bedford Park, South Australia 5042, Australia
* Corresponding author. Adelaide Institute for Sleep Health, College of Medicine and Public Health, Flinders University, Mark Oliphant Building, 5 Laffer Drive, Bedford Park, South Australia 5042, Australia.
E-mail address: ChingLi.Chai-Coetzer@sa.gov.au

Sleep Med Clin 16 (2021) 1–10
https://doi.org/10.1016/j.jsmc.2020.10.001
1556-407X/21/© 2020 Elsevier Inc. All rights reserved.

DISCUSSION
Excessive Daytime Sleepiness

Excessive daytime sleepiness (EDS) is a frequent symptom of OSA and commonly assessed using the Epworth Sleepiness Scale (ESS).[7] The ESS subjectively assesses sleep propensity, with a score greater than 10 often interpreted as EDS.[8] One study examined multiple markers of sleepiness before and after 3 months of PAP for moderate–severe OSA[9]; 66% of participants with EDS normalized their ESS after treatment, with higher PAP use noted in those who were successful versus those who were not (mean 5.1 [SD 2.1] hours/night vs 4.0 [SD 2.3] hours/night, respectively). There was a dose-dependent effect of PAP on ESS: 41.2% with use 0 hours/night to 2 hours/night had a post-treatment ESS of less than or equal to 10, rising to 92.9% in those using PAP greater than 7 hours/night. Analysis showed that further improvements in ESS was not expected above 4 hours/night use.

A study published in 2011 analyzed data from a randomized controlled trial (RCT) to assess PAP adherence against ESS at 0 months and 3 months in moderate–severe OSA.[10] The mean (SD) baseline ESS was 13.4 (SD 4.0). ESS scores also showed a dose-dependent improvement with PAP. Normalization of ESS at 3 months occurred in 71.4% of patients using PAP greater than 7 hours/night, 70.6% using PAP 5 hours/night to 6 hours/night, and only 41.2% using PAP 2 hours/night to 4 hours/night. Despite differences in methodology, the overall results from these 2 studies are similar: it seems that the tipping point for PAP adherence in sleepy patients with moderate–severe OSA is 4 hours/night to 5 hours/night.

Does this mean that those with less than 4 hours/night PAP use may as well give up PAP? The answer is no. In the first study, 41% of participants normalized their ESS despite average PAP use of 0 hours/night to 2 hours/night, and 25% of patients from the second study normalized their ESS with less than or equal to 2 hours/night of PAP use. A recent double-blind, sham-controlled RCT demonstrated worsening EDS in moderate–severe OSA patients with poor PAP adherence (mean PAP use 3–4 hours/night in the prior 12 months) when their therapy was replaced by sham PAP—ESS rose 2.4 points (95% CI, 0.6–4.2; $P = .01$) in those receiving sham PAP after just 2 weeks compared with those randomized to therapeutic PAP.[11] This demonstrates that suboptimal PAP use still can provide benefit in terms of ESS improvements in moderate–severe OSA. This benefit, however, becomes less apparent in mild–moderate OSA, with a meta-analysis (7 trials, n = 418) showing a decrease in ESS of only 1.2 points (95% CI, 0.6–1.9) with mean PAP use of 2.8 hours/night to 4.9 hours/night.[12]

The 2005 American Academy of Sleep Medicine (AASM) guidelines examined the clinical utility of the multiple sleep latency test (MSLT) and maintenance of wakefulness test (MWT), 2 commonly performed sleep laboratory tests used to objectively assess for hypersomnolence, in OSA. Only 2 studies[13,14] were found that showed improvements in mean sleep latency (MSL) in OSA patients using PAP versus placebo. The weighted MSL on PAP was 9.8 (SD 4.5) minutes, compared with 8.3 (SD 4.7) minutes on placebo. Mean PAP adherence was 3.4 (SD 0.4) hours/night and 2.8 (SD 2.0) hours/night. Only 1 article was included for examination of the effect of the PAP treatment compared with placebo on the MWT with 40-minute trials (MWT-40) and did not show a significant increase in MSL.[15] No articles examining PAP effect on the MWT with 20-minute trials (MWT-20) were found.

Since then, 2 studies have assessed the effect of PAP adherence on MSLT and MWT results. One study[9] found that 62.5% of moderate–severe OSA patients had abnormal MLST results at baseline—and only 35.3% successfully normalized their MSLT after 3 months of PAP. ESS also was assessed alongside MSLT in this study: there was less benefit with PAP for MSLT compared with ESS, and the threshold for PAP adherence above which further substantial improvement in MSL was not expected was 6 hours. A study by Antic and colleagues[10] explored the effect of 3 months of PAP use on MWT-40 and found that approximately 30% of patients had an abnormal result after 3 months of PAP, with no relationship between PAP adherence and the likelihood of a normal MWT result.

Finally, a post hoc analysis of data from an RCT analyzed the effect of greater than 4 or less than or equal to 4 hours/night PAP use on MWT-20 results.[16] MWT-20 was performed at baseline and after 6 months of PAP use; 52% of participants had EDS at baseline, and there were significant improvements in MSL at 6 months in those using PAP greater than 4 hours/night compared with less than or equal to 4 hours/night (18.5 [SD 2.8] minutes vs 17.5 [SD 3.8] minutes, respectively; $P = .01$). Logistic regression confirmed significantly lower odds of an abnormal MSL at 6 months with PAP use greater than 4 hours/night (odds ratio 0.55; $P = .008$).

The authors interpret these results several ways. The MSLT has a poor track record for measuring sleepiness in OSA: when used as a metric to assess PAP treatment in OSA (vs placebo), improvements in MSL, although statistically significant, still are within 1 SD of normal, suggesting that the MSLT is not suited to discriminating a treatment response.[17] Budhiraja and colleagues'[16] finding that only 35% of participants normalized their MSLT with PAP also casts doubt on the utility of the MSLT in this setting. The MSLT is not recommended by the AASM for assessing change after PAP or in the initial evaluation and diagnosis of OSA—a recommendation that the authors echo, given the state of play in the literature.

The MWT has clinical utility for discerning residual EDS post-treatment; however, the lack of dose-response effect of PAP on the MWT-40 in the study by Antic and colleagues[10] suggests that the MWT-40 protocol may not be suited for assessing improvement post-PAP. What about the MWT-20 then? Although these positive results reported are encouraging, they should be interpreted with caution because the MWT-20 has been shown to be relatively insensitive for detecting difficulties in maintaining wakefulness compared with the MWT-40.[18] At this point, the authors are unable to give a recommendation for MWT to be used as a clinically meaningful metric for assessing PAP adherence.

Quality of Life

The impact of PAP also can be assessed using health-related quality of life (HRQL) instruments. HRQL scales are by nature subjective tools that incorporate a broad overview of physical well-being, psychological health, social relationships, and interactions with the environment. This article focuses on 3 tools: Short Form 36-Item Survey (SF-36),[19] Functional Outcomes of Sleep Questionnaire (FOSQ),[20] and Calgary Sleep Apnea Quality of Life Index (SAQLI).[21]

The SF-36 is a generic 36-item survey divided into 8 subscales: vitality, physical functioning, bodily pain, general health perceptions, physical role, emotional role, social role, and mental health. Lower scores indicate a greater impact on HRQL. The FOSQ was designed to measure the impact of EDS on activities of daily living. An FOSQ score less than 17.9 points suggests a negative impact on quality of life, although there is no consensus regarding this.[20] The SAQLI assesses the impact of OSA on HRQL, with lower scores indicating a greater negative impact on daily living.

PAP has not been shown to consistently improve all SF-36 subscale scores in OSA compared with placebo. A Cochrane review found that in parallel and partial crossover PAP studies (3 studies, n = 188), only physical function and general health subscales had consistent and significant improvements in favor of PAP; and there was significant statistical heterogeneity for vitality, physical role, emotional role, and mental health subscales.[22] In crossover studies (3 studies, n = 91), the vitality subscale showed consistent and significant improvements in favor of PAP.

A linear relationship has been seen between increased PAP adherence and improvement in FOSQ score after 3 months in patients with moderate–severe OSA in 1 study,[9] with no further functional gains in FOSQ scores above 7 hours/night of PAP use. Another study simultaneously assessed the effect of PAP adherence on FOSQ and SF-36 at 3 months in moderate–severe OSA,[10] and found discordant results for the 2 instruments. The FOSQ showed progressive improvement with greater PAP use—the proportion of normal FOSQ scores rose from 13.9% of patients at baseline to 48.4% at 3 months for the group using PAP greater than or equal to 7 hours/night (treatment-by-adherence interactions; $P = .021$). Of the SF-36 subscales, only vitality showed significant improvements in patients with greater adherence. These differences may stem from the design intent of the HRQL instruments—SF-36 is a generic tool, whereas the FOSQ was designed specifically for sleep disorders.

Finally, post hoc analysis of data from an RCT studied the impact of PAP on HRQL. Participants had moderate–severe OSA, and baseline ESS greater than or equal to 12.[23] The SF-36, FOSQ, and SAQLI were performed concurrently at baseline and after 3 months of PAP. FOSQ and SAQLI were evaluated for their psychometric properties and associations of responsiveness to PAP adherence (using a 4-hour threshold) and correlated when possible with SF-36 domains. Both the FOSQ and SAQLI showed excellent internal reliability, and both were responsive to PAP intervention. The FOSQ was more sensitive to differences in PAP adherence than the SAQLI.

It is clear from the literature that PAP adherence also has a dose-dependent effect on functional status improvement. The SF-36, despite being the oldest HRQL tool, is limited by its generic nature, which has led to inconsistent results. The SAQLI, although promising as an HRQL scale for OSA, is not yet widely used. The authors believe that the FOSQ has shown the greatest consistency and thus recommend an adherence target of 4 hours/night to 7 hours/night of PAP for a clinically meaningful improvement in quality of life.

Neurocognitive Outcomes

The impact of PAP on neurocognitive function also is important to consider when determining an optimal target for PAP therapy. A recent systematic review of 68 studies exploring the relationship between OSA and cognition, mild cognitive impairment, and Alzheimer's disease[24] found an association between OSA and impaired cognition, particularly in young and middle-aged adults, and considerable interest in the impact of PAP on neurocognitive performance, memory, and attention is apparent within the literature.[10,25–30] Various assessment tools have been used within these studies, with the Hopkins Verbal Learning Test–Revised (HVLT-R)[31] and the Psychomotor Vigilance Task[32] the most common; however, there is little consistency in assessment approaches.

A recent study by Jackson and colleagues[26] explored the impact of PAP on neurobehavioral function in mild–moderate OSA and found no improvement in 7 neurocognitive outcomes assessed, even when PAP use was greater than 5.8 hours/night.[26] Three studies also have explored the impact of PAP in moderate–severe OSA. An RCT by Antic and colleagues[10] discovered that 3 months of PAP therapy resulted in improvements in both verbal memory and executive function, although these improvements were not associated with hours of PAP use per night. Similarly, a recent study exploring the effects of PAP on cognitive and psychomotor outcomes in severe OSA reported improvements in both psychomotor and cognitive function in participants considered "optimal" users of PAP (mean usage 6.2 hours/night); however, they did not report the impact of differing hours of use on the treatment effect.[25] Deering and colleagues,[25] in their study of attention within patients with moderate–severe OSA, also demonstrated a reduction in minor lapses of attention within the Psychomotor Vigilance Task in relation to PAP use, reporting that increased hours of PAP use were associated with a reduction in lapses but they were not specific about the hours of use required for this effect.[25] Within this study, mean PAP use was 3.3 (2.5) hours/night.

Three studies have explored the role of PAP in normalizing or slowing cognitive decline in patients with comorbid OSA and cognitive impairment or established Alzheimer's disease. An observational study showed that optimal PAP users (median 6.4 hours/night) were 7.9 times more likely to have normal memory, as assessed by the HVLT-R, than poor users (median 0.9 hours/night) after 3 months.[28] Recently a similar study was conducted by Richards and colleagues,[29] who found improvements in psychomotor and cognitive processing speeds of people with mild cognitive impairment using PAP for OSA but did not find significant changes to HVLT-R. Again, this study did not report the impact of specific hours of use,

instead comparing adherent (≥4 hours/night use) versus nonadherent individuals. An RCT exploring the impact of 3 weeks of PAP on memory in comorbid Alzheimer's disease and OSA demonstrated small improvements in cognitive function with mean 5 hours/night PAP use; however, the investigators suggested that future studies exploring longer periods of therapy in this population were warranted.[30]

Variation in the assessment tools, outcomes, and target populations within studies makes it difficult to directly compare results. With demonstrated benefits in moderate–severe OSA, however, and those with memory impairment with average usage of approximately 6 hours/night of PAP use, 6 hours may be a reasonable target for PAP use to optimize neurocognitive outcomes. Given the lack of effect in patients with mild–moderate OSA[26] at more than 5.8 hours/night, however, this target may not apply to those with milder OSA severities. Further investigation into the impact of PAP on people with mild OSA and those with comorbid OSA and Alzheimer's disease is needed before an optimal PAP adherence target can be determined for those groups.

Depression

Several studies have investigated the effect of the hours of PAP use on depressive symptoms. A nonrandomized study explored the effects of PAP on the Beck Depression Inventory[33] in individuals with an apnea-hypopnea index (AHI) greater than 10 events/hour. After both 1 month and 3 months of treatment, there were statistically significant improvements in the Beck Depression Inventory with average PAP use of 5.51 ($P = .04$) hours and 5.81 ($P = .015$) hours, respectively.[34] Similarly, a pre–post intervention study demonstrated improvement in depressive symptoms, as measured by the Patient Heath Questionnaire (PHQ)-9 depression scale,[35] with greater than or equal to 5 hours/night PAP use after 12 weeks in participants with moderate–severe OSA.[36] A recent study by Bhat and colleagues[37] also demonstrated improvements in the PHQ-8 depression scale for patients with both mild–moderate and severe OSA. Participants in this study were treated with PAP for greater than or equal to 4 hours/night and greater than or equal to 60% of nights for greater than or equal to 1 month.

A small study (n = 17) from Japan explored the impact of 2 months of PAP therapy on comorbid depression and OSA and found a significant improvement in depressive symptoms in 11 participants but found that 6 were nonresponders to treatment,[38] with both groups using PAP for means of 5.3 hours/night and 5.4 hours/night, respectively. The investigators proposed that these results may be linked to a strong correlation between improvements in subjective daytime sleepiness and depressive symptoms, suggesting that improvements in daytime sleepiness of patients medicated for major depression could improve their symptoms of depression. Another study conducted by Lee and colleagues[39] explored the impact of 3 weeks of PAP therapy on mood and found that PAP had no impact on mood and that hours of use had no effect on treatment outcomes.

Two studies have explored the effect of PAP on mood in individuals with comorbid cardiovascular disease (CVD) and OSA.[40,41] The Sleep Apnea Cardiovascular Endpoints (SAVE) study, the largest international, multicenter trial of PAP in patients with comorbid moderate–severe OSA and CVD, demonstrated a significant reduction in the rates of clinical depression with mean (SD) PAP usage of 3.4 (SD 2.6) hours/night at 24 months.[3,40] A prospective study from Taiwan (n = 79) found a significant improvement in depression symptoms in patients who used PAP greater than or equal to 4 hours/night for greater than or equal to 70% nights for 6 months, but only in those who did not have comorbid CVD.[41]

There appear to be marked improvements in depressive symptoms in some studies with approximately 5 hours of use; however, new findings from the large SAVE study demonstrated improvements in depression with a mean of only 3.4 hours/night PAP use. It may be suggested then that for improvements in symptoms of depression, the target for PAP use should be greater than or equal to 3.5 hours/night to 5 hours/night.

Hypertension

Studies have shown the effect of PAP therapy on blood pressure (BP) in patients with OSA to be modest, with reductions in systolic and/or diastolic BP of approximately 2 mm Hg to 3 mm Hg. A meta-analysis by Montesi and colleagues[42] involving 29 studies (n = 1948) showed improvements in diurnal systolic BP (−2.58 mm Hg; 95% CI, −3.57 to −1.59 mm Hg) and diastolic BP (−2.01 mm Hg; 95% CI, −2.84 to −1.18 mm Hg) as well as nocturnal systolic BP (−4.09 mm Hg; 95% CI, −6.24 mm Hg to −1.94 mm Hg) and diastolic BP (−1.85 mm Hg, 95% CI, −3.53 mm Hg to −0.17 mm Hg) in OSA patients on PAP treatment compared with controls. Subgroup analyses showed significant reductions in diurnal BP only in studies with mean PAP

adherence greater than or equal to 4 hours/night. A more recent meta-analysis conducted by Hu and colleagues,[43] which included 7 RCTs (n = 794) and assessed 24-hour ambulatory BP changes in patients randomized to either PAP or control showed significant reductions in systolic BP (−2.32 mm Hg [95% CI, −3.65 to −1.00]) and diastolic BP (−1.98 [95% CI, −2.82 to −1.14]) with PAP. Meta-regression revealed that PAP adherence was positively correlated with the improvement in 24-h ambulatory diastolic BP but not systolic BP. A dose-response relationship between PAP adherence and decreases in BP was seen in an RCT by Barbe and colleagues,[44] which evaluated the effects of PAP therapy on BP response in hypertensive, nonsleepy patients with OSA. The study found a significant reduction in diastolic BP (−2.19 mm Hg; 95% CI, −0.93 to −3.46; $P<.001$) after 12 months' follow-up. Significant reductions in systolic BP and diastolic BP were evident only in patients using PAP for more than 5.65 hours/night.

Larger effects on BP with PAP have been seen in OSA patients with resistant or refractory hypertension. A meta-analysis by Iftikhar and colleagues[45] examining the effects of PAP on BP in patients with OSA and resistant hypertension included 6 studies (n = 329) and showed a mean change in systolic BP of −7.21 mm Hg (95% CI, −5.38 to −9.04) and diastolic BP of −4.99 mm Hg (95% CI, −3.96 to −6.01). In the Hipertensión Arterial Resistente Control con CPAP (HIPARCO) study by Martínez-García and colleagues,[46] which randomized 194 patients with resistant hypertension to PAP or no treatment of OSA, positive linear correlations between the hours of PAP use and the decrease in 24-hour mean BP, systolic BP, and diastolic BP were demonstrated. Linear regression analyses revealed reductions in mean BP of 1.3 mm Hg (95% CI, 0.4–2.2), systolic BP of 1.9 mm Hg (95% CI, 0.6–3.3), and diastolic BP of 1.0 mm Hg (95% CI, 0.1–1.8) for every 1-hour increase in PAP use. In this study, mean (SD) PAP use was 5.0 (SD 1.9) hours/night, with 71 patients (72.4%) using PAP greater than or equal to 4 hours/night.

Finally, the absence of comorbid EDS may mitigate somewhat the effect of PAP on BP reduction. A meta-analysis by Bratton and colleagues[47] examined the effect of PAP on BP in patients within minimally symptomatic OSA. Four eligible RCTs were included (n = 1206) and a slight increase in systolic BP of 1.1 mm Hg (95% CI, −0.2–2.3; $P = .086$) and a slight reduction in diastolic BP of 0.8 mm Hg (95% CI, −1.6–0.1; $P = .083$) were seen, although these results were not statistically significant. When PAP adherence was taken into account, a statistically significant reduction in only diastolic BP was found with PAP use greater than 4 hours/night (-1.4 mm Hg; 95% CI, -2.5 to -0.4; $P = .008$).

The studies, discussed previously, suggest that the evidence for PAP use in OSA is strongest for those with resistant hypertension and EDS and that at least 4 hours/night to 5.5 hours/night use is recommended to improve BP. PAP cannot be recommended, however, as a replacement for antihypertensive medications and lifestyle changes for treatment of hypertension in OSA patients.

Cardiovascular Disease and Mortality

Observational studies have reported strong associations between OSA and CVD and that PAP use in OSA patients is associated with improved rates of CVD morbidity and mortality.[48–52] Unfortunately, subsequent RCTs have failed to demonstrate an improvement in CVD outcomes with PAP use on intention-to-treat analyses.[53–56] The earliest RCT published in 2012 by Barbé and colleagues[53] randomized 725 nonsleepy patients with moderate–severe OSA (AHI $\geq$20 events/h) to PAP or no active treatment and showed no significant reduction in the incidence of hypertension or cardiovascular (CV) events after a median of 4.0 years' follow-up. Post hoc analyses, however, did reveal a significant reduction in the incidence of hypertension and CV events for patients using PAP greater than or equal to 4 hours/night compared with controls (incidence density ratio 0.69; 95% CI, 0.50–0.94). A subsequent RCT by Peker and colleagues[54] (Randomized Intervention with Continuous Positive Airway Pressure in CAD and OSA [RICCADSA] study), which recruited 244 nonsleepy OSA patients with newly revascularized coronary artery disease, also failed to show a significant improvement in adverse CV outcomes with PAP. Similar to the study by Barbé and colleagues,[53] post hoc analyses revealed a significant CV risk reduction in patients using PAP greater than or equal to 4 hours/night versus less than 4 hours/night or no treatment (hazard ratio [HR] 0.29; 95% CI, 0.10–0.86), whilst no significant risk reduction was seen for use greater than or equal to 3 hours/night.

The SAVE study, by McEvoy and colleagues,[55] randomized 2717 adults aged 45 years to 75 years with moderate–severe OSA and coronary artery or cerebrovascular disease to either PAP or usual care and found no significant difference in the primary composite CV endpoint after a median follow-up of 3.7 years. Mean PAP use in the intervention arm was only 3.3 hours/night. Propensity score-matched analyses showed that patients using PAP greater than or equal to 4 hours/night had a lower risk of stroke than those in the usual-care group (HR 0.56; 95% CI, 0.32–1.00; $P = .05$), but a post hoc PAP dose–response analysis of the primary and secondary CV endpoints showed no significant association. A more recent RCT by Sánchez-de-la-Torre and colleagues[56] (Impact of Sleep Apnea syndrome in the evolution of Acute Coronary syndrome [ISAACC] study) randomized 1264 nonsleepy patients with moderate–severe OSA and acute coronary syndrome to either PAP therapy or usual care for a median follow-up of 3.35 years. This study also showed no significant difference in the rate of CV events with PAP versus usual care. PAP adherence was very low in the study, with mean usage of only 2.78 hours/night. No significant difference in CVD outcomes were seen for patients with mean adherence greater than or equal to 4 hours/night compared with the usual care group on propensity score–matched analyses (HR 0.80; 95% CI, 0.52–1.23; $P = .32$).

Although multiple longitudinal studies have shown a clear association between untreated OSA and increased mortality,[57–60] the literature is mixed regarding the impact of PAP on mortality. A large prospective registry study of moderate–severe OSA patients on PAP stratified into fully adherent ($\geq$4 hours/night), partially adherent (<4 hours/night), and nonadherent arms. A mortality analysis was performed with a median follow-up of 2.4 years.[61] Although there were no significant differences in mortality between fully and partially adherent participants, the HR for nonadherent participants was nearly 2-fold that of all adherent participants (HR 1.73 [1.30–2.29]; $P<.001$). Previous cohort studies that have shown a mortality benefit with PAP have not looked at PAP adherence with this level of granularity, instead classifying patients as either treated or untreated.[50,62]

This mortality benefit derived from PAP appears to be unevenly spread. Another large registry study (n = 22,135) retrospectively evaluated the impact of an OSA diagnosis on all-cause mortality.[63] Overall all-cause mortality actually increased in the PAP arm (HR 1.84; 95% CI, 1.14–2.97; $P = .013$)—accounted for by a greater proportion of men, the elderly, and a higher comorbidity burden in the PAP arm. When these factors were adjusted for, PAP treatment produced a positive effect in middle-aged (aged 40–59 years; HR 0.60; 95% CI, 0.37–0.97; $P = .038$) and elderly persons (aged $\geq$60 years; HR 0.45; 95% CI, 0.28–0.73; $P<.001$) but did not affect all-cause mortality for women (HR 1.18; 95% CI, 0.94–1.48; $P = .149$). This gender disparity remains unexplained and has also been found using data from another population registry analysis.[64]

Although the results from cohort studies are encouraging, the lack of clear benefit shown by large RCTs, such as the SAVE and ISAAC studies, preclude the authors from concluding that PAP produces a clear and consistent CVD and mortality benefit in OSA. As such, the authors are unable to give a PAP adherence recommendation for CVD or mortality outcomes.

SUMMARY

It is now understood that clinically meaningful PAP adherence can vary markedly with the outcome in question, providing good reason to challenge the commonly used and rigidly applied 4-hour rule that has evolved in relation to the definition of good PAP adherence. PAP has a dose-dependent benefit on ESS in moderate–severe OSA with gains diminishing after the 4-hour to 5-hour mark; however, the evidence is less clear for patients with mild–moderate OSA. Like ESS scores, PAP has a dose-dependent effect on HRQL as assessed via the FOSQ, although the tipping point appears higher at 7 hours/night. Objective tests are poor tools to assess PAP response. Similar to ESS, the impact of PAP on neurocognitive outcomes in patients with mild–moderate OSA is unclear, although for those with moderate–severe OSA, benefit is apparent at approximately 6 hours/night use. For depressive symptoms, this target is lower at 3.5 hours/night to 5 hours/night. For BP reduction, PAP therapy should be targeted at those with existing hypertension (in particular, those with resistant or refractory disease), with usage aimed at greater than or equal to 4 hours/night to 5.5 hours/night, but PAP should not be offered as a substitute for antihypertensive medications or lifestyle modifications. At this point in time, current evidence does not support the use of PAP to reduce CVD risk or mortality in patients with OSA.

The varying responses to PAP according to patient outcomes raise the prospect that the sleep clinician of the future potentially may recommend PAP adherence targets based on a patient's presenting complaint(s), comorbidities or even their gender. The bulk of the literature examining the impact of PAP adherence consists of nonrandomized studies, introducing bias into the equation. Many observational trials have follow-up times measured in short months, or even weeks. Enrollment numbers generally are low. There clearly is more work to be done to clearly define these subtleties in PAP response.

Finally, the authors would like to acknowledge as well that although they have collated and drawn conclusions from the present state of the literature, they have not questioned the present concept of adherence as a time-based value. Might PAP adherence be better defined as a proportion of total sleep time? Furthermore, given the frequent preponderance and greater adverse physiologic consequences of OSA in rapid-eye-movement (REM) sleep, should PAP adherence in the latter half of the night (when REM sleep is more predominant) be given more clinical weight than PAP in the first half of the night? Is more consistent adherence to PAP on a nightly basis more clinically impactful than intermittent adherence with overall acceptable mean PAP use? These all are questions that are at present not satisfactorily addressed in the literature and that present exciting avenues for future research.

CLINICS CARE POINTS

- EDS in OSA is improved by PAP in a dose-dependent fashion, with diminishing improvements to ESS scores after 4 hours/night of PAP use.
- No single HRQL instrument is widely used for evaluating the effect of PAP adherence in OSA; increasing PAP use in general improves HRQL instrument scores—the magnitude and consistency of this improvement vary from scale to scale. HRQL instruments that are more specific to sleep disorders, like the FOSQ, show improvement with PAP in a dose-dependent fashion—adherence of 4 hours/night to 7 hours/night is recommended.
- The literature on neurocognitive function has widely varying study methodology, making interpretation and clinical correlation difficult. In patients with preexisting cognitive impairment and moderate–severe OSA, PAP adherence of greater than or equal to 6 hours/night may improve neurocognitive outcomes—this benefit has not been shown in mild–moderate OSA.
- PAP use in OSA improves depressive symptoms, and this benefit is evident in comorbid CVD—adherence to PAP greater than or equal to 3.5 hours/night to 5 hours/night is recommended.
- In hypertension, both systolic BP and diastolic BP are modestly improved by PAP use of greater than or equal to 4 hours/night, to 5.5 hours/night, with greater benefit seen in resistant/refractory hypertension.
- Although observational studies show a strong association between OSA and CVD and mortality, RCTs have thus far failed to demonstrate a benefit for either outcome with

PAP—a PAP adherence recommendation is not possible at this time.

DISCLOSURE

N. Grivell and C.L. Chai-Coetzer are currently involved in research for a Centres of Research Excellence in Health Services Research (Primary Health Care) that has been funded by the National Health and Medical Research Council of Australia (ID1134954). A. Oh has nothing to disclose.

REFERENCES

1. Schwab RJ, Badr SM, Epstein LJ, et al. An official American Thoracic Society statement: continuous positive airway pressure adherence tracking systems. The optimal monitoring strategies and outcome measures in adults. Am J Respir Crit Care Med 2013;188(5):613–20.
2. Patil S, Ayappa I, Caples S, et al. Treatment of adult obstructive sleep apnea with positive airway pressure: an American Academy of Sleep Medicine clinical practice guideline. Sleep 2019;15(2):335–43.
3. Van Ryswyk E, Anderson CS, Antic NA, et al. Predictors of long-term adherence to continuous positive airway pressure in patients with obstructive sleep apnea and cardiovascular disease. Sleep 2019; 42(10):zsz152.
4. Nadal N, de Batlle J, Barbé F, et al. Predictors of CPAP compliance in different clinical settings: primary care versus sleep unit. Sleep Breath 2018; 22(1):157–63.
5. Cistulli PA, Armitstead J, Pepin JL, et al. Short-term CPAP adherence in obstructive sleep apnea: a big data analysis using real world data. Sleep Med 2019;59:114–6.
6. Krakow B, Ulibarri VA, Foley-Shea MR, et al. Adherence and subthreshold adherence in sleep apnea subjects receiving positive airway pressure therapy: a retrospective study evaluating differences in adherence versus use. Respir Care 2016;61(8): 1023.
7. Johns MW. A new method for measuring daytime sleepiness: the Epworth sleepiness scale. Sleep 1991;14(6):540–5.
8. Johns M, Hocking B. Daytime sleepiness and sleep habits of Australian workers. Sleep 1997;20(10): 844–9.
9. Weaver TE, Maislin G, Dinges DF, et al. Relationship between hours of CPAP use and achieving normal levels of sleepiness and daily functioning. Sleep 2007;30(6):711–9.
10. Antic NA, Catcheside P, Buchan C, et al. The effect of CPAP in normalizing daytime sleepiness, quality of life, and neurocognitive function in patients with moderate to severe OSA. Sleep 2011;34(1):111–9.
11. Gaisl T, Rejmer P, Thiel S, et al. Effects of suboptimal adherence of CPAP therapy on symptoms of obstructive sleep apnoea: a randomised, double-blind, controlled trial. Eur Respir J 2020;55(3): 1901526.
12. Marshall NS, Barnes M, Travier N, et al. Continuous positive airway pressure reduces daytime sleepiness in mild to moderate obstructive sleep apnea: a meta-analysis. Thorax 2006;61(5):430–4.
13. Engleman HM, Martin SE, Douglas NJ, et al. Effect of continuous positive airway pressure treatment on daytime function in sleep apnoea/hypopnoea syndrome. Lancet 1994;343(8897):572–5.
14. Engleman HM, Martin SE, Kingshott RN, et al. Randomised placebo controlled trial of daytime function after continuous positive airway pressure (CPAP) therapy for the sleep apnoea/hypopnoea syndrome. Thorax 1998;53(5):341.
15. Engleman HM, Kingshott RN, Wraith PK, et al. Randomized placebo-controlled crossover trial of continuous positive airway pressure for mild sleep Apnea/Hypopnea syndrome. Am J Respir Crit Care Med 1999;159(2):461–7.
16. Budhiraja R, Kushida CA, Nichols DA, et al. Predictors of sleepiness in obstructive sleep apnoea at baseline and after 6 months of continuous positive airway pressure therapy. Eur Respir J 2017;50(5): 1700348.
17. Arand D, Bonnet M, Hurwitz T, et al. The clinical use of the MSLT and MWT. Sleep 2005;28(1):123–44.
18. Arzi L, Shreter R, El-Ad B, et al. Forty- versus 20-minute trials of the maintenance of wakefulness test regimen for licensing of drivers. J Clin Sleep Med 2009;5(1):57–62.
19. Ware JE, Sherbourne CD. The MOS 36-item short-form health survey (SF-36). I. Conceptual framework and item selection. Med Care 1992;30(6):473–83.
20. Weaver TE, Laizner AM, Evans LK, et al. An instrument to measure functional status outcomes for disorders of excessive sleepiness. Sleep 1997;20(10): 835–43.
21. Flemons W, Reimer MA. Development of a disease-specific health-related quality of life questionnaire for sleep apnea. Am J Respir Crit Care Med 1998; 158(2):494–503.
22. Giles TL, Lasserson TJ, Smith BH, et al. Continuous positive airways pressure for obstructive sleep apnoea in adults. Cochrane Database Syst Rev 2006;(3):CD001106.
23. Billings ME, Rosen CL, Auckley D, et al. Psychometric performance and responsiveness of the functional outcomes of sleep questionnaire and sleep apnea quality of life instrument in a randomized trial: the HomePAP study. Sleep 2014;37(12):2017–24.
24. Bubu OM, Andrade AG, Umasabor-Bubu OQ, et al. Obstructive sleep apnea, cognition and Alzheimer's disease: a systematic review integrating three

decades of multidisciplinary research. Sleep Med Rev 2019;50:101250.

25. Pecotic R, Dodig IP, Valic M, et al. Effects of CPAP therapy on cognitive and psychomotor performances in patients with severe obstructive sleep apnea: a prospective 1-year study. Sleep Breath 2019; 23(1):41–8.

26. Jackson ML, McEvoy RD, Banks S, et al. Neurobehavioral impairment and CPAP treatment response in mild-moderate obstructive sleep apnea. J Clin Sleep Med 2018;14(1):47–56.

27. Deering Liu L, Zamora T, Hamilton J, et al. CPAP adherence is associated with attentional improvements in a group of primarily male patients with moderate to severe OSA. J Clin Sleep Med 2017; 13(12):1423–8.

28. Zimmerman ME, Arnedt JT, Stanchina M, et al. Normalization of memory performance and positive airway pressure adherence in memory-impaired patients with obstructive sleep apnea. Chest 2006; 130(6):1772–8.

29. Richards KC, Gooneratne N, Dicicco B, et al. CPAP adherence may slow 1-year cognitive decline in older adults with mild cognitive impairment and apnea. J Am Geriatr Soc 2019;67(3):558–64.

30. Ancoli-Israel S, Palmer BW, Cooke JR, et al. Cognitive effects of treating obstructive sleep apnea in Alzheimer's disease: a randomized controlled study. J Am Geriatr Soc 2008;56(11):2076–81.

31. Benedict RHB, Schretlen D, Groninger L, et al. Hopkins verbal learning test - revised: normative data and analysis of inter-form and test-retest reliability. Clin Neuropsychol 1998;12(1):43–55.

32. Dinges D, Powell J. Microcomputer analyses of performance on a portable, simple visual RT task during sustained operations. Behav Res Methods Instrum Comput 1985;17(6):652–5.

33. Beck AT, Ward CH, Mendelson M, et al. An inventory for measuring depression. Arch Gen Psychiatry 1961;4(6):561–71.

34. Sánchez AI, Buela-Casal G, Bermúdez MP, et al. The effects of continuous positive air pressure treatment on anxiety and depression levels in apnea patients. Psychiatry Clin Neurosciences 2001;55(6): 641–6.

35. Spitzer RL, Kroenke K, Williams JB, et al. Validation and utility of a self-report version of PRIME-MD: the PHQ primary care study. JAMA 1999;282(18):1737–44.

36. Edwards C, Mukherjee S, Simpson L, et al. Depressive symptoms before and after treatment of obstructive sleep apnea in men and women. J Clin Sleep Med 2015;11(9):1029–38.

37. Bhat S, Gupta D, Akel O, et al. The relationships between improvements in daytime sleepiness, fatigue and depression and psychomotor vigilance task testing with CPAP use in patients with obstructive sleep apnea. Sleep Med 2018;49:81–9.

38. Habukawa M, Uchimura N, Kakuma T, et al. Effect of CPAP treatment on residual depressive symptoms in patients with major depression and coexisting sleep apnea: contribution of daytime sleepiness to residual depressive symptoms. Sleep Med 2010;11(6): 552–7.

39. Lee IS, Bardwell W, Ancoli-Israel S, et al. Effect of three weeks of continuous positive airway pressure treatment on mood in patients with obstructive sleep apnoea: a randomized placebo-controlled study. Sleep Med 2012;13(2):161–6.

40. Zheng D, Xu Y, You S, et al. Effects of continuous positive airway pressure on depression and anxiety symptoms in patients with obstructive sleep apnoea: results from the sleep apnoea cardiovascular Endpoint randomised trial and meta-analysis. EClinicalMedicine 2019;11:89–96.

41. Lee MC, Shen YC, Wang JH, et al. Effects of continuous positive airway pressure on anxiety, depression, and major cardiac and cerebro-vascular events in obstructive sleep apnea patients with and without coronary artery disease. Tzu Chi Med J 2017;29(4):218–22.

42. Montesi SB, Edwards BA, Malhotra A, et al. The effect of continuous positive airway pressure treatment on blood pressure: a systematic review and meta-analysis of randomized controlled trials. J Clin Sleep Med 2012;8(5):587–96.

43. Hu X, Fan J, Chen S, et al. The role of continuous positive airway pressure in blood pressure control for patients with obstructive sleep apnea and hypertension: a meta-analysis of randomized controlled trials. J Clin Hypertens 2015;17(3):215–22.

44. Barbé F, Durán-Cantolla J, Capote F, et al. Long-term effect of continuous positive airway pressure in hypertensive patients with sleep apnea. Am J Respir Crit Care Med 2010;181(7):718–26.

45. Iftikhar I, Valentine C, Bittencourt L, et al. Effects of continuous positive airway pressure on blood pressure in patients with resistant hypertension and obstructive sleep apnea: a meta-analysis. Am J Respir Crit Care Med 2014;32(12):2341–50 [discussion: 2350].

46. Martínez-García M-A, Capote F, Campos-Rodríguez F, et al. Effect of CPAP on blood pressure in patients with obstructive sleep apnea and resistant hypertension: the HIPARCO randomized clinical trial. JAMA 2013;310(22):2407–15.

47. Bratton DJ, Stradling JR, Barbé F, et al. Effect of CPAP on blood pressure in patients with minimally symptomatic obstructive sleep apnoea: a meta-analysis using individual patient data from four randomised controlled trials. Thorax 2014;69(12): 1128–35.

48. Gottlieb DJ, Yenokyan G, Newman AB, et al. Prospective study of obstructive sleep apnea and incident coronary heart disease and heart failure: the

sleep heart health study. Circulation 2010;122(4): 352–60.

49. Yaggi HK, Concato J, Kernan WN, et al. Obstructive sleep apnea as a risk factor for stroke and death. N Engl J Med 2005;353(19):2034–41.

50. Young T, Finn L, Peppard PE, et al. Sleep disordered breathing and mortality: eighteen-year follow-up of the Wisconsin sleep cohort. Sleep 2008;31(8):1071.

51. Marin JM, Carrizo SJ, Vicente E, et al. Long-term cardiovascular outcomes in men with obstructive sleep apnoea-hypopnoea with or without treatment with continuous positive airway pressure: an observational study. Lancet 2005;365(9464):1046–53.

52. Campos-Rodriguez F, Martinez-Garcia MA, de la Cruz-Moron I, et al. Cardiovascular mortality in women with obstructive sleep apnea with or without continuous positive airway pressure treatment: a cohort study. Ann Intern Med 2012;156(2):115.

53. Barbé F, Durán-Cantolla J, Sánchez-de-La-Torre M, et al. Effect of continuous positive airway pressure on the incidence of hypertension and cardiovascular events in nonsleepy patients with obstructive sleep apnea: a randomized controlled trial. JAMA 2012; 307(20):2161–8.

54. Peker Y, Glantz H, Eulenburg C, et al. Effect of positive airway pressure on cardiovascular outcomes in coronary artery disease patients with nonsleepy obstructive sleep apnea. The RICCADSA randomized controlled trial. Am J Respir Crit Care Med 2016;194(5):613–20.

55. McEvoy RD, Antic NA, Heeley E, et al. CPAP for prevention of cardiovascular events in obstructive sleep apnea. N Engl J Med 2016;375(10):919–31.

56. Sánchez-de-la-Torre M, Sánchez-de-la-Torre A, Bertran S, et al. Effect of obstructive sleep apnoea and its treatment with continuous positive airway pressure on the prevalence of cardiovascular events in patients with acute coronary syndrome (ISAACC study): a randomised controlled trial. Lancet Respir Med 2019;8(4):359–67.

57. Gami AS, Olson EJ, Shen WK, et al. Obstructive sleep apnea and the risk of sudden cardiac death: a longitudinal study of 10,701 adults. J Am Coll Cardiol 2013;62(7):610–6.

58. Doherty LS, Kiely JL, Swan V, et al. Long-term effects of nasal continuous positive airway pressure therapy on cardiovascular outcomes in sleep apnea syndrome. Chest 2005;127(6):2076–84.

59. Young T, Palta M, Dempsey J, et al. Burden of sleep apnea: rationale, design, and major findings of the Wisconsin Sleep Cohort study. WMJ 2009;108(5): 246–9.

60. Marshall NS, Wong KK, Liu PY, et al. Sleep apnea as an independent risk factor for all-cause mortality: the Busselton Health Study. Sleep 2008;31(8):1079–85.

61. Palm A, Midgren B, Theorell-Haglöw J, et al. Factors influencing adherence to continuous positive airway pressure treatment in obstructive sleep apnea and mortality associated with treatment failure – a national registry-based cohort study. Sleep Med 2018;51:85–91.

62. Yuan X, Fang J, Wang L, et al. Adequate continuous positive airway pressure therapy reduces mortality in Chinese patients with obstructive sleep apnea. Sleep Breath 2015;19(3):911–20.

63. Jennum P, Tønnesen P, Ibsen R, et al. Obstructive sleep apnea: effect of comorbidities and positive airway pressure on all-cause mortality. Sleep Med 2017;36:62–6.

64. de Batlle J, Bertran S, Turino C, et al. Mortality in patients treated with continuous positive airway pressure at the population level. Am J Respir Crit Care Med 2018;197(11):1486–8.

Adherence to Sleep Therapies in Children and Adolescents

Rakesh Bhattacharjee, DABP(SM), FRCPC, CBSM, DBSM, RPSGT[a,b]

KEYWORDS

- Obstructive sleep apnea • Positive airway pressure • Pediatric sleep-disordered breathing
- Adherence

KEY POINTS

- Positive airway pressure (PAP) therapy in children has become mainstay to treat sleep-disordered breathing in children.
- Adherence to PAP therapy in children is lower than reported in adults; however, there are several modifiable factors associated with PAP adherence in children.
- Monitoring adherence early with early intervention strategies including patient engagement programs or other behavioral interventions may optimize adherence in children.

INTRODUCTION

Any discussion regarding childhood sleep-disordered breathing disorders and adherence to therapy must consider that in children there is a marked influence of age on both disease presentation and response to therapy, which includes adherence to therapy. For example, an indication for treatment of obstructive sleep apnea (OSA) may be less obvious in younger children than older children. Further, when positive airway pressure therapy (PAP) is indicated, the efficacy of PAP therapy differs when comparing a toddler with an adolescent. Finally, factors promoting adherence in young children is quite distinct from adolescents, likely related to the increasing autonomy associated during adolescence. Thus, when discussing the adherence of PAP therapy in children, it is always important to acknowledge that the age of the child may have a marked influence.

One of the primary indications for PAP therapy in children is for OSA. In children, OSA is highly prevalent, affecting 2% to 3% of all children.[1–4] Hypertrophy of adenotonsillar tissue is considered the main contributor to the pathogenesis of pediatric OSA,[5,6] particularly in young children. Adenotonsillar hypertrophy in the upper airway reduces the anatomic patency of the airway and leads to exponential increases in pharyngeal resistance, which can result in episodic airway collapse during sleep, characteristic of OSA.[5,6] In children with OSA, particularly young children, daytime symptoms related to OSA such as excessive daytime sleepiness are not typical but are related mostly to neurocognitive and behavioral disturbances,[4,7–12] which include inattention and hyperactivity, impaired executive functioning, impulsive or aggressive behaviors, poor communication, and/or diminished adaptive skills.[13,14] In contrast, in older children, particularly obese children, symptoms of daytime sleepiness and social withdrawal are more typical.[15] In addition, recent studies have shown that OSA in children is also associated with cardiovascular disease[16] including hypertension,[17–19] endothelial dysfunction,[20–22] and left ventricular dysfunction.[23] Cumulatively, the risks associated with pediatric OSA calls for prompt treatment.

In children, the American Academy of Pediatrics clinical practice guideline recommends that

a Division of Respiratory Medicine, Department of Pediatrics, University of California-San Diego, 9500 Gilman Drive MC 0731, San Diego, CA 92093-0731, USA; b Rady Children's Hospital, 3020 Children's Way, San Diego, CA 92120, USA
E-mail address: r1bhattacharjee@ucsd.edu

Sleep Med Clin 16 (2021) 11–21
https://doi.org/10.1016/j.jsmc.2020.10.002
1556-407X/21/© 2020 Elsevier Inc. All rights reserved.

barring no contraindication to surgery, adenoton-sillectomy should be considered the first line of treatment of pediatric OSA.[24] Overall rates of adenotonsillectomy have increased over time[25] related to improved awareness of this disease in children. Notwithstanding, the efficacy of adeno-tonsillectomy is not uniform, and indeed many children may have residual OSA following surgery.[26,27] Evidence has identified several risk factors for residual OSA following surgery,[26,27] including older age, severity of underlying OSA, and the presence of obesity. In fact, adenotonsil-lectomy may be contraindicated in children with morbid obesity.[24]

Obesity is of particular relevance because it now follows adenotonsillar hypertrophy as the next major contributor for pediatric OSA. With obesity rates ranging as high as 7% to 22% of children in various Western countries,[28,29] there is an observed increase in the prevalence of pediatric OSA.[30] Finally, at any level of OSA severity, the magnitude of adenotonsillar hypertrophy is less relevant in obese children.[31]

Several other risk factors increase the risk of OSA independent of adenotonsillar hypertrophy. These include congenital diseases that affect normal craniofacial development such as Treacher Collins disease or Pierre Robin Sequence, neuro-muscular diseases that include cerebral palsy, and syndromes that may affect both craniofacial and neuromuscular development such as Turner syndrome or Down syndrome. Although the efficacy of adenotonsillectomy in these groups is understudied, there is evidence suggesting reduced efficacy in children with Down syndrome.[32,33]

When adenotonsillectomy is contraindicated, particularly in the case of morbidly obese children, or when OSA is refractory following surgery, PAP then becomes the mainstay for therapy. With the increase in prevalence of childhood obesity, it is anticipated that more and more children will require PAP therapy to treat OSA effectively. The earliest report of PAP efficacy was in 1986 by Guil-leminault and colleagues, where nasal continuous positive airway pressure (CPAP) represented a novel alternative to tracheostomy in 10 young children with OSA.[34] Since this study, there have been more than 50 studies assessing effectiveness and adherence of PAP therapy in children. Although PAP therapy resolves OSA as shown using poly-somnography, adherence to PAP therapy in children is particularly challenging raising the concern as to whether PAP therapy is an effective treatment strategy in pediatric OSA.[35] Recently, several studies have also sought to identify risk factors associated with PAP adherence, including

the influence of disease severity, psychosocial factors, socioeconomic status, parental education levels, mask type, pressure discomfort, and the perceived benefit.[36–38]

It is also important to acknowledge that PAP is often indicated in several other sleep-related breathing disorders in children, including central sleep apnea and sleep related hypoventilation. Although several studies evaluate the efficacy of PAP therapy in these disease settings,[39,40] few studies have examined adherence to PAP in these patient populations. Generally, it is thought that adherence is in fact higher in patients with sleep-related hypoventilation (eg, neuromuscular disease, central alveolar hypo-ventilation syndromes) compared with other sleep-related breathing disorders, as these devices support ventilation rather than just maintaining airway patency as would be the case for OSA.

ADHERENCE TO POSITIVE AIRWAY PRESSURE IN CHILDREN
Definition

Before reviewing the existing evidence pertaining to children and adherence to PAP therapy, it is imperative to recognize the absence of consensus that exists defining adequate adherence in the pediatric population. As has been discussed elsewhere in this issue, adequate adherence among adult PAP users is defined as greater than 4 hours of usage per night for greater than 70% of nights for 30 consecutive days within the first 90 days of treatment.[41] This criterion is largely used by insurance companies to determine if adult patients are nonadherent, ultimately leading to therapy termination, which includes removal of PAP machines and supplies.[41]

In children, a threshold defining adequate adherence is not established. Complicating the issue is the fact that sleep duration changes considerably as children grow older and although the goal is for patients to wear PAP most of the night, setting a threshold for 4 hours could be considered too low in a young child in whom sleep duration is typically 10 hours or more. Further, there is a dearth of studies identifying adequate adherence thresholds that equates to positive outcomes, such as improving neurocognitive dysfunction and the potential for reversing or preventing end organ morbidity including cardiovascular disease.[42]

The lack of consensus of adherence criteria in children renders it difficult to interpret published studies examining PAP adherence in children. The heterogeneous criteria used to define adequate adherence in children limits the generalizability of the findings from these studies.

Adherence and Existing Evidence

When reviewing the literature regarding adherence to PAP therapy, it is noted that the bulk of the literature is in adults rather than in pediatric patients. Although there are many studies evaluating adherence in pediatric patients with PAP, it is important to acknowledge that most studies are retrospective with small sample sizes, ranging from 29 to 140 patients.[38,43–50]

In one of the earliest single center studies,[51] originating from Australia, the investigators evaluated the effectiveness of PAP therapy in a case series of 80 pediatric patients and reported that CPAP was mostly effective and well tolerated. Subsequently, the earliest multicenter study[52] examining PAP therapy in children with OSA was very favorable with high levels of adherence. Despite involvement of 9 academic pediatric sleep centers, the sample size of 94 was relatively small. Nonetheless, using physician questionnaires, the investigators reported that in 81 of 94 patients (86%), CPAP was effective to treat OSA and in only 12 patients (13%) was adherence inadequate. This early report of CPAP usage in children was largely limited to subjective questionnaire-based data rather than objective adherence data that have become available only recently.

Since these early studies, more than 50 studies have been published on this subject manner. In the first published review of PAP adherence and children with OSA, Watach and colleagues[53] evaluated pooled data of 2216 children from 46 studies that met inclusion criteria. In their analysis, the investigators only identified 20 of 46 studies that reported complete data as frequency of adherence and/or reported hours of PAP usage. Further complicating their analysis, there were 24 unique definitions of PAP adherence such as mean or median hours of usage or percentage of nights uses, which were used across all of the studies, reflecting the heterogeneous nature of these studies. Although the investigators were able to report adherence data on 1079 of 2216 children (49%), the analysis revealed that less than 60% of participants met adequate adherence based on varying definitions of adequate adherence. Using objective data, the investigators reported PAP usage ranged from 4.0 to 5.2 hours per night. One of the pertinent findings from their analysis was that hourly usage did depend on whether PAP users were naïve or non-naïve to PAP therapy, with naïve patients having lower reported prevalence. Although this could imply that

PAP adherence may improve over time, the reality is that those who were non-naïve to PAP therapy and adherent were using their PAP device at the time of data collection, whereas those who were "non-naïve" and nonadherent were likely selected out because of therapy termination.

The largest study to date in children assessed PAP adherence cross-sectionally using data collected from proprietary cloud-based adherence monitoring technology[54] in the United States. Bhattacharjee and colleagues evaluated children aged 4 to 18 years who were using CPAP or automated CPAP therapy (APAP). Bilevel PAP therapy was excluded given the likelihood that many patients use bilevel PAP to treat sleep-related hypoventilation, and the investigators targeted only children with OSA. Although the primary outcome for the study was the percentage of patients who did not have their therapy terminated due to 30 consecutive nights of nonusage over a 90-day observation period, the investigators did also report the number of patients who met adult-based adherence criteria ($\geq$4 hours of usage per night for $\geq$70% of nights for 30 consecutive days within the first 90 days of treatment). Of 20,533 patients examined in this study, 12,699 (61.8%) did not have therapy terminated due to 30 consecutive nights of non-usage. However, in this large cohort of children, only 9504 (46.3%) of patients met adult-based adherence criteria. Notwithstanding, when PAP was used, the mean average usage per session was 5.2 ± 2.6 hours in children reflecting the greater duration of total sleep time that is expected in children.

Collectively, the pooled data from numerous small and mostly single center studies, coupled with the large cross-sectional analysis by Bhattacharjee and colleagues, report that about half of children adequately achieve adherence and that average hourly usage of PAP ranged from 4.0 to 5.2 hours. Given that children are expected to sleep between 8 and 12 hours per night, the current evidence suggests that even when children are wearing PAP, very rarely do they wear it most of the night. Although the cross-sectional study by Bhattacharjee and colleagues implies most of the children did not have therapy terminated due to nonusage, there are many hurdles to achieve a high level of PAP adherence for children, and a better understanding of these obstacles will only serve to enhance clinicians in developing strategies to optimize adherence.

Predictors of Positive Airway Pressure Adherence in Children

As stated earlier, several retrospective studies have critically evaluated the influence of several risk factors that are positively and negatively associated with PAP adherence in children. Risk factors evaluated range from specific demographic factors to disease severity to device mode. For example, in the study of 56 children, DiFeo and colleagues[38] reported the influence of race and maternal education level rather than OSA severity on PAP adherence in children (aged 2–16 years). In another study, female sex was identified as being positively predictive for PAP adherence in children.[49] It has also been reported that children with developmental disabilities have better adherence to PAP.[49,55] Notwithstanding, several demographic factors predictive of adherence are not necessarily consistent across the literature. For example, although age was reported to significantly influence adherence[38,56] in some studies, in other studies, there was no association.[43,45] Other factors such as disease severity, caregiver concern, factors related to PAP device, and the presence of comorbidities may also have an influence on adherence.

In the pooled analysis of mostly sleep centers across Europe, North America, and Australia by Watach and colleagues,[53] the investigators identified 43 factors associated with PAP adherence across 16 of the included studies. Their analysis identified that 19 met statistically significance when associated with PAP adherence, although the findings were not uniform across all studies. Among 13 studies, age was significantly associated with PAP in 5 (38%) studies with younger children, as opposed to adolescence, being found to be positively associated with PAP adherence. Female sex was also significantly associated in 2 of 11 studies (18%). Of note, the only other factor significantly associated with PAP adherence in this pooled analysis across 2 or more studies was the presence of developmental delay in 2 of 5 (40%) studies, where children with developmental delay were found to be more adherent, which is likely related to these children requiring more parental support. Other demographic factors including race, socioeconomic status, and disease factors including severity of disease and duration of PAP were not consistently associated with PAP adherence. In addition, the device mode (bilevel vs continuous positive airway pressure), device pressures, and mask type were also not consistently associated with PAP adherence. The lack of uniformity of all 19 factors across the 16 included studies is very likely related to the heterogeneous nature of these studies including heterogeneous definitions of adherence. Further, although certainly these studies were relatively small in sample size, there is limited generalizability in these studies, as health care delivery

including access to multidisciplinary clinics is quite variable across all sites.

In the cross-sectional study of by Bhattacharjee and colleagues[54] of 20,533 US children using CPAP and APAP, the investigators reported that age had a significant effect on adherence and termination of PAP therapy, with the age group of 15 to 18 years found to have the lowest adherence, whereas those children aged 6 to 12 years having the highest adherence. As expected, the age group of 15 to 18 years was also most likely to have their therapy terminated. This study did not evaluate the effect of sex on adherence. Evaluation of therapy efficacy parameters collected in PAP devices nightly and stored in cloud-based monitoring revealed several interesting associations with PAP adherence in children. The presence of residual sleep apnea as determined by the PAP device had marked effects on PAP usage with a residual apnea hypopnea index (AHI) greater than 5/hour having the lowest reported PAP usage (55.6%, $P<.001$). An elevated residual AHI, which could suggest subtherapeutic airway pressures and subsequent inadequate therapy, likely culminates in secondary sleep fragmentation and greater intolerance to PAP therapy in children. In fact, the study did confirm that low average 95th percentile pressure level over 90 days also affected usage significantly, with the lowest 95th percentile pressure range (4–6 cm H2O) being associated with the lowest PAP usage (52.0%, $P<.001$). Finally, median PAP detected mask leak averaged over 90 days was also significantly associated with PAP usage with average median leaks exceeding 24 L/min having the lowest observed usage at 90 days (43.7%, $P<.001$). The findings from this large cohort of children certainly support the rational of routinely monitoring therapy efficacy parameters collected nightly in the cloud database as an important strategy to improve adherence in children. However, one must caution that it is unclear regarding the accuracy of PAP devices at measuring these parameters in children, as all values have been validated in adults only. For example, thresholds for mask leak and residual AHI detection in small children is likely very different than in adults, given children have reduced tidal volumes and expiratory flow rates.

Taken together, although it is challenging to draw inferences from several single-site studies, the addition of the aforementioned large cross-sectional dataset does seem to confirm that age is a significant factor on PAP adherence in children, with adolescents seeming to have lowest reported PAP adherence. Considering that adolescents also have lower reported adherence with chronic medical therapies among all children,[57] this finding should not be surprising. Few studies seem to also suggest that female sex and a history of developmental delay result in greater PAP adherence, although these should be confirmed using larger datasets. Other demographic factors such as race and socioeconomic status, including household income, patient insurance type, and maternal education level may have an influence on PAP adherence, but these findings were not consistent across all studies making the case that more studies, particularly studies with large sample sizes, are needed to conclude on these demographic factors. Finally, both small sample size studies and a large dataset do support that certain technical factors assessing device efficacy such as mask leak and residual AHI have significant influences on PAP adherence (**Table 1**).

Intervention studies and positive airway pressure adherence

Few studies have evaluated the efficacy of specific interventions or modifications to improve PAP adherence in children. Again, limiting the generalizability of the findings is the heterogeneous definition of adherence but also the variability that is observed in clinical practice, ranging from the frequency of follow-up for patients with PAP to

Table 1
Predictors of pediatric positive airway pressure adherence

Data from n >1000 Study[54]	
Demographic	
	Age
Patient Engagement Program	
Device Parameters	
	Mask leak
	Residual AHI
	Average 95th percentile pressure
Consistent[a] Data from n <1000 Studies[53]	
Demographic	
	Sex
	Developmental delay
Inconsistent[b] Data from n <1000 Studies[68]	
Demographic	
	Race
	BMI
	Comorbidities
	Socioeconomic status
	Maternal education
	Insurance status
	Parent using PAP
Disease	
	Duration of PAP use
	Disease severity
	Disease symptoms
Technological	
	Device mode
	Mask type

Abbreviation: BMI, body mass index.
[a] Denotes factors found to be significantly associated with adherence in 2 or more studies.
[b] Denotes factors not found to be significantly associated with adherence in 2 or more studies.
Adapted from Watach AJ, Xanthopoulos MS, Afolabi-Brown O, et al. Positive airway pressure adherence in pediatric obstructive sleep apnea: A systematic scoping review. Sleep medicine reviews. 2020;51:101273; with permission.

access to multiple disciplines including respiratory therapists[58] and sleep psychologists.[59]

The efficacy of several interventions in improving PAP adherence is well established from adult studies. Techniques such as systematic desensitization,[60] patient education,[61] motivational interviewing,[62] and cognitive behavioral interventions[63] have all shown to promise to increase PAP adherence in adults. In children, there are fewer studies evaluating the efficacy of these interventions in PAP adherence. In fact, most studies addressing adherence in pediatrics have focused mostly on children with chronic illnesses and long-term medication usage. In a systematic review of medication adherence,[57] Dean and colleagues conclude that although educational strategies are often indicated, these are often insufficient and that the addition of a behavioral intervention may further optimize adherence in children. This rational has led several groups to evaluate the efficacy of behavioral interventions to optimize adherence to PAP therapy in children.

Before reviewing this evidence, it is important to emphasize that enhancing the physician-patient relationship generally yields improvements in patient adherence, including the notion to abandon the paternalistic approach of physicians and replacing this with a partnership between the physician and the patient/family.[64] In doing so, the physician and patient are sharing decision-making and creating a negotiated treatment plan. Such an approach should have a role in pediatric PAP clinics in order to optimize PAP adherence.

In one of the few studies assessing behavioral interventions and PAP adherence in children, Koontz and colleagues[65] retrospectively evaluated 20 nonadherent pediatric patients with PAP (aged 1–17 years) who were subdivided into 3 groups: (1) a group receiving a 1.5-hour consultation and recommendation session, (2) a group receiving consultation and recommendations plus a course of behavior therapy, and (3) a group for whom behavior therapy was recommended but the family did not follow-up (negative control). Behavioral therapy consisted of positive reinforcement, graduated exposure, or implementing PAP gradually, counter-conditioning, and avoidance prevention strategies. These investigators reported that the consultation and behavior therapy groups led to 75% of nonadherent patients now successfully tolerating PAP with increased hours of documented usage compared with 0% of children who did not receive these therapies. Although the negative control group of nonfollow-up patients likely selected unmotivated families, this pilot study supported a role for behavioral interventions to rescue nonadherent children.

Slifer and colleagues[66] incorporated similar intensive behavioral therapy in 4 preschool studies nonadherent to PAP therapy and showed that using these approaches, all 4 children eventually became adherent to PAP, albeit some took longer than others.

In another small pilot study[67] comparing 6 nonadherent children to 9 adherent PAP users (mean age: 5 years), Mendoza-Ruiz and colleagues showed evidence that using a monitoring table that integrates tokens on a daily calendar for positive reinforcement improved PAP nightly usage following 1 month, although not necessarily the hourly usage of PAP, in the nonadherent group. Taken together, despite the limitations of very small sample sizes, the findings from these pilot studies seem to support a role for behavioral therapy for rescuing children identified with poor PAP adherence.

The major challenge to integrating approaches such as education and/or behavioral interventions in children using PAP is that most centers lack the resources and personnel. Specialized behavioral therapists and sleep psychologists are generally scarce and only exist in a few tertiary pediatric sleep programs. Further, in one of the few tertiary pediatric sleep centers with these resources, the application of an intensive program, which included device consignment, behavioral psychology counseling, and follow-up telephone calls to routine care of pediatric patients with PAP, Riley and colleagues[68] reported that although improvements in follow-up of pediatric patients with PAP was observed, the program was not necessarily cost-effective.

Therefore, methods to implement behavioral interventions in a simple, cost-effective and easily accessible manner could be more effective to improve PAP adherence to a larger group of patients. Recent development of a patient engagement program (PEP) developed for smart phones has delivered significant traction in optimizing adherence in adult patients using PAP therapy in a large group of patients.[69] Similarly, in the cloud-based cross-sectional study of 20,533 children on PAP therapy,[54] these investigators evaluated the efficacy of PEP to optimize adherence in children. PEP accesses cloud-based data while providing real-time feedback to patients and families, which includes a score that incorporates usage hours, mask seal indicating leak level, residual respiratory events per hour of usage, and the number of times the mask was taken on/off. Integrating these measures, patients are given real-time feedback as well as constructive suggestions through personalized coaching messages. The overarching goal of PEP is to enhance self-management, recognize success through awards, and identify and resolve basic treatment issues on their own. In the study,[54] participation to PEP was voluntary and likely introduced a selection bias, as those patients who signed up for PEP were likely to be more motivated or educated than other groups, thereby contributing to better PAP usage. Notwithstanding, when PEP use was compared with non-PEP users, PAP usage was significantly higher in PEP users, with 79.1% of PEP users remaining on PAP therapy at 90 days compared with 57.5% of non-PEP users (P<.001). Although confirming the efficacy of PEP will require a randomized clinical trial, this preliminary evidence in a large cross-sectional study of children on PAP therapy does seem to support its use in optimizing adherence.

Future Goals for Positive Airway Pressure Care in Children

The available evidence suggests that about half of children prescribed PAP therapy will have reduced adherence, with many children having their therapy terminated due to nonusage. Given the high likelihood of children with residual sleep apnea following adenotonsillectomy, coupled with the impact of obesity on the increasing prevalence of pediatric OSA, clinicians should anticipate that a large population of children will be prescribed PAP devices. If nearly half of these children will have reduced or inadequate adherence to PAP, it is imperative then for clinicians to identify at-risk children and tailor therapy to try and optimize PAP adherence.

Numerous studies have identified risk factors, both negative and positive, that can also help clinicians identify children at risk for reduced adherence (see **Table 1**). Consistently across all studies, adolescent children seem to have the most reduced adherence to PAP and are at highest risk for therapy termination. This is of concern for 2 reasons: this group is least likely to respond to adenotonsillectomy[26] and least likely to "outgrow" OSA, as growth is near completion during adolescence. Thus, among children, adolescents are most likely to be prescribed PAP therapy[54] and most likely to need PAP long term. Other demographic factors such as sex, developmental status, race, and socioeconomic status may also be relevant to assessing risk for PAP adherence.

The study by Nixon and colleagues[45] made it apparent that an "adherence phenotype" can be identified early, in which children who have suboptimal adherence to PAP therapy can be identified right off the gate. Because of the advent of cloud-based monitoring, access to adherence data can begin as early as day one of implementation of PAP therapy. Thus, regardless of potential

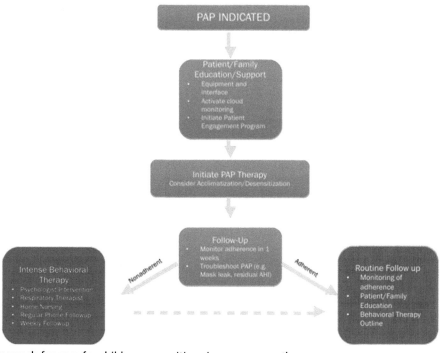

Fig. 1. Framework for care for children on positive airway pressure therapy.

demographic risk factors, clinicians are certainly able to identify adherence patterns following the first week of therapy and stratify risk immediately using cloud-based data. Cloud-based data may in fact provide the framework for how best to treat children prescribed PAP therapy (**Fig. 1**). In addition, cloud-based monitoring allows clinicians to trouble shoot PAP therapy instantaneously, because measures such as mask leak and residual AHI are significantly associated with PAP adherence[54]; these potentially actionable items, if identified and rectified early, could yield improvements in adherence.

The nature of PEP could also allow patients to take more control of their therapy and intervene in their management earlier, either independently or in tandem with their health care providers. PEP also introduces behavioral intervention strategies, and if these strategies are implemented earlier, these may yield better outcomes.[54] Although not yet confirmed in a prospective randomized clinical trial, the existing evidence[54,69] seems to strongly support its use in both adults and children. Given the positive influence of also having a family member use PAP therapy on adherence in children,[46] one could justify the creation of specific support groups, which would integrate children and families who themselves are using PAP therapy.

Apart from these postulated early intervention strategies, if anything the early identification of an adherence phenotype allows for tailored therapy, including implementation of intensive behavioral therapy programs with consultations by sleep psychologists, respiratory therapists, and behavioral therapists for nonadherent patients. For example, this may help in determining whether it would be appropriate to consider PAP mask acclimatization or desensitization.[42] Although it remains to be seen whether such a program is cost-effective, restricting access to these programs to those who are in need may be more realistic. Finally, ongoing monitoring of cloud-based data may help clinicians decide the nature (see **Fig. 1**) and frequency of follow-up. Decision-making could include whether follow-up should take place in person or via telemedicine or whether patients should restart or modify their formalized behavioral intervention programs.

SUMMARY

With improvements in recognition of sleep-disordered breathing in children, it is likely that more and more children will require PAP therapy as an intervention to eradicate sleep-disordered breathing. Existing evidence seems to identify that although many children succeed with adequate PAP adherence, there does remain many children with suboptimal adherence. Future studies addressing both the timing and the efficacy of intervention strategies, including child specific behavioral interventions, are needed. With evolving technology including the nature of cloud-based monitoring and integration of PEP, it is very possible that adherence to PAP therapy in children will only improve in the not-so-distant future.

CLINICS CARE POINTS

- Recent evidence has identified adherence rates in children using positive airway pressure therapy.
- Awareness of factors improving adherence rates are prudent to enhancing care.

DISCLOSURE

The author has no disclosures of financial relationships related to the subject matter of this article.

REFERENCES

1. Lumeng JC, Chervin RD. Epidemiology of pediatric obstructive sleep apnea. Proc Am Thorac Soc 2008;5(2):242–52.
2. Montgomery-Downs HE, O'Brien LM, Holbrook CR, et al. Snoring and sleep-disordered breathing in young children: subjective and objective correlates. Sleep 2004;27(1):87–94.
3. Gislason T, Benediktsdottir B. Snoring, apneic episodes, and nocturnal hypoxemia among children 6 months to 6 years old. An epidemiologic study of lower limit of prevalence. Chest 1995;107(4):963–6.
4. Ali NJ, Pitson DJ, Stradling JR. Snoring, sleep disturbance, and behaviour in 4-5 year olds. Arch Dis Child 1993;68(3):360–6.
5. Marcus CL, McColley SA, Carroll JL, et al. Upper airway collapsibility in children with obstructive sleep apnea syndrome. J Appl Physiol (1985) 1994;77(2):918–24.
6. Arens R, Marcus CL. Pathophysiology of upper airway obstruction: a developmental perspective. Sleep 2004;27(5):997–1019.
7. Gozal D. Sleep-disordered breathing and school performance in children. Pediatrics 1998;102(3 Pt 1):616–20.
8. Gozal D, Crabtree VM, Sans Capdevila O, et al. C-reactive protein, obstructive sleep apnea, and cognitive dysfunction in school-aged children. Am J Respir Crit Care Med 2007;176(2):188–93.

9. Chervin RD, Archbold KH, Dillon JE, et al. Inattention, hyperactivity, and symptoms of sleep-disordered breathing. Pediatrics 2002;109(3):449–56.

10. Chervin RD, Dillon JE, Bassetti C, et al. Symptoms of sleep disorders, inattention, and hyperactivity in children. Sleep 1997;20(12):1185–92.

11. Marcotte AC, Thacher PV, Butters M, et al. Parental report of sleep problems in children with attentional and learning disorders. J Dev Behav Pediatr 1998;19(3):178–86.

12. Owens J, Spirito A, Marcotte A, et al. Neuropsychological and behavioral correlates of obstructive sleep apnea syndrome in children: a preliminary study. Sleep Breath 2000;4(2):67–78.

13. Perfect MM, Archbold K, Goodwin JL, et al. Risk of behavioral and adaptive functioning difficulties in youth with previous and current sleep disordered breathing. Sleep 2013;36(4):517–525B.

14. Kheirandish L, Gozal D. Neurocognitive dysfunction in children with sleep disorders. Dev Sci 2006;9(4):388–99.

15. Dayyat E, Kheirandish-Gozal L, Gozal D. Childhood obstructive sleep apnea: one or two distinct disease entities? Sleep Med Clin 2007;2(3):433–44.

16. Bhattacharjee R, Kheirandish-Gozal L, Pillar G, et al. Cardiovascular complications of obstructive sleep apnea syndrome: evidence from children. Prog Cardiovasc Dis 2009;51(5):416–33.

17. Amin R, Somers VK, McConnell K, et al. Activity-adjusted 24-hour ambulatory blood pressure and cardiac remodeling in children with sleep disordered breathing. Hypertension 2008;51(1):84–91.

18. Marcus CL, Greene MG, Carroll JL. Blood pressure in children with obstructive sleep apnea. Am J Respir Crit Care Med 1998;157(4 Pt 1):1098–103.

19. Kohyama J, Ohinata JS, Hasegawa T. Blood pressure in sleep disordered breathing. Arch Dis Child 2003;88(2):139–42.

20. Gozal D, Kheirandish-Gozal L, Serpero LD, et al. Obstructive sleep apnea and endothelial function in school-aged nonobese children: effect of adenotonsillectomy. Circulation 2007;116(20):2307–14.

21. Bhattacharjee R, Kim J, Alotaibi WH, et al. Endothelial dysfunction in children without hypertension: potential contributions of obesity and obstructive sleep apnea. Chest 2012;141(3):682–91.

22. Kheirandish-Gozal L, Etzioni T, Bhattacharjee R, et al. Obstructive sleep apnea in children is associated with severity-dependent deterioration in overnight endothelial function. Sleep Med 2013;14(6):526–31.

23. Amin RS, Kimball TR, Kalra M, et al. Left ventricular function in children with sleep-disordered breathing. Am J Cardiol 2005;95(6):801–4.

24. Marcus CL, Brooks LJ, Draper KA, et al. Diagnosis and management of childhood obstructive sleep apnea syndrome. Pediatrics 2012;130(3):576–84.

25. Erickson BK, Larson DR, St Sauver JL, et al. Changes in incidence and indications of tonsillectomy and adenotonsillectomy, 1970-2005. Otolaryngol Head Neck Surg 2009;140(6):894–901.

26. Bhattacharjee R, Kheirandish-Gozal L, Spruyt K, et al. Adenotonsillectomy outcomes in treatment of obstructive sleep apnea in children: a multicenter retrospective study. Am J Respir Crit Care Med 2010;182(5):676–83.

27. Marcus CL, Moore RH, Rosen CL, et al. A randomized trial of adenotonsillectomy for childhood sleep apnea. N Engl J Med 2013;368(25):2366–76.

28. Wang Y, Lobstein T. Worldwide trends in childhood overweight and obesity. Int J Pediatr Obes 2006;1(1):11–25.

29. Lobstein T, Jackson-Leach R. Child overweight and obesity in the USA: prevalence rates according to IOTF definitions. Int J Pediatr Obes 2007;2(1):62–4.

30. Tauman R, Gozal D. Obesity and obstructive sleep apnea in children. Paediatr Respir Rev 2006;7(4):247–59.

31. Dayyat E, Kheirandish-Gozal L, Sans Capdevila O, et al. Obstructive sleep apnea in children: relative contributions of body mass index and adenotonsillar hypertrophy. Chest 2009;136(1):137–44.

32. Nation J, Brigger M. The efficacy of adenotonsillectomy for obstructive sleep apnea in children with down syndrome: a systematic review. Otolaryngol Head Neck Surg 2017;157(3):401–8.

33. Hurvitz MS, Lesser DJ, Dever G, et al. Findings of routine nocturnal polysomnography in children with Down syndrome: a retrospective cohort study. Sleep Med 2020;76:58–64.

34. Guilleminault C, Nino-Murcia G, Heldt G, et al. Alternative treatment to tracheostomy in obstructive sleep apnea syndrome: nasal continuous positive airway pressure in young children. Pediatrics 1986;78(5):797–802.

35. Marcus CL, Beck SE, Traylor J, et al. Randomized, double-blind clinical trial of two different modes of positive airway pressure therapy on adherence and efficacy in children. J Clin Sleep Med 2012;8(1):37–42.

36. O'Donnell AR, Bjornson CL, Bohn SG, et al. Compliance rates in children using noninvasive continuous positive airway pressure. Sleep 2006;29(5):651–8.

37. Simon SL, Duncan CL, Janicke DM, et al. Barriers to treatment of paediatric obstructive sleep apnoea: development of the adherence barriers to continuous positive airway pressure (CPAP) questionnaire. Sleep Med 2012;13(2):172–7.

38. DiFeo N, Meltzer LJ, Beck SE, et al. Predictors of positive airway pressure therapy adherence in

children: a prospective study. J Clin Sleep Med 2012;8(3):279–86.

39. Fauroux B, Boffa C, Desguerre I, et al. Long-term noninvasive mechanical ventilation for children at home: a national survey. Pediatr Pulmonol 2003; 35(2):119–25.

40. Fauroux B, Boffa C, Desguerre I, et al. Long-term noninvasive mechanical ventilation for children at home: a national survey. Pediatric Pulmonology 2003;35(2):119–25.

41. Services CfMM. Decision memo for continuous positive airway pressure (CPAP) therapy for obstructive sleep apnea (OSA) (CAG-00093N). Available at: https://wwwcmsgov/medicare-coverage-database/details/nca-decision-memoaspx?NCAId=19&fromdb=true. 100.

42. King MS, Xanthopoulos MS, Marcus CL. Improving positive airway pressure adherence in children. Sleep Med Clin 2014;9(2):219–34.

43. Marcus CL, Rosen G, Ward SL, et al. Adherence to and effectiveness of positive airway pressure therapy in children with obstructive sleep apnea. Pediatrics 2006;117(3):e442–51.

44. Machaalani R, Evans CA, Waters KA. Objective adherence to positive airway pressure therapy in an Australian paediatric cohort. Sleep Breath 2016; 20(4):1327–36.

45. Nixon GM, Mihai R, Verginis N, et al. Patterns of continuous positive airway pressure adherence during the first 3 months of treatment in children. J Pediatr 2011;159(5):802–7.

46. Puri P, Ross KR, Mehra R, et al. Pediatric positive airway pressure adherence in obstructive sleep apnea enhanced by family member positive airway pressure usage. J Clin Sleep Med 2016;12(7): 959–63.

47. Ramirez A, Khirani S, Aloui S, et al. Continuous positive airway pressure and noninvasive ventilation adherence in children. Sleep Med 2013;14(12): 1290–4.

48. Uong EC, Epperson M, Bathon SA, et al. Adherence to nasal positive airway pressure therapy among school-aged children and adolescents with obstructive sleep apnea syndrome. Pediatrics 2007;120(5): e1203–11.

49. Hawkins SM, Jensen EL, Simon SL, et al. Correlates of pediatric CPAP adherence. J Clin Sleep Med 2016;12(6):879–84.

50. Perriol MP, Jullian-Desayes I, Joyeux-Faure M, et al. Long-term adherence to ambulatory initiated continuous positive airway pressure in non-syndromic OSA children. Sleep Breath 2019;23(2):575–8.

51. Waters KA, Everett FM, Bruderer JW, et al. Obstructive sleep apnea: the use of nasal CPAP in 80 children. Am J Respir Crit Care Med 1995;152(2):780–5.

52. Marcus CL, Ward SL, Mallory GB, et al. Use of nasal continuous positive airway pressure as treatment of

childhood obstructive sleep apnea. J Pediatr 1995; 127(1):88–94.

53. Watach AJ, Xanthopoulos MS, Afolabi-Brown O, et al. Positive airway pressure adherence in pediatric obstructive sleep apnea: a systematic scoping review. Sleep Med Rev 2020;51:101273.

54. Bhattacharjee R, Benjafield AV, Armitstead J, et al. Adherence in children using positive airway pressure therapy: a big-data analysis. The Lancet Digital Health 2020;2(2):e94–101.

55. Kang EK, Xanthopoulos MS, Kim JY, et al. Adherence to positive airway pressure for the treatment of obstructive sleep apnea in children with developmental disabilities. J Clin Sleep Med 2019;15(6): 915–21.

56. Avis KT, Gamble KL, Schwebel DC. Effect of positive airway pressure therapy in children with obstructive sleep apnea syndrome: does positive airway pressure use reduce pedestrian injury risk? Sleep Health 2019;5(2):161–5.

57. Dean AJ, Walters J, Hall A. A systematic review of interventions to enhance medication adherence in children and adolescents with chronic illness. Arch Dis Child 2010;95(9):717–23.

58. Jambhekar SK, Com G, Tang X, et al. Role of a respiratory therapist in improving adherence to positive airway pressure treatment in a pediatric sleep apnea clinic. Respir Care 2013;58(12): 2038–44.

59. Harford KL, Jambhekar S, Com G, et al. Behaviorally based adherence program for pediatric patients treated with positive airway pressure. Clin Child Psychol Psychiatry 2013;18(1):151–63.

60. Edinger JD, Radtke RA. Use of in vivo desensitization to treat a patient's claustrophobic response to nasal CPAP. Sleep 1993;16(7):678–80.

61. Likar LL, Panciera TM, Erickson AD, et al. Group education sessions and compliance with nasal CPAP therapy. Chest 1997;111(5):1273–7.

62. Aloia MS, Arnedt JT, Riggs RL, et al. Clinical management of poor adherence to CPAP: motivational enhancement. Behav Sleep Med 2004;2(4): 205–22.

63. Aloia MS, Di Dio L, Ilniczky N, et al. Improving compliance with nasal CPAP and vigilance in older adults with OAHS. Sleep Breath 2001; 5(1):13–21.

64. Vermeire E, Hearnshaw H, Van Royen P, et al. Patient adherence to treatment: three decades of research. A comprehensive review. J Clin Pharm Ther 2001; 26(5):331–42.

65. Koontz KL, Slifer KJ, Cataldo MD, et al. Improving pediatric compliance with positive airway pressure therapy: the impact of behavioral intervention. Sleep 2003;26(8):1010–5.

66. Slifer KJ, Kruglak D, Benore E, et al. Behavioral training for increasing preschool children's

adherence with positive airway pressure: a preliminary study. Behav Sleep Med 2007;5(2):147–75.

67. Mendoza-Ruiz A, Dylgjeri S, Bour F, et al. Evaluation of the efficacy of a dedicated table to improve CPAP adherence in children: a pilot study. Sleep Med 2019;53:60–4.

68. Riley EB, Fieldston ES, Xanthopoulos MS, et al. Financial analysis of an intensive pediatric continuous positive airway pressure program. Sleep 2017;40(2):1–8.

69. Malhotra A, Crocker ME, Willes L, et al. Patient engagement using new technology to improve adherence to positive airway pressure therapy: a retrospective analysis. Chest 2018;153(4): 843–50.

Socioeconomic Disparities in Positive Airway Pressure Adherence: An Integrative Review

Earl Charles Crew, PhD[a,b], William K. Wohlgemuth, PhD[c,d],
Amy M. Sawyer, PhD, RN[e,f,g], Natasha J. Williams, EdD, MPH[h],
Douglas M. Wallace, MD[d,i],*

KEYWORDS

- Sleep • Sleep apnea • Positive airway pressure • Socioeconomic status
- Socioeconomic disparities • Adherence • Compliance

KEY POINTS

- Lower socioeconomic status (SES) is associated with reduced adherence to positive airway pressure (PAP) therapy.
- Aspects of low SES may interact with biomedical, psychological, social, and health care system factors to promote or impede PAP adherence.
- The current body of literature on SES and PAP adherence is limited and does not explain why disparities exist, possible pathways/mechanisms to explain these relationships, or the level at which interventions could be most effective (eg, at the level of the individual patient, sleep clinic/hospital, or health care system/government).
- Future investigations should apply a biopsychosocial framework, would benefit from obtaining as much SES data as possible to explain relationships between SES variables and PAP adherence, and should consider reporting PAP use relative to total sleep time.

INTRODUCTION

Obstructive sleep apnea (OSA) is a significant public health concern given the immediate (eg, daytime sleepiness and deficits in cognitive function)[1,2] and longer-term (eg, risk for motor vehicle accidents, myocardial infarction/stroke, depression, and dementia)[3–6] sequelae when untreated. The societal costs of untreated OSA also are significant. Prior to diagnosis, patients with OSA accrue about double the medical expenses than they would if treated sooner (due primarily to cardiovascular disease morbidity), and cost-

a Behavioral Health Program, Mental Health Care Line, Michael E. DeBakey VA Medical Center, Building 108-A Room 224, 2002 Holcombe Boulevard, Houston, TX 77030, USA; b Psychology Division, Menninger Department of Psychiatry and Behavioral Sciences, Baylor College of Medicine, Houston, TX, USA; c Psychology Service, Bruce W. Carter Medical Center, Miami VA Healthcare system, Sleep Disorders Center, Room A212, 1201 NW 16th ST, Miami, FL 33125, USA; d Neurology Service, Bruce W. Carter Medical Center, Miami VA Healthcare system, Sleep Disorders Center, Room A212, 1201 NW 16th ST, Miami, FL 33125, USA; e University of Pennsylvania, School of Nursing, Clair Fagin Hall, Room 349, 418 Curie Boulevard, Philadelphia, PA 19104, USA; f Perelman School of Medicine Center for Sleep and Circadian Neurobiology, Philadelphia, PA, USA; g Corporal Michael J. Crescenz VA Medical Center, Philadelphia, PA, USA; h Department of Population Health, Division of Health and Behavior, Center for Healthful Behavior Change, New York University Grossman School of Medicine, 180 Madison Avenue, 7th Floor, New York, NY 10016, USA; i Department of Neurology, University of Miami Miller School of Medicine, Miami, FL, USA
* Corresponding author. Bruce W. Carter Medical Center, Miami VA Healthcare system, Sleep Disorders Center, Room A212, 1201 NW 16th ST, Miami, FL 33125, USA.
E-mail address: Dwallace@med.miami.edu

Sleep Med Clin 16 (2021) 23–41
https://doi.org/10.1016/j.jsmc.2020.10.003
1556-407X/21/Published by Elsevier Inc.

effectiveness evaluations of current therapies suggest that it costs more not to treat OSA than to treat it.[7,8] The gold standard for management of OSA is pressurized air to pneumatically splint the airway, known as positive airway pressure therapy (PAP).[9] Despite decades of accumulating advancements in PAP technology focused on improving individuals' experience with the device, PAP nonadherence remains rampant.[10] Up to 50% of patients initially refuse PAP therapy, whereas an additional 12% to 25% have discontinued PAP use by 3 years.[11] Following diagnosis of OSA, adherence with PAP therapy has been found to reduce health care utilization (ie, outpatient visits and hospital admissions) among patients by up to 25%, compared with just 5% in those with OSA that eventually discontinue PAP.[12] Given the mortality risks associated with untreated OSA, adherence with efficacious therapies like PAP is critical.[13]

Socioeconomic Disparities in Positive Airway Pressure Adherence

The issue of poor treatment adherence in the management of OSA is hardly distinctive among other chronic medical conditions. It is estimated that more than 50% of all individuals with a chronic illness fail to adhere to their prescribed therapies.[14] In the broader field of medicine, disparities in access and health outcomes often are considered in terms of 2 primary factors: race/ethnicity and socioeconomic status (SES). SES is a complex construct that can be measured in several ways. Commonly used metrics of SES include years of education, individual or family income, area of residence (ie, area-based composite indices, median neighborhood income based on census data), and access to health care resources.[15]

Members of the authors' group conducted a recent scoping review of PAP adherence among minority populations in the United States and observed relatively poorer adherence for black patients compared with white patients and equivalent use among US Hispanic patients compared with whites.[16] The authors' conclusions with regard to the role of SES were less clear, which they attributed to small sample sizes and the high intercorrelation reported between race/ethnicity and lower SES among the included studies. Therefore, understanding for how SES factors may have an impact on individuals' engagement with PAP in combination with other variables remains uncertain. One likely reason for this is that SES metrics often are utilized only as covariates within analyses of other racial/ethnic

predictors of adherence, as opposed to SES being the primary variable of interest. Similarly, SES and race/ethnicity often are examined as a single unique index, which precludes knowledge about the individual effects. These are acknowledged limitations of most investigations of SES on health research outcomes[17]; the extent to which this is present within the current literature on SES effects on PAP adherence has not been explored.

Purpose of Review

Currently, understanding of how SES factors affect PAP adherence is limited due to numerous within-study issues (eg, representativeness of SES groups, sample size/power, and statistical adjustment for confounders) and across-study variation (eg, designs, adherence outcome definitions, and operationalization of SES). This integrative review aims to provide a structured summary of the current body of literature regarding whether SES factors have an impact on adherence to PAP therapy. Through this, the authors hope to highlight factors that contribute to disparities among adult PAP users and identify future directions to improve equity in the management of OSA.

METHODS
Selection Criteria

All primary research publications written in English investigating socioeconomic factors and relationships with objectively assessed PAP adherence in adults with OSA were considered relevant for inclusion. Studies that analyzed individual-level socioeconomic variables (eg, income level) or contexts (eg, neighborhood location) were the main focus of this review. Studies that examined a broader range of factors associated with PAP adherence and included socioeconomic variables, however, also were eligible for inclusion.

Search Strategy

The lead author (ECC) performed a literature search in PubMed (Medline), Embase, and Web of Science Plus using combinations of the following search terms: "sleep apnea," "sleep-disordered breathing," "sleep-related breathing," "CPAP," or "positive airway pressure" AND "socioeconomic" or "SES" AND "adherence," "compliance," "acceptance," or "use." Although the authors were interested only in studies of PAP adherence, search terms to identify studies of initial PAP "use" or "acceptance" were included to increase the initial yield, given overlap between these studies. Because PAP technology has included only the capability to record objective device usage since the early 1990s,[18] the search date was restricted to span January 1990 to February 2020. The search targeted articles that met the following criteria: (1) primary studies, (2) published in peer review articles (no abstracts), (3) written in English, and included (4) adults (≥18 years old), (5) objective PAP adherence, (6) measure(s) of SES (eg, income, education, occupation, composite index, health insurance status) as an independent variable, and (7) samples greater than or equal to 100 with complete PAP adherence data. A list of all relevant articles then was compiled, with each full-text article read by the lead author to confirm inclusion based on selection criteria. For all retrieved articles that met criteria, ancestry search of each full-text reference list was performed to identify additional articles meeting these criteria for inclusion in the review.

RESULTS
Search Results

A total of 407 unique articles initially were retrieved across databases (**Fig. 1**). With title review, 315 articles were excluded immediately (eg, not about OSA or PAP and sample included only children); 92 articles underwent abstract review, of which 81 were eliminated. Ancestry search of the references lists for these retrieved articles identified 5 additional articles, resulting in a list of 16 articles that were included for full text review and reporting.

Study Characteristics

Characteristics of the retrieved studies (n = 16) investigating effects of SES factors on PAP adherence (defined as objectively derived recording of daily PAP use at home) are presented in **Table 1**. Most of the included studies were observational and prospective (n = 11) or retrospective (n = 4) cohort studies. One article was an experimental investigation with 2 experimental groups.[19] Sample sizes ranged from 101 to 170,641. Regarding clinical severity of sampled participants, half of the reviewed studies included all severity levels of OSA (n = 8) whereas some restricted their sample to only moderate-to-severe OSA (n = 8). All retrieved studies were exclusively composed of—or also included—data from individuals who were PAP-naïve; only 4 studies included data for individuals who were PAP-experienced at time of enrollment.[20–23] Among modalities of PAP utilized in the included studies, most were continuous PAP (CPAP) only (n = 9).

How adherence was reported varied across articles and generally included mean daily use in minutes/h (n = 8) or grouping individuals as adherent versus nonadherent based on whether their use met or exceeded 4 hours per day (n = 10), with 2 of these studies[21,23] also stipulating use of greater than or equal to 4 hours per day on 70% of days during a 30-day period (in-line with definitions set by the Centers for Medicare & Medicaid Services [CMS]).[24] Regarding measurement intervals for adherence, 4 studies (25.0%) assessed adherence at multiple time points after initiation.[25–28] Three studies assessed adherence during the first week,[28–30] 4 articles (25.0%) assessed adherence during the first 30 days/4 weeks/1 month,[26,31,32] 5 studies (31.3%) assessed adherence during the first 30 days to 90 days,[26–28,30,32] 5 studies (31.3%) looked at average use after the first 3 months,[20,25,27,33,34] 1 study looked at use during

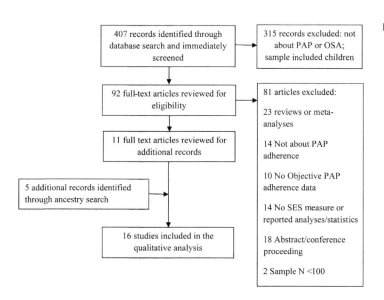

Fig. 1. Search flow diagram.

Table 1
Primary studies assessing positive airway pressure adherence as a function of socioeconomic status variables

Study Citation	Design/Location	Sample with Positive Airway Pressure Data; Pertinent Demographics	Outcome Interval(s)	Adherence Outcome(s)	Socioeconomic Status Variable(s)	Analysis Methods	Covariates	Findings for Socioeconomic Status Variables
Aloia et al,[25] 2007	Prospective, single sleep center; Providence, Rhode Island, USA	N = 140, 66% men; CPAP-naïve	Initial 6 mo	M use group: consistent users (≥6 nights); intermittent users (<6 nights) M use h/night	Years of education	Student t test Pearson bivariate correlation	None	Intermittent users less educated than consistent users; t(140) = 2.61, P<.01 Years of education uncorrelated with M use h/night
Bakker et al,[31] 2011	Prospective, single sleep laboratory; Wellington, New Zealand	N = 126, 79% men; 19.8% Māori; CPAP-naïve	Initial 4 wk	Group: adherent ≥4 h/ night vs not adherent	Health care eligibility (government vs private) Area-based SES deprivation score (1–5; 5 = high deprivation) Individual SES deprivation score (1–5; 5 = high deprivation) Annual income (<20k; ≥20 k<60k; ≥60k NZ dollars)	Univariate logistic regression Multivariate logistic regression	None Ethnicity (Māori vs non-Māori); health care eligibility, education, income, area-based and individual deprivation score	No differences: higher education, area-based deprivation score, employment type Predictors of adherence <4 h: Lower education OR 0.25 (95% CI, 0.08–0.83); P = .02 Highest individual deprivation

Source	Design, setting	Sample	Duration	PAP use outcome	SES measure	Statistical analysis	None (no association)	Results
					Highest education (primary/secondary vs tertiary) Employment type (full time, part time, unemployed)			score OR 0.10 (95% CI, 0.02–0.86; $P = .02$)
Billings et al,[26] 2011	Prospective, 7 sleep centers; 5 US cities (Seattle, WA; Chicago, IL; Madison, WI; Minneapolis, MN; Cleveland, OH)	N = 191, 65% men; 11.5% black, 4.9% Hispanic; CPAP-naïve	First month, initial 3 mo	M use min/night % d >4 h Group: adherent (>4 h) vs nonadherent (<4 h)	ZIP code SES z score (median household income, % HS and college graduates age 25+; % families < poverty level; % unemployed; % in managerial/professional occupations); higher score = higher SES (stratified into quartiles)	Student t test Multivariate linear regression	None black race, Hispanic, AHI, study arm (home vs in-laboratory study)	No differences: % d >4 h or M use min/night Lowest ZIP code SES quartile predicts lower use at 3 mo; $P<.10$
Campbell et al,[37] 2012	Prospective, single sleep laboratory; Wellington, New Zealand	N = 214, 73% men; 22% Maori, 15.4% Pacific peoples; CPAP-naïve	Initial 4 wk	M use h/night	Area-based SES deprivation score (1–10; 10 = high deprivation)	ANOVA	None Ethnicity (Asian, Maori, Pacific peoples, European)	Lower vs higher deprivation associated with increased usage; F (4209) = 15.2; $P = .02$; $r = 0.23$

(continued on next page)

Table 1
(continued)

Study Citation	Design/Location	Sample with Positive Airway Pressure Data; Pertinent Demographics	Outcome Interval(s)	Adherence Outcome(s)	Socioeconomic Status Variable(s)	Analysis Methods	Covariates	Findings for Socioeconomic Status Variables
								No differences after adjusting for ethnicity
Chai-Coetzer et al,[33] 2013	Prospective; 50 sleep centers in China (n = 37), Australia (n = 9), and New Zealand (n = 4)	N = 275, 80% men; 100% hx of CVD; CPAP-naïve	During 7–12 mo follow-up period after initiation	M use h/night	GDP of region of recruitment	Hierarchical linear regression	Site of data collection	No differences
Gagnadoux et al,[20] 2011	Prospective, 7 sleep centers; Western region of France	N = 1141%; 76% men; 76% married or living with partner; CPAP/APAP-experienced (3+ mo)	Since initiating treatment (minimum 90 d)	Group: adherent (>4 h) vs nonadherent (<4 h)	Education (less vs more than full-time education) Employment status (full time/ part time, unemployed, retired) Last occupation	Chi-square test Logistic regression	None BMI, AHI, marital status, employment status.	No effect of education or occupation Predict adherence: retired (vs employed) OR 1.414 (95% CI, 1.097–1.821); P = .007

Study	Design/Setting	Sample	Timing	Outcome	SES measure	Statistical test		Findings
Gulati et al,[27] 2017	Prospective, single sleep center; Wolverhampton, West Midlands, UK	N = 265, 77% men; PAP-naïve; 97% CPAP, 3% BiPAP	First follow-up (6–10 wk); second follow-up (6 mo)	M use h/night Group: adherent (≥4 h/night) vs nonadherent	National statistics socioeconomic classification for employment status (6 levels) Level of education (no formal, school certificate, higher school certificate or bachelor degree)	Mann-Whitney U test	None	No differences for level of education At 6–10 wk Long-term unemployed used PAP 2.1 h less ($P = .028$) and ≥4 h 26% less ($P = .046$) than in-work/retired At 6 mo Long-term unemployed used PAP 3.4 h less ($P = .016$) and ≥4 h 38% less ($P = .011$) than in-work/retired
Hui et al,[32] 2001	Prospective, single respiratory clinic; Shatin, New Territories, Hong Kong	N = 112, 90% men	First month, initial 3 mo	M use h/night	Rented/paid for device vs reimbursed by government Education level	ANOVA	None	No differences

(continued on next page)

Table 1
(*continued*)

Study Citation	Design/Location	Sample with Positive Airway Pressure Data; Pertinent Demographics	Outcome Interval(s)	Adherence Outcome(s)	Socioeconomic Status Variable(s)	Analysis Methods	Covariates	Findings for Socioeconomic Status Variables
Liou et al,[21] 2018	Prospective, single sleep center; Seattle, Washington, USA	N = 119, 57.1% men, 56.3% white non-Hispanic, PAP-naïve; 55% APAP, 34% CPAP, 9.4% BiPAP, 2% ASV	Most recent 30 d	Group: adherent (≥4 h/night for ≥70% d in a 30-d period; CMS criteria) vs nonadherent	Education (high school or less, some college/ associate's degree, college or graduate degree)	Multivariate logistic regression	Frequently changing sleeping location (≥1/mo); race/ ethnicity, marital status, and obesity.	Relative to HS or less: greater adherence with Some college/ associate: OR 3.0 (95% CI, 0.8–10.5); college or graduate degree: OR 6.4 (95% CI, 1.7–24.5)
May et al,[28] 2018	Prospective randomized clinical trial of sham vs active CPAP, 2 academic sleep clinics; Cleveland, Ohio, USA	N = 143, 55% men, 55% white; 100% moderate-to-severe OSA; PAP-naïve	First week, initial 8-wk	M use min/night 8-wk M use h/night first week only	Income >$50k (dichotomous) Education (HS or less, any college/ vocational, bachelor's degree or above) Subjective social status (1–10 NRS)	Univariate linear regression Multivariable logistic regression (α = .10 for interactions)	None Treatment arm, age, race, sex, BMI, CVD, ESS, FOSQ, CESD, PANAS, AHI, T90, CPAP pressure, first week M use h/ night	Initial 8 wk: no differences for income, education, or social status First week: M use h/night predicted by self-reported social status (P = .06) and education: bachelor or above (P = .09)

Study	Design/Setting	N / Sample	Timing	Group	SES measure	Analysis	Covariates	Results
Pandey et al,[23] 2020	Retrospective database study (EncoreAnywhere) database; all US participants; completed in Tucson, AZ, USA	N = 170,641%, 49% men; 35%–40% CPAP	All initial use	Group: adherent (≥4 h/night for ≥70% d in a 30-d period; CMS criteria) vs nonadherent	ZIP code household income (aggregated into quartiles)	Multivariate logistic regression Cox proportional hazards regression	Age, sex, race, ethnicity, device type, altitude elevation, residual apneic events, year of PAP set-up (2000–2016)	Increasing odds of meeting CMS criteria adherence with higher median income (*P<.0001*) Highest income group achieved CMS criteria for adherence faster than all other income quartiles (*P<.0001*)
Platt et al,[29] 2009	Retrospective, single VA sleep center; Philadelphia, Pennsylvania, USA	N = 266, 93.6% men, 49.6% black; PAP-naïve; 100% APAP	First week of therapy	Group: adherent (≥4 h/night) vs nonadherent	Neighborhood of residence Socioeconomic index (z score; includes median household income, % male and female employment, % of adults with a high school degree, and (inversely) % nonwhite)	Multivariable logistic regression	Age, race, marital status, employment status, Charlson index, first-day CPAP use vs all other days	Adherence: higher odds for higher neighborhood SES; OR 1.4 (95% CI, 1.2–1.7; *P<.001*) Probability: 34.1% (95% CI, 26.4–42.7) for low SES (fifth percentile) to 62.3% (95% CI, 53.8–70.1) for high SES (95th percentile)

(continued on next page)

Table 1
(continued)

Study Citation	Design/Location	Sample with Positive Airway Pressure Data; Pertinent Demographics	Outcome Interval(s)	Adherence Outcome(s)	Socioeconomic Status Variable(s)	Analysis Methods	Covariates	Findings for Socioeconomic Status Variables
Soltaninejad et al,[30] 2017	Prospective, single sleep center; Isfahan, Iran	N = 106, 55.6% men; PAP-naïve	Initial 7 and 90 d	M use h/night	Living area (urban vs rural) Education (under diploma, diploma, higher than diploma)	Repeated measures ANOVA	None	No differences for living area Use was higher for most educated group at 7 (0.86 h) and 90 d (4.12 h) relative to the lowest educated group at 7 (0.52 h) and 90 d (2.38 h); both $P<.001$
Tanahashi et al,[34] 2012	Prospective, single sleep clinic; Fukuoka, Japan	N = 101; 91.1% men; PAP-naïve	Initial 6 mo	Group: nonadherent (quit CPAP within 6 mo); poor adherence ($\leq$4 h/night); good adherence ($\geq$4 h daily)	Years of education Individual income (<5 million yen/y; 5–10 million yen/y; $\geq$10 million yen/y)	Multiple logistic regression	None	No differences

Source	Design/Setting	Sample	PAP Use Measure	M use h/night	Predictor	Analysis	Covariates	Findings
Wallace et al,[35] 2013	Retrospective; single VA sleep center; Miami, Florida, USA	N = 248, 94% men; 38% black, 25% Hispanic; PAP-naive and existing users	All initial use through study clinic visit (mean 1.4 y ± 1.3 y)		Education (high school or lower, some college, college graduate, or higher)	Multivariable linear regression	Race-ethnicity, age, race-ethnicity × age, marital status, BMI	No effect of education on daily use (β = 0.11; P = .08)
Yang et al,[38] 2013	Retrospective, single sleep center; New Taipei City, Taiwan	N = 315, grouped by age: 11% young (25–40 y), 54% middle-aged (41–65 y), 35% elderly (n = 111); PAP-naive CPAP, APAP, and BiPAP	First month, initial use through most recent follow-up (3.0–16.0 mo after titration)	Group: high adherence (≥4 h/night for ≥70% of nights) vs low adherence	Work status (unemployed, retired, employed, homemaker)	Univariate logistic regression	None	No differences

Abbreviations: AHI, apnea hypopnea index; ASV, adaptive servo-ventilation; BiPAP, bilevel PAP; CESD, Center for Epidemiologic Studies Depression Scale; Charlson index, measure of medical comorbidity; CV, cardiovascular disease; ESS, Epworth sleepiness scale; F, F-statistic; FOSQ, functional outcomes of sleep questionnaire; HS, High School; NRS, numeric rating scale; NZ, New Zealand; PANAS, positive and negative affect schedule; T90, duration arterial pressure is desaturated below 90%; U, Mann Whitney U-test statistic.

the most recent 30-day period,[21] and 2 studies looked at all usage data following PAP distribution.[23,35] Regarding measurement of SES, the included studies were relatively split between those that included only 1 measure of SES resulting in 1 research variable for analysis (n = 9)[21,23,26,29,33,35–38] and studies that included multiple measures of SES and thereby more than 1 SES research variable for analysis (n = 7).[20,27,28,30–32,34]

Overview of Findings: Socioeconomic Status Effects on Positive Airway Pressure Adherence

Among the 16 retrieved studies, 11 (68.8%) found evidence of reduced daily adherence as a function of SES factors. Two studies looked at effects of health care/insurance eligibility (eg, public vs private) or insurance reimbursement status (n = 2)[31,32]; this was the only SES-related variable that was found unassociated with adherence among the studies reviewed. Three studies examined individual or family income[28,31,34]; only Bakker and colleagues[31] found that this was related to PAP adherence in univariate analyses but not in covariate-adjusted models. Although 11 studies (68.8.%) assessed level or years of education, only 4 observed that PAP adherence was affected significantly.[21,25,28,30] Of 4 four studies that looked at effects of occupational status (eg, full-time employed vs unemployed vs retired), 2 observed that employment status was a significant predictor of adherence.[20,27] Some effect on PAP adherence was observed in 4[23,26,29,30,37] out of the 7 retrieved studies that used area-based SES metrics. The 3 studies that did not observe area-based effects used either broader definitions, such as urban versus rural area of residence[30] or gross domestic product (GDP) of the country of recruitment[33] or also included an individual composite index of SES in adjusted models that may have better captured differences in PAP adherence at the individual level.[31] Both studies which utilized a composite index of SES (n = 2; "subjective socioeconomic status" or "individual deprivation" score) found that this was the only SES variable associated with PAP adherence.[28,31]

Upon qualitative synthesis of the findings, those studies that found significant effects seemed to fall within 2 categories: (1) analyses focused on assessing effects of socioeconomic attainment (eg, education or employment status), which were included along with other predictors of PAP adherence (n = 4),[20,25,27,30] and (2) included analyses that were focused on investigating SES and other contributors to disparities in PAP adherence within racially/ethnically heterogeneous samples

(n = 7).[21,23,26,28,29,31,37] These subcategories are used to group summaries of the findings.

Socioeconomic Attainment and Positive Airway Pressure Adherence

Aloia and coauthors[25] found that individuals prescribed CPAP/auto-adjusting PAP (APAP) were more likely to be classified as intermittent versus consistent users (based on use ≥6 d/wk) if they had fewer years of education; $t(140) = 2.61$, $P<.01$. Within individuals treated for OSA at their sleep center in Isfahan, Iran, Soltaninejad and coauthors[30] observed that individuals who were the most educated (more than a diploma) demonstrated significantly longer nightly use at 7 days and 90 days (7 d: 0.86 h; 90 d: 4.12 h) relative to the lowest-educated groups (7 d: 0.52 h; 90 d: 2.38 h); both $P<.001$.

Gulati and colleagues[27] investigated daily use as well as adherence (≥4 h) at participants' first follow-up (6–10 wk after initiation) and at 6 months in 265 individuals who were mostly prescribed CPAP (all devices provided free of charge). Compared with those individuals who reported being employed or retired, individuals who identified as long-term unemployed used PAP 2.1 hours less ($P = .028$) at 6 weeks to 10 weeks and 3.4 hours less at 6 months ($P = .016$). Unemployed individuals also used their devices 26% and 38% less than retired/employed individuals at 6 weeks to 10 weeks ($P = .046$) and 6 months ($P = .011$), respectively. In contrast, Gagnadoux and coauthors[20] observed that adherent individuals (all experienced with PAP for at least 3 mo) were more likely to be retired versus employed, odds ratio [OR] 1.41 (95% CI, 1.097–1.821; $P = .007$), in their large, multisite cohort in France.

Socioeconomic Status and Positive Airway Pressure Adherence in Racially/Ethnically Representative Samples

After adjusting for age, race, marital status, and employment status, Charlson comorbidity index, and first-day CPAP use, Platt and colleagues[29] observed that, relative to the population mean, veterans living in the lowest SES neighborhoods (fifth percentile) were 34.1% less likely to be adherent with PAP (use >4 h/d) during the first week (95% CI, 26.4–42.7), whereas veterans who lived in the highest SES neighborhoods (95th percentile) were 62.3% more likely to be adherent (95% CI, 53.8–70.1). For these veterans, all services were reimbursed by the Department of Veterans Affairs (VA). May recruited a cohort of 143 individuals (45% nonwhite) from 2 sleep centers in Cleveland, Ohio, for a randomized clinical trial comparing active and sham PAP for moderate-to-severe OSA (all devices provided free of charge).[28] After adjusting for design (treatment arm), demographics (age, race, and sex), health factors, daytime functioning scores, and OSA variables, they found a significant interaction (comparing predictors of adherence between active vs sham CPAP, when $\alpha = 0.10$), indicating that higher subjective social status ($P = .09$) and more education (bachelor's degree or greater; $P = .06$) predicted mean nightly CPAP use during the first week of treatment. In Billings and colleagues'[26] investigation of 191 white, black, and Hispanic CPAP-naïve individuals recruited from sleep centers in 5 metropolitan US cities, the investigators examined whether SES based on ZIP code (aggregate of multiple SES factors and separated into quartiles) as a predictor of adherence. When assessing use greater than 4 hours per day at 1 month ($\alpha = 0.10$), those in the lowest quartiles were less likely to be adherent ($\beta = -.22$; $P<.10$).

In the largest and most recently published study reviewed, Pandey and colleagues[23] obtained user data from 170,641 US individuals to investigate CMS criteria adherence as a function of estimated household income based on ZIP code. In adjusted logistic regression models, the investigators observed that an individual's odds of being adherent increased at higher income quartiles (highest OR 1.18; 95% CI, 1.14–1.21; $P<.0001$), whereas Cox proportional hazards regression indicated that the highest income group also met criteria for adherence earlier after treatment initiation than the lower income quartiles (highest hazard ratio [HR] 1.12; 95% CI, 1.10–1.15; $P<.0001$). Data for this study were collected from 2000 to 2016; in subsequent post hoc analyses, the investigators found no evidence that the Affordable Care Act (ACA) going into effect in 2014 (which increased access to private health insurance) reduced inequities in adherence between income quartiles ($P = .07$). In multivariate analyses—after adjusting for frequently changing sleeping location greater than or equal to 1/month, race/ethnicity, marital status, and obesity—Liou and colleagues[21] found that individuals with the most education (college/graduate degree) were most likely to meet CMS criteria for adherence (≥ 4 h/night for $\geq 70\%$ d during the last 30 d) relative to individuals with a high school diploma or less (OR 6.4; 95% CI, 1.7–24.5; $P<.05$).

Bakker and colleagues[31] looked at multiple SES factors, including employment status, level of education, annual income, health care eligibility, and relative deprivation based on area-based (New Zealand Deprivation Index [NZDep06])[19] and individual (New Zealand Individual Deprivation Index

[NZiDep06]),[39] as composite metrics of relative deprivation in a New Zealand–based sample of 126 CPAP-naïve individuals (19.8% Māori; 80.3% had services reimbursed by government health care).[40,41] In multivariate regression models adjusted for ethnicity (Māori vs non-Māori), health care eligibility, education, income, NZDep06, and NZiDep06 scores, individuals with lower SES based on individual factors—those with lower education (OR 0.25; 95% CI, 0.08–0.83; $P = .02$) and with the highest individual deprivation score (OR 0.10; 95% CI, 0.02–0.86; $P = .02$)—were least likely to meet criteria for adherence (use ≥ 4 h/night). Campbell and colleagues[37] used the same area-based metric (NZDep06) to assess effects on mean PAP use/night within an ethnically diverse sample of 214 CPAP-naïve individuals (22.2% Māori; 15.4% Pacific peoples). Individuals representing the lower deprivation areas had more use relative to individuals in the highest deprivation areas statistical F test($F_{[4209]} = 15.2$; $P = .02$; $r = 0.23$). After adjusting for ethnicity (Asian, Māori, Pacific peoples, or European [ie, New Zealand European, European, Australian, or American]), however, significant differences no longer were observed.[37]

DISCUSSION

The aim of this review is to identify and summarize studies that assessed the effects of SES factors on objective adherence to PAP therapy. The main findings are summarized in **Box 1**. Of the 16 included articles, 11 found disparities in PAP adherence as a function of SES factors (68.8%). This provides evidence that some, but not all, individuals who are prescribed PAP therapy may have lower adherence due to the circumstances and associated features of their SES. Four of these studies that found differences in PAP use were less focused on SES disparities (ie, these were secondary analyses and may have been underpowered) but included metrics of socioeconomic attainment (eg, education and employment status). Seven of the studies were more focused on identifying disparities in PAP adherence and included more racially/ethnically diverse samples while prioritizing analysis of SES-related factors.

In their comprehensive review article, Crawford and colleagues[42] posit an integrative framework that strives to explain barriers and facilitators of PAP adherence in terms of the complex interactions of biomedical, psychological, and social factors; this model may be used to devise potential pathways for intervention. The authors have chosen to frame the discussion in terms of this model to illustrate avenues for future investigation

Box 1
Summary of findings
• There is evidence that lower SES is related to objective adherence with PAP therapy in 69% of retrieved studies.
• There is no evidence that health insurance eligibility/coverage or income can affect adherence.
• There is some evidence that higher educational attainment is linked with greater PAP adherence in 36% of reviewed studies that utilized this SES variable.
• There is mixed evidence that occupational status (working vs unemployed) is related to greater PAP adherence in 50% of studies that utilized this SES variable.
• There is moderate evidence, depending on the quality of measurement used, that individual or area-based composite indices of SES are associated with adherence in 57% of studies that utilized this SES variable.

Box 2
Summary of remaining questions
• How do unexplored measures of SES, such as financial strain or wealth (eg, financial assets and home ownership) affect adherence to PAP therapy?
• How do health care system factors (eg, full coverage vs required copayment, and national health services vs alternative models) affect adherence (eg, need to be assessed via larger international comparison studies)?
• What are the pathways linking SES with racial/ethnic disparities in PAP use?
o Is the relationship linking SES and adherence mediated by health literacy or other SES-related constructs?
• What physical and/or social features of low SES neighborhoods affect PAP adherence?
• What impact do telemedicine technologies have on SES-related disparities in PAP adherence?
• At what level, or combination of levels, would interventions to address disparities in PAP adherence as a function of SES be most effective (eg, the individual patient, sleep clinic/hospital, or health care system/government)?

(summarized in **Box 2**), while also emphasizing systemic/health care organization factors.

Interactions with Health Care/Insurance Systems

The authors did not find evidence that individuals' eligibility for government health care assistance or receipt of reimbursement for their device had a significant impact on adherence. This finding certainly is limited, however, by the few studies that addressed this relationship that were included in the review (n = 2).[31,32] Government assistance programs may be important in lower SES contexts where individuals experience greater levels of financial strain[19] or are without access to resources (eg, individual/family wealth). These SES variables (financial strain and wealth) were not used as predictors of PAP adherence in any of the included studies. This is a limitation which could be addressed by future research.

It also does not appear, however, that expanding health care access can mitigate other effects of low SES. For example, Pandey and colleagues[23] did not find support that enactment of the ACA in 2014 (which mostly expanded access to private insurance for low-income to middle-income individuals) reduced income-related disparities in adherence while also controlling for race/ethnicity and pertinent disease/treatment-related factors. Data were only available, however, only from 2014 to 2016, whereas possible

influence of the ACA on PAP adherence may take longer to emerge. Additionally, access to cost-free or subsidized care did not appear to eliminate disparities because it still was observed that patients with lower SES were less adherent among veterans seen in VA settings[29] and when services were offered free of charge to participants.[26–28] It, therefore, is likely that other factors underlying low SES may better explain disparities in PAP adherence.

Although the focus of this article is on SES predictors of PAP adherence, there is additional evidence that improving access to sleep medicine services/treatment might not improve likelihood to adhere to PAP, based on previous studies which investigated predictors of initial acceptance (ie, initiation of treatment and/or purchase of a PAP device). For example, several studies have found that insurance eligibility or type of coverage/reimbursement does not predict purchase of a device and/or initiation of PAP therapy.[39,43,44] Other factors, such as individual or neighborhood income, seem to be better predictors of PAP acceptance and deserve additional attention.[26,45,46]

Another limitation of the included studies is that only 1 included SES comparisons across individuals in different countries (China, New Zealand, and Australia).[33] To further disentangle whether the features of some national health care systems' policies with regard to coverage for PAP therapy (eg, require copayment, full out-of-pocket costs, or devices are offered free of charge), further research via international comparison studies is warranted.

Interactions with Biomedical Factors

Biomedical variables are among the most widely discussed factors thought to have an impact on PAP adherence and were the covariates used most frequently within adjusted analyses of the studies reviewed. Biomedical factors include demographic (eg, age, gender, race, and ethnicity), symptom severity (eg, OSA severity and daytime sleepiness/functioning), health factors (eg, body mass index [BMI] and comorbid conditions), and/or treatment-specific (eg, PAP modality, mask interface, humidification, and pressure setting) variables.[42] Overall, 9 (56.3%) of the retrieved studies reported analyses adjusted for biomedical and other factors, among which only 2 did not find SES differences in PAP use.[35,37] Studies (n = 7) that reported univariate results of SES-PAP adherence effects seemed to be less likely to observe significant findings, with 2 studies observing differences in PAP use within unadjusted analyses.[25,27,30] This reiterates that controlling for other individual-level factors is important to determine the unique effects of SES/context on PAP adherence, particularly given the prominent role of biomedical variables in affecting adherence within the extant literature.[47]

Within the studies reviewed, effects of SES were assessed within analyses, which adjusted for race (n = 5) and ethnicity (n = 6), both of which have been found to be related to PAP adherence outcomes in previous review studies.[16,48] The review did observe some trends for there being a greater risk of nonadherence for those individuals representing the lowest SES bands after controlling for race/ethnicity,[26,31] but these were inconsistent across studies and therefore insufficient to conclude how SES factors may differentially confer additional risk for lower adherence (eg, in the Campbell and colleagues[37] study, differences in adherence as a function of SES disappeared when ethnicity was added).[37] Additionally, when area-based metrics are used, as in Billings and colleagues'26 study, racial/ethnic minorities are confounded with SES in that most minorities reside in lower SES ZIP codes. This confounding limits overall conclusions regarding race/ethnicity by SES interactions.[26] Additionally, many of the

articles featured in the review contained samples representing only a single racial/ethnic group based on geographic location (or racial-ethnic comparisons were not reported). For these reasons, more definitive answers as to how individual and neighborhood-level socioeconomic features differentially impede PAP adherence across/between different racial-ethnic groups is unavailable from this analysis. Greater attention in this area is sorely needed.

Interactions with Psychological Factors

The psychological factors highlighted by Crawford and colleagues[42] can include cognitive-motivational knowledge, coping styles, and psychological morbidity. The probable role of education to affect PAP adherence was the most frequently assessed within studies reviewed. Only 1 study reviewed included measures of psychological functioning within multivariate models, which observed disparities in PAP adherence due to SES after correcting for depression and daily negative/positive affect.[28] Given reports of increased mental health symptoms among socioeconomically deprived persons relative to those with higher SES, this finding suggests that features aside from psychiatric morbidity may have an impact on PAP adherence.[49] One interesting finding was that, when composite measures of subjective SES were used (eg, "rate your SES from 1–10" and use of the NZiDEP06 variable, which is based on self-reported levels of relative deprivation), scores indicating lower SES were associated more strongly with poorer adherence relative to other SES variables.[28,31] This suggests that an individual's perception of their socioeconomic standing, and possibly the extent to which this poses more barriers to initial/longer-term PAP use, may explain 1 aspect of the SES-PAP adherence relationship. Future investigations that utilize multiple objective and subjective measures of SES appear to be warranted.

Although education is easy to measure and typically correlated with other SES factors like income and occupation, there are several limitations to using education as a metric of SES, particularly in countries where access to higher education may not increase SES for individuals of different racial/ethnic and gender groups.[15] This utility as an "easy" measure is demonstrated in how frequently it was included across all studies of PAP adherence that the authors retrieved (68.8%), with 4 studies reporting significant differences in adherence as a function of educational attainment. Although integrated educational programs now are standard components of comprehensive sleep medicine clinics, most of these interventions have been found to be ineffective to augment adherence beyond other aspects of usual care.[50] Although health literacy (the degree to which individuals have the capacity to obtain, process, and understand basic health information and services needed to make appropriate health decisions) may be an important mediator in the education-PAP use relationship, none of the reviewed studies examined this variable.[51] Perhaps those individuals with lower educational attainment have lower health literacy and, therefore, lack relative knowledge (about cognitive, social, psychological, and material resources); this then inhibits them from fully understanding and then applying the content covered in these educational programs. Such hypotheses need to be explored in future studies as personalizing OSA education based on health literacy levels may help reduce SES-PAP use disparities.

Interactions with Social Context

The most consistent predictor that the authors observed was the use of area-based metrics for SES, which predicted PAP adherence in 4 of 7 investigations.[23,26,29,37] The authors noted that some of these investigations utilized area-based variables that were broad and, therefore, less likely to detect individual differences in adherence (eg, country GDP and urban vs rural residence).[30,33] Multiple studies included aggregate metrics to characterize individuals' SES based on features of their neighborhood/ZIP code from recent census data, which may provide some of the richest evidence for how SES may affect adherence after controlling for the effects of race and other clinical features (although also a limitation given observed concentration of black participants in low SES neighborhoods/ZIP codes).

Neighborhood economics can affect access to transportation (to attend clinic appointments), reliable utilities like electricity (to power their PAP device), environmental pollutants like noise, light, air pollution (interfere with sleep quality), and increase experience of recurrent threats to safety/health, which may worsen anxiety/insomnia (and impede tolerance of PAP). Liou and colleagues[21] observed that lower education predicted nonadherence, while they also examined the frequency with which sleeping location changed $\geq 1 \times$/month and found this significantly related to adherence. Given that multiple competing socioeconomic factors may be interacting to have an adverse impact on initiation and maintenance of PAP adherence, continuing to look only at summary/composite SES variables may not be sufficient to address

the full scope of the issue. Future investigations should pursue similar lines of research and examine the more nuanced aspects of the social and physical environment of lower SES individuals to identify new pathways for PAP adherence interventions. Additionally, recent advancements in technology have allowed for virtual appointments and remote monitoring of PAP usage, which can improve access to diagnostic and treatment services for management of OSA.[52] Although this was not explored as a facilitator of adherence within the studies reviewed, investigation of whether these telemedicine technologies can affect SES-related disparities in usage certainly is warranted.

In 3 of 4 analyses where marital status was included in multivariate models, higher SES was linked to adherence with PAP therapy.[20,21,29] Recent investigations have targeted aspects of the marital relationship toward improving engagement with PAP therapy,[53] whereas these findings suggest that factors beyond having/lacking a partner may affect adherence with treatment.

Recommendations

A summary of the recommendations for future directions is presented in **Box 3**. It is evident that the current body of research on SES predictors of PAP adherence is severely limited by its ability to explain (1) why these discrepancies exist, (2) what pathways/mechanisms facilitate these relationships, and (3) where interventions could be most effective (eg, at the level of the individual patient, sleep clinic/hospital, or health care system/

Box 3
Summary of recommended future directions

- Apply the biopsychosocial model when designing investigations to examine interactions of SES with biomedical, psychological, and other social factors

- Investigate direct relationships between SES and PAP adherence outcomes, as well as outcomes as a function of different group levels (eg, low vs high SES among racial/ethnic minority groups)

- Obtain multiple measures of SES, including subjective and objective sources of data, and measurement of individual and area-based SES factors

- Objective PAP use should be reported as a proportion of total sleep time, requiring measurement and reporting of sleep duration in PAP adherence studies

government). A large reason for this is the emphasis on designs that include SES factors as covariates as opposed to the variable of main interest, and widespread use of single-assay SES metrics, which incompletely capture the socioeconomic circumstances of these individuals. Additionally, objective assessment of PAP adherence historically has been reported independent from nightly total sleep time, which may confound interpretation of adherence for individuals with shorter sleep durations who actually use PAP nightly and for the entire sleep episode. This is a particularly salient concern because lower SES and minority race/ethnicity also have been linked to shorter sleep durations,[54] whereas interventions might be designed which encourage sleep duration extension rather than just increasing PAP use.

Based on these critiques, the authors present the following broad recommendations for future investigations on associations of SES with PAP therapy outcomes. (1) Consider the bio-psychosocial model when designing investigations to examine how SES may interact with biomedical, psychological, and other social factors to affect PAP adherence.[42] Given that aspects of SES may be less modifiable than other variables, understanding of the factors that indirectly impede/enhance PAP therapy outcomes in the context of lower SES may represent the most effective pathway to increase adherence. (2) In accordance with recommendations by Braveman and colleagues[17] for investigations of SES in health research, future investigations of PAP adherence should utilize outcome-based and group-based designs, which (a) consider pathways/mechanisms to explain SES-PAP adherence relationships, (b) utilize multiple measures of SES to obtain a breadth of information, (c) specify all particular SES factors measured, and (d) acknowledge whether SES factors that are not measured may confound conclusions. Finally, the authors recommend (3) that PAP use be reported as a proportion of total sleep time, which would require integration of additional measures of sleep duration into PAP adherence studies.

Limitations

The authors utilized an extensive search that was intended to identify only articles investigating how SES factors may affect individuals' interactions with PAP. Due to stipulations of the search criteria that investigations must report analyses of SES factors on objective PAP adherence outcomes, it is possible that there are studies that were not captured by the search strategy. Additionally, given the focus of this review on investigating objectively assessed adherence to treatment over time, some investigations that assessed factors affecting PAP purchase/acceptance, long-term use versus discontinuation, or included only self-report data were eliminated from our review and were not reported herein.

SUMMARY

Several well-established, individual-level factors have been identified as contributing to PAP nonadherence, which largely have informed the development of proactive solutions to address these barriers to enhance the likelihood of PAP uptake and long-term use. This review sought to provide a comprehensive summary of the current literature on disparities in PAP adherence based on socioeconomic factors at the individual and system levels. Although some patterns emerged through the synthesis, there still is little consensus to be reached from these findings, which might suggest that any 1 socioeconomic variable could be targeted to reliably improve treatment outcomes. For this reason, the authors encourage continued investigation into PAP-SES relationships.

DISCLOSURE

The views expressed in this article are those of the authors and do not necessarily reflect the position or policy of the Department of Veterans Affairs or the United States government. Dr A.M. Sawyer has received grant funding from the National Institutes of Health, American Lung Association and American Nurses Foundation and currently is in receipt of grant support from VA HSR&D. Dr N.J. Williams was supported by the National Heart, Lung, and Blood Institute K23HL125939. The authors have nothing else to disclose.

CLINICS CARE POINTS

- Most studies show that lower SES individuals are at greater risk for poor PAP adherence and may potentially benefit from closer clinical follow up.
- As opposed to single measures, multi-dimensional assessments of SES may be more helpful in predicting trajectories of PAP use.

REFERENCES

1. Weaver TE, Maislin G, Dinges DF, et al. Relationship between hours of CPAP use and achieving normal levels of sleepiness and daily functioning. Sleep 2007;30(6):711–9.
2. Antic NA, Catcheside P, Buchan C, et al. The effect of CPAP in normalizing daytime sleepiness, quality

of life, and neurocognitive function in patients with moderate to severe OSA. Sleep 2011;34(1):111–9.

3. Martínez-García M-A, Campos-Rodríguez F, Catalán-Serra P, et al. Cardiovascular mortality in obstructive sleep apnea in the elderly: role of long-term continuous positive airway pressure treatment: a prospective observational study. Am J Respir Crit Care Med 2012;186(9):909–16.

4. Yaffe K, Laffan AM, Harrison SL, et al. Sleep-disordered breathing, hypoxia, and risk of mild cognitive impairment and dementia in older women. JAMA 2011;306(6):613–9.

5. Tregear S, Reston J, Schoelles K, et al. Obstructive sleep apnea and risk of motor vehicle crash: systematic review and meta-analysis. J Clin Sleep Med 2009;5(6):573–81.

6. Schröder CM, O'Hara R. Depression and obstructive sleep apnea (OSA). Ann Gen Psychiatry 2005;4(1):13.

7. Streatfeild J, Hillman D, Adams R, et al. Cost-effectiveness of continuous positive airway pressure therapy for obstructive sleep apnea: health care system and societal perspectives. Sleep 2019;42(12): zsz181.

8. Wickwire EM, Tom SE, Vadlamani A, et al. Older adult US Medicare beneficiaries with untreated obstructive sleep apnea are heavier users of health care than matched control patients. J Clin Sleep Med 2020;16(1):81–9.

9. Calik MW. Treatments for obstructive sleep apnea. J Clin Outcomes Manag 2016;23(4):181.

10. Rotenberg BW, Murariu D, Pang KP. Trends in CPAP adherence over twenty years of data collection: a flattened curve. J Otolaryngol Head Neck Surg 2016;45(1):43.

11. Engleman HM, Wild MR. Improving CPAP use by patients with the sleep apnoea/hypopnoea syndrome (SAHS). Sleep Med Rev 2003;7(1):81–99.

12. Walter RJ, Hagedorn SI, Lettieri CJ. Impact of diagnosing and treating obstructive sleep apnea on healthcare utilization. Sleep Med 2017;38:73–7.

13. Marshall NS, Wong KK, Liu PY, et al. Sleep apnea as an independent risk factor for all-cause mortality: the Busselton Health Study. Sleep 2008;31(8):1079–85.

14. World Health Organization. Adherence to long-term therapies: evidence for action. Geneva (Switzerland): World Health Organization; 2003.

15. Shavers VL. Measurement of socioeconomic status in health disparities research. J Natl Med Assoc 2007;99(9):1013.

16. Wallace DM, Williams NJ, Sawyer AM, et al. Adherence to positive airway pressure treatment among minority populations in the US: a scoping review. Sleep Med Rev 2018;38:56–69.

17. Braveman PA, Cubbin C, Egerter S, et al. Socioeconomic status in health research: one size does not fit all. JAMA 2005;294(22):2879–88.

18. Kribbs NB, Pack AI, Kline LR, et al. Objective measurement of patterns of nasal CPAP use by patients with obstructive sleep apnea. Am Rev Respir Dis 1993;147(4):887–95.

19. Aldana SG, Liljenquist W. Validity and reliability of a financial strain survey. J Fin Couns Plann 1998; 9(2):11.

20. Gagnadoux F, Le Vaillant M, Goupil F, et al. Influence of marital status and employment status on long-term adherence with continuous positive airway pressure in sleep apnea patients. PloS one 2011; 6(8):e22503.

21. Liou HYS, Kapur VK, Consens F, et al. The effect of sleeping environment and sleeping location change on positive airway pressure adherence. J Clin Sleep Med 2018;14(10):1645–52.

22. Wallace D, Vargas S, Schwartz SJ, et al. Determinants of continuous positive airway pressure adherence in a sleep clinic cohort of South Florida Hispanic veterans. Sleep Breath 2013;17(1):351–63.

23. Pandey A, Mereddy S, Combs D, et al. Socioeconomic inequities in adherence to positive airway pressure therapy in population-level analysis. J Clin Med 2020;9(2):442.

24. Centers for Medicare & Medicaid Services (CMS). Positive Airway Pressure (PAP) devices: complying with documentation and coverage requirements. In: DoHaH Service, editor. U.S. centers for medicare & medicaid services. Baltimore (MD): Medicare Learning Network; 2016.

25. Aloia MS, Arnedt JT, Stanchina M, et al. How early in treatment is PAP adherence established? Revisiting night-to-night variability. Behav Sleep Med 2007; 5(3):229–40.

26. Billings ME, Auckley D, Benca R, et al. Race and residential socioeconomics as predictors of CPAP adherence. Sleep 2011;34(12):1653–8.

27. Gulati A, Ali M, Davies M, et al. A prospective observational study to evaluate the effect of social and personality factors on continuous positive airway pressure (CPAP) compliance in obstructive sleep apnoea syndrome. BMC Pulm Med 2017;17(1):56.

28. May AM, Gharibeh T, Wang L, et al. CPAP adherence predictors in a randomized trial of moderate-to-severe OSA enriched with women and minorities. Chest 2018;154(3):567–78.

29. Platt AB, Field SH, Asch DA, et al. Neighborhood of residence is associated with daily adherence to CPAP therapy. Sleep 2009;32(6):799–806.

30. Soltaninejad F, Sadeghi A, Amra B. Compliance with continuous positive airway pressure in Persian patients with obstructive sleep apnea. J Res Med Sci 2017;22.

31. Bakker JP, O'Keeffe KM, Neill AM, et al. Ethnic disparities in CPAP adherence in New Zealand: effects of socioeconomic status, health literacy and self-efficacy. Sleep 2011;34(11):1595–603.

32. Hui DS, Choy DK, Li TS, et al. Determinants of continuous positive airway pressure compliance in a group of Chinese patients with obstructive sleep apnea. Chest 2001;120(1):170–6.

33. Chai-Coetzer CL, Luo Y-M, Antic NA, et al. Predictors of long-term adherence to continuous positive airway pressure therapy in patients with obstructive sleep apnea and cardiovascular disease in the SAVE study. Sleep 2013;36(12):1929–37.

34. Tanahashi T, Nagano J, Yamaguchi Y, et al. Factors that predict adherence to continuous positive airway pressure treatment in obstructive sleep apnea patients: a prospective study in Japan. Sleep Biol Rhythms 2012;10(2):126–35.

35. Wallace DM, Shafazand S, Aloia MS, et al. The association of age, insomnia, and self-efficacy with continuous positive airway pressure adherence in black, white, and Hispanic US Veterans. J Clin Sleep Med 2013;9(09):885–95.

36. Aloia MS, Arnedt JT, Riggs RL, et al. Clinical management of poor adherence to CPAP: motivational enhancement. Behav Sleep Med 2004;2(4):205–22.

37. Campbell A, Neill A, Lory R. Ethnicity and socioeconomic status predict initial continuous positive airway pressure compliance in New Zealand adults with obstructive sleep apnoea. Intern Med J 2012; 42(6):e95–101.

38. Yang M-C, Lin C-Y, Lan C-C, et al. Factors affecting CPAP acceptance in elderly patients with obstructive sleep apnea in Taiwan. Respir Care 2013; 58(9):1504–13.

39. Bouscoulet LT, Escárcega EL, Maldonado AC, et al. Continuous positive airway pressure used by adults with obstructive sleep apneas after prescription in a public referral hospital in Mexico City. Arch Bronconeumol 2007;43(1):16–21.

40. Salmond C, Crampton P, King P, et al. NZiDep: a New Zealand index of socioeconomic deprivation for individuals. Soc Sci Med 2006;62(6):1474–85.

41. White P, Gunston J, Salmond C, et al. Atlas of Socioeconomic Deprivation in New Zealand, NZDep 2006. Wellington: Ministry of Health; 2008.

42. Crawford MR, Espie CA, Bartlett DJ, et al. Integrating psychology and medicine in CPAP adherence–new concepts? Sleep Med Rev 2014; 18(2):123–39.

43. Goyal A, Agarwal N, Pakhare A. Barriers to CPAP use in India: an exploratory study. J Clin Sleep Med 2017;13(12):1385–94.

44. Zonato AI, Bittencourt L, Martinho FL, et al. A comparison of public and private obstructive sleep apnea clinics. Braz J Med Biol Res 2004; 37(1):69–76.

45. Brin YS, Reuveni H, Greenberg S, et al. Determinants affecting initiation of continuous positive airway pressure treatment. Therapy 2005;9:11.

46. Simon-Tuval T, Reuveni H, Greenberg-Dotan S, et al. Low socioeconomic status is a risk factor for CPAP acceptance among adult OSAS patients requiring treatment. Sleep 2009;32(4):545–52.

47. Sawyer AM, Gooneratne NS, Marcus CL, et al. A systematic review of CPAP adherence across age groups: clinical and empiric insights for developing CPAP adherence interventions. Sleep Med Rev 2011;15(6):343–56.

48. Woods CE, Usher K, Maguire GP. Obstructive sleep apnoea in adult indigenous populations in high-income countries: an integrative review. Sleep Breath 2015;19(1):45–53.

49. Reijneveld SA, Schene AH. Higher prevalence of mental disorders in socioeconomically deprived urban areas in The Netherlands: community or personal disadvantage? J Epidemiol Community Health 1998;52(1):2–7.

50. Wozniak DR, Lasserson TJ, Smith I. Educational, supportive and behavioural interventions to improve usage of continuous positive airway pressure machines in adults with obstructive sleep apnoea. Cochrane Database Syst Rev 2014;(1):CD007736.

51. Baker DW. The meaning and the measure of health literacy. J Gen Intern Med 2006;21(8):878–88s3.

52. Hwang D. Monitoring progress and adherence with positive airway pressure therapy for obstructive sleep apnea: the roles of telemedicine and mobile health applications. Sleep Med Clin 2016;11(2): 161–71.

53. Luyster FS, Aloia MS, Buysse DJ, et al. A couples-oriented Intervention for positive airway pressure therapy adherence: a pilot study of obstructive sleep apnea patients and their partners. Behav Sleep Med 2018;17:1–12.

54. Grandner MA, Williams NJ, Knutson KL, et al. Sleep disparity, race/ethnicity, and socioeconomic position. Sleep Med 2016;18:7–18.

Adherence to Positive Airway Pressure Therapy in Obesity Hypoventilation Syndrome

Jeremy Wearn, MD[a], Bimaje Akpa, MD[b], Babak Mokhlesi, MD, MSc[c],*

KEYWORDS

- Pickwickian • Hypercapnia • Sleep apnea • Noninvasive ventilation • CPAP • Compliance
- Pressure support • Hypercarbia

KEY POINTS

- Compared with eucapnic patients with obstructive sleep apnea (OSA), patients with obesity hypoventilation syndrome (OHS) are more symptomatic, have increased morbidity and mortality, and have worse socioeconomic outcomes.
- In patients with OHS, long-term adherence to continuous positive airway pressure (CPAP) and noninvasive ventilation (NIV) improves outcomes.
- CPAP and NIV are equally effective in patients with OHS who have severe concomitant OSA (~70% of patients with OHS).
- There is no difference in long-term adherence to CPAP or NIV.
- Compared with patients with moderate to severe OSA, positive airway pressure adherence is better in patients with OHS, likely driven by higher severity of sleepiness and other symptoms associated with OHS.

INTRODUCTION

Although the association of obesity and increased daytime sleepiness has been well established, the term Pickwickian syndrome was first used by Burwell and colleagues[1] in a case report in which they described similar phenotypic characteristics between their patient and the character fat boy Joe in the classic Charles Dickens book *The Posthumous Papers of the Pickwick Club*.

Obesity hypoventilation syndrome (OHS) is defined as daytime hypercapnia (partial pressure of carbon dioxide in the arterial blood or [Pa_{CO_2}] >45 mm Hg) in an obese patient (body mass index [BMI] $\geq$30 kg/m^2) with sleep-disordered breathing, after all known causes of hypoventilation, such as obstructive lung disease, restrictive chest wall disease, interstitial lung disease, neuropathic and myopathic conditions, and severe hypothyroidism, have been excluded.[2] The term sleep-disordered breathing in the definition of OHS includes either obstructive sleep apnea (OSA) or sleep hypoventilation (10-mm Hg increase in CO_2 during sleep compared with awake CO_2 or P_{CO_2}>55 mm Hg during sleep for 10 minutes).[3]

Severe obesity is an important risk factor for developing OHS. The prevalence of severe obesity (class III or BMI $\geq$40 kg/m^2) is increasing. The Centers for Disease Control and Prevention estimated

[a] Sleep Medicine and Internal Medicine, Oregon Health & Science University and Portland VAMC, 3710 SW US Veterans Hospital Rd, PULM3/Sleep, Portland OR 97239, USA; [b] Division of Pulmonary, Allergy, Critical Care and Sleep Medicine, University of Minnesota, 420 Delaware Street SE, MMC 276, Minneapolis, MN 55455, USA; [c] Sleep Disorders Center, University of Chicago, 5841 South Maryland Avenue, MC6076/Room M630, Chicago, IL 60637, USA
* Corresponding author.
E-mail address: bmokhles@medicine.bsd.uchicago.edu

Sleep Med Clin 16 (2021) 43–59
https://doi.org/10.1016/j.jsmc.2020.10.009
1556-407X/21/© 2020 Elsevier Inc. All rights reserved.

that 9.2% of the adult United States population has a BMI greater than or equal to 40 kg/m^2.[4] The prevalence of OHS in the general population is unknown, but, with increasing prevalence of severe obesity, it is likely that the prevalence of OHS will increase.[5] In contrast, the prevalence of OHS in obese patients referred to sleep centers for evaluation of sleep-disordered breathing has been reported to be between 8% and 20%.[6]

Patients with OHS are typically severely obese (BMI $\geq$ 40 kg/m^2), have severe OSA (apnea-hypopnea index [AHI] $\geq$30 events/h), and are sleepy during the day.[7] Compared with obese patients with eucapnic OSA, patients with OHS are more likely to report symptoms such as dyspnea, manifest cor pulmonale, and have worse quality of life, all of which lead to increased use of health care resources.[8,9] In the Pickwick trial, the prevalence of pulmonary hypertension at baseline, defined as systolic pulmonary artery pressure greater than or equal to 40 mm Hg measured by echocardiography, was 52%.[10] Not surprisingly, the significant cardiometabolic comorbidities observed in patients with OHS leads to increased mortality compared with eucapnic OSA.[11,12]

TREATMENT OF OBESITY HYPOVENTILATION SYNDROME
Weight Loss

The treatment of OHS includes weight loss and positive airway pressure (PAP) therapy during sleep. Weight loss has been shown to improve sleep-disordered breathing, improve nocturnal and diurnal gas exchange, and reduce cardiovascular morbidity.[13,14] Recent guidelines suggest that weight loss of 25% to 30% of actual body weight is required to reverse OHS. However, achieving and sustaining this degree of weight loss is difficult with lifestyle interventions alone.[14,15] Comprehensive and intensive weight loss programs (incorporating diet, exercise, and motivational interviewing) have been shown to reduce weight by 6% to 7%.[15] However, compared with usual care, intensive lifestyle interventions did not confer a clinically significant effect on the management of OHS.[16] In contrast, bariatric surgery has been shown to reduce weight by 15% to 65%, depending on the interventional modality. Furthermore, bariatric surgery is associated with a reduction of OSA severity (AHI decrease by 18%–44%), improved gas exchange (Pa$_{CO_2}$ decrease of 17%–20%), and improved daytime sleepiness.[14] Importantly, many patients with OHS are not interested in bariatric surgery or may be deemed at high surgical risk because of chronic respiratory failure or the presence of

pulmonary hypertension.[14] Given the difficulty of initiating and sustaining weight loss for many patients with OHS, PAP therapy during sleep has become the mainstay of therapy for patients with OHS.

Positive Airway Pressure Therapy

Because OHS is always accompanied by sleep-disordered breathing, the use of PAP therapy during sleep is a clinically sound intervention. PAP treatment modalities include continuous PAP (CPAP) or noninvasive ventilation (NIV). NIV is most commonly delivered as bilevel PAP therapy, which can be implemented with or without a respiratory back-up rate. In addition, NIV can be provided in modalities with more complex pressure-cycle algorithms such as volume-targeted pressure support. Both CPAP and NIV alleviate upper airway obstruction, increase functional residual capacity, and improve microatelectasis in obese patients, thereby facilitating clearance of CO$_2$ during sleep.[17] The proposed advantage to NIV is that, with the use of pressure support (greater inspiratory pressure than expiratory pressure), it can further augment alveolar ventilation to assist with CO$_2$ removal and oxygenation.

Impact of Positive Airway Pressure Therapy

PAP improves quality of life, daytime sleepiness, sleep-disordered breathing, diurnal and nocturnal hypoxemia and hypercapnia, health care resource use, and mortality in patients with OHS.[13,18]

Symptoms
Patients with OHS experience significant symptoms and reduction in quality of life compared with patients with eucapnic OSA.[2,8] In the largest randomized clinical trial to date, PAP improved daytime sleepiness, quality of life, and dyspnea, with no significant difference in the degree of improvement between the NIV and CPAP groups.[19] Sleepiness, measured by the Epworth Sleepiness Scale (ESS), decreased from a baseline average of 11 (out of a maximum of 24, with scores >10 suggesting hypersomnia) at the time of randomization to an average ESS score of 5 at the completion of the trial after 3 years of PAP use. Similarly, this study showed that the percentage of patients experiencing clinically significant dyspnea (MRC scale $\geq$2; eg, short of breath when activity is equal to or exceeds hurrying on level ground or walking up a slight hill) decreased from 58% at baseline to 28% at the completion of the trial. In addition, both CPAP and NIV improved quality of life.[19]

Gas exchange

Given that approximately 70% of patients with OHS have concomitant severe OSA, any modality of PAP therapy that splints the upper airway can improve sleep-disordered breathing and, thereby, gas exchange during sleep. Multiple trials have shown that CPAP and NIV therapy are equally effective in improving sleep-disordered breathing, ventilation, and oxygenation during sleep in ambulatory patients with stable OHS and concomitant severe OSA.[19–22] Moreover, these studies have shown that CPAP and NIV lead to a similar degree of improvement in gas exchange during wakefulness in these patients.[23] Despite not providing additional ventilatory support compared with NIV, CPAP improves lung volume, thereby preventing small airway closure or microatelectasis in severely obese patients. Moreover, the application of CPAP even at low pressures can reduce the work of breathing in supine obese patients.[24] As such, adequately titrated CPAP in the sleep laboratory can improve sleep-disordered breathing, oxygenation, and ventilation, particularly in most patients with OHS who also have concomitant severe OSA. Short-term[20–22] and long-term studies[19,25] have shown that, in the subgroup of patients with OHS and severe OSA, daytime gas exchange, symptoms, and quality of life improve similarly between those treated with CPAP and NIV. Collectively, these studies suggest that patients with OHS and severe OSA phenotype, in whom upper airway obstruction is the primary driver for development of hypercapnia, tend to respond well to long-term CPAP therapy.[23] However, it is important to consider that there is clinical heterogeneity in patients with OHS. Those without severe concomitant OSA, more severe hypercapnia, recent acute-on-chronic hypercapnic respiratory failure, or CPAP intolerance may benefit from NIV.[15]

Health care resource use

Compared with patients with eucapnic OSA[12,26] or eucapnic obesity,[9,27] patients with OHS have a higher burden of respiratory and cardiovascular comorbidities leading to increased health care cost and resource use.[28] In a Danish registry, the cost of caring for patients with OHS was 7.5 times more than matched controls and 2.5 times more than patients with eucapnic OSA.[29] In a retrospective study of 20 patients, PAP therapy was associated with a reduction in hospital resource use during the 2 years after initiating therapy compared with the 5 years before treatment.[9] Well-designed prospective studies assessing whether long-term PAP therapy leads to a reduction in health care resource use compared with no therapy are lacking. However, in a recent analysis of the Pickwick trial, in which 202 patients with OHS and severe OSA were randomized to CPAP or NIV and followed for a median of 3 years, NIV cost per patient was €857.6 ± €105.5 higher than CPAP therapy each year. Therefore, CPAP therapy is more cost-effective than NIV and should be the preferred treatment of patients with OHS with severe OSA.[30]

Mortality

Patients with OHS have high rates of mortality. All-cause mortality has been reported at 18% to 31% at 1 to 3 years in observational studies that enrolled hospitalized patients with acute-on-chronic hypercapnic respiratory failure who survived hospitalization but were mostly discharged without therapy.[31–33] A high 2-year mortality of 24% was also reported in ambulatory patients with untreated OHS.[28] In contrast, a recent meta-analysis showed that, in patients with OHS who experienced an episode of acute-on-chronic hypercapnic respiratory failure, those discharged on PAP therapy had a lower mortality at 3 and 6 months.[34] Moreover, studies of ambulatory patients with OHS who are adherent to NIV therapy have reported much lower mortalities, between 5% and 13%, after 2 to 5 years of follow-up.[19,25,35] One study, with up to 7 years of follow-up in patients who were mostly adherent to NIV, reported a mortality of 24.5%.[12] A recent randomized controlled trial showed that patients with OHS who were adherent to CPAP and NIV had better outcomes compared with their less adherent counterparts. The subgroup analysis in this study revealed that patients with higher PAP adherence had lower rates of hospitalization, ICU admissions, emergency department visits, and mortality.[19]

Collectively, these studies suggest that patients with OHS who are adherent to PAP therapy have lower rates of mortality. Accordingly, identifying patients with OHS, instituting adequate PAP therapy, and ensuring adherence to PAP therapy in a timely manner is important in order to prevent adverse outcomes such as hospital readmissions, acute-on-chronic hypercapnic respiratory failure, and death.

Treatment Impact of Noninvasive Ventilation Versus Continuous Positive Airway Pressure in Obesity Hypoventilation Syndrome

Until recently, there was no consensus with regard to the optimal mode of PAP therapy for the initial treatment of OHS. The American Thoracic Society recently developed clinical practice guidelines that provided a conditional recommendation based on low-quality evidence that CPAP rather than NIV should be provided as first-line therapy to stable ambulatory patients with OHS and concurrent severe OSA.[15,23] Based on an extensive literature review of the limited available trials that compared NIV with CPAP, there was no difference in the degree of improvement in symptoms, quality of life, daytime sleepiness, health care resource use, cardiovascular events, and mortality between patients with OHS who were treated with CPAP or NIV.[23] Furthermore, CPAP is more cost-effective than NIV.[19,30] The recommendation included a caveat that patients with poor lung function, advanced age, more advanced ventilatory failure, and without coexistent severe OSA may not respond adequately to CPAP.[15] However, as stated in the American Thoracic Society guidelines, the recommendation to use CPAP rather than NIV as initial therapy is conditional/weak based on very-low-quality evidence. As such, high-quality and adequately powered clinical trials with long observation periods are still needed in order to provide further clarity on long-term management of patients receiving PAP therapy.

The Impact of Positive Airway Pressure Adherence on the Management of Obesity Hypoventilation Syndrome

The effectiveness of PAP therapy in the management of OHS is strongly related to patient adherence to PAP. PAP adherence seems to be better in patients with OHS compared with patients with eucapnic OSA, as shown in **Fig. 1**. Even with behavioral interventions (**Table 1**) and telemedicine interventions (**Table 2**) in eucapnic patients with OSA, individuals with OHS tend to have better PAP adherence (**Table 3**) compared with their eucapnic peers with OSA.

In a retrospective cohort study of 75 patients with OHS, the daytime $Paco_2$ decreased by 1.84 mm Hg for each hour of nightly PAP therapy, the effect of which plateaued at 7 hours of daily PAP use. Similarly, the Pao_2 improved by approximately 3 mm Hg for each hour of nightly PAP therapy, and its beneficial effect plateaued at 4.5 hours of daily PAP therapy.[36] In a prospective study of 252 patients initiated on PAP for OHS (37% on CPAP and 63% on bilevel PAP) and followed for a median of 30 months, there were significant improvements in gas exchange, sleepiness, and quality of life for those participants who were more adherent to PAP therapy.[25] Furthermore, this study showed that patients who used PAP for greater than 6 h/night compared with those that used if for less than 6 h/night experienced an increase in wake Pao_2 (mean increase of 10.7 mm Hg vs 4.9 mm Hg), a reduction in wake $Paco_2$ (median reduction of 10.7 mm Hg vs 3.0 mm Hg), and decreased mortalities (8.7% vs 2.5%).[25]

In aggregate, 3 medium-term randomized clinical trials,[20–22] a long-term randomized clinical trial,[19] and a long-term observational study[25] have compared CPAP with NIV and have not shown any significant difference in outcomes. Moreover, there was no significant difference in adherence between the 2 PAP modalities in these clinical trials (summarized in **Table 3** and shown in **Fig. 1**). The average PAP adherence in these prospective trials ranged from 4.2 to 6.3 h/night, with

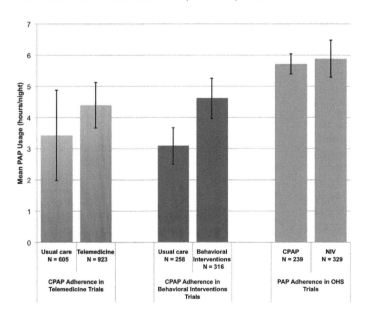

Fig. 1. Adherence to PAP therapy in patients with OSA enrolled in clinical trials designed to enhance adherence to therapy using telemedicine or behavioral interventions and in patients enrolled in clinical trials of OHS. For studies that had multiple intervention arms, data from all intervention arms were combined and appropriately weighted into the aggregated intervention data represented earlier. Whiskers represent standard deviation. NIV includes bilevel PAP in spontaneous mode, bilevel PAP in spontaneous-timed mode, and volume-targeted pressure support.

Table 1
Overview of studies assessing the impact of behavioral interventions on continuous positive airway pressure adherence for the treatment of obstructive sleep apnea

Study/ Year	Study Design	Age (y)	BMI (kg/m²)	ESS	AHI/RDI (Events/h)	Intervention	Inclusion/ Exclusion Criteria	Usual Care Adherence (h/Night)	Intervention Adherence (h/Night)
Aloia et al,[37] 2001	Parallel, 2-arm RCT Duration 3 mo N = 12 Completed study: Intervention = 6 Usual care = 6	Intervention 63.4 ± 4.5 Usual care 67.6 ± 4.7	—	—	Intervention 46.1 ± 11.1 Usual care 46.1 ± 25.2	Two 45-min therapy sessions involving education on the severity of OSA and the efficacy of CPAP	Inclusion: age ≥55, RDI>10, MMSE ≥ 25, and no history of other treatment of apnea Exclusion: claustrophobia, panic while using CPAP on the CPAP PSG night	4.65	7.76
Richards et al,[38] 2007	Parallel, 2-arm RCT Duration 1 mo N = 100 Completed study: Intervention = 48 Usual care = 48	Intervention 53.1 ± 11.8 Usual care 56.2 ± 12.5	Intervention 30.4 ± 5.1 Usual care 30.1 ± 4.9	Intervention 10.3 ± 5.0 Usual care 10.6 ± 5.4	Intervention 27.6 ± 21.2 Usual care 25.3 ± 23.1	Two, 60-min, CBT sessions (involving videos of real CPAP users)	Inclusion: diagnosis with OSA and referral for CPAP titration Exclusion: inability to understand English and previous use of CPAP	2.51 ± 2.70	5.38 ± 2.55

(continued on next page)

Table 1
(continued)

Study/Year	Study Design	Age (y)	BMI (kg/m²)	ESS	AHI/RDI (Events/h)	Intervention	Inclusion/Exclusion Criteria	Usual Care Adherence (h/Night)	Intervention Adherence (h/Night)
Olsen et al,[39] 2012	Parallel, 2-arm RCT Duration 3 mo N = 106 Completed study: Intervention = 50 Usual care = 50	Intervention 55.1 ± 12.6 Usual care 57.7 ± 9.5	Intervention 34.3 ± 6.7 Usual care 34.7 ± 7.1	Intervention 10.8 ± 4.4 Usual care 11.1 ± 5.3	Intervention 36.2 ± 27.8 Usual care 32.4 ± 20.3	Three sessions of motivational interviewing	Inclusion: age ≥ 18 y, diagnosis of OSA by clinical PSG, recommended CPAP use and CPAP naive Exclusion: required bilevel PAP because of CSA, did not complete a CPAP titration, or unable to give informed consent	3.16 ± 2.69	4.63 ± 2.69
Aloia et al,[40] 2013	Parallel, 3-arm RCT Duration 12 mo N = 227 Completed study: Intervention = 47 Education = 53 Usual care = 49	Intervention 51.7 ± 10.0 Education 47.0 ± 11.4 Usual care 52.4 ± 11.8	Intervention 11.6 ± 5.2 Education 12.6 ± 4.9 Usual care 11.9 ± 5.1	Intervention 11.9 ± 5.1 Education 12.6 ± 4.9 Usual care 11.6 ± 5.2	Intervention 45.7 ± 23.8 Education 46.1 ± 23.2 Usual care 48.2 ± 26.2	MET involved assessing readiness to change, effects of sleep apnea and PAP on health, perceived benefits of PAP and goal settings	Inclusion: moderate to severe OSA and naive to PAP therapy Exclusion: diagnosis by split PSG, severe neurologic condition, unstable psychiatric illness, sleep disorder other than OSA (including CSA), CHF, and ESRD	3.73 ± 2.50	Motivational enhancement therapy 3.86 ± 2.61 Education 4.36 ± 2.45

Study	Design					Intervention	Inclusion/Exclusion		
Partha-sarathy et al,[41] 2013	Parallel, 2-arm RCT Duration 3 mo N = 39 Completed study: Intervention = 22 Usual care = 12	Intervention 53 ± 14 Usual care 50 ± 14	Intervention 35 ± 6 Usual care 33 ± 5	Intervention 10.5 ± 5.3 Usual care 11.2 ± 3.8	Intervention 36.7 ± 28.6 Usual care < 37.5 ± 36.9	Two one-on-one peer support sessions involving sharing of coping strategies and 8 30-min follow-up calls	Inclusion: AHI ≥5, age between 21 and 85 y, stable medical history with no change in medications Exclusion: CSA, required oxygen or bilevel PAP for treatment of OSA or hypoventilation, decompensated cardiac or pulmonary disease	4.0 ± 2.4	5.2 ± 2.0
Lai et al,[42] 2014	Parallel, 2-arm RCT Duration 3 mo N = 100 Completed study: Intervention = 49 Usual care = 51	Intervention 53 ± 10 Usual care 51 ± 10	Intervention 28.6 ± 5.5 Usual care 29.3 ± 5.4	Intervention 9.5 ± 5.8 Usual care 9.0 ± 5.0	Intervention 30.7 (20.6-52.2) Usual care 28.2 (20.3-53.6)	Motivation enhancement education involved 25-min video providing information on OSA and CPAP; included experiences from current CPAP users	Inclusion criteria: age >18 y with newly diagnosed OSA (AHI>5), receiving in-laboratory auto-CPAP titration for the first time, and no prior OSA or CPAP education classes Exclusion: CSA, periodic leg movement disorders, COPD, pregnancy, psychiatric illness on treatment, cognitive impairment, illiteracy, unstable health conditions such as ESRD	2.4 ± 2.3	4.4 ± 1.8

(continued on next page)

Table 1
(continued)

Study/Year	Study Design	Age (y)	BMI (kg/m²)	ESS	AHI/RDI (Events/h)	Intervention	Inclusion/Exclusion Criteria	Usual Care Adherence (h/Night)	Intervention Adherence (h/Night)
Bakker et al,[43] 2016	Parallel, 2-arm RCT Duration 6 mo N = 83 Completed study: Intervention = 41 Usual care = 42	Intervention 53 ± 10 Usual care 51 ± 10	Intervention 31.6 ± 5.9 Usual care 30.6 ± 4.5	Intervention 8.4 ± 4.8 Usual care 7.7 ± 4.2	Intervention 21.8 (17.4–31.0) Usual care 23.7 (15.9–31.4)	Each session involved an evaluation of the subject's readiness to begin CPAP, understanding of the health risk associated with untreated OSA, and the benefit of CPAP	Inclusion: 4% AHI ≥ 10 or 3% AHI ≥ 15, 45–75 y-old with established CVD or cardiometabolic disease Exclusion: prior CPAP, ESS score > 14, drowsy driving within 2 y, commercial driving, or an uncontrolled medical condition	3.3 ± 2.7	4.4 ± 2.9

Only prospective trials that assessed the impact of behavioral therapies on CPAP adherence were included.

Values represent mean ± standard deviation, or median (25th–75th percentile).

Abbreviations: CBT, cognitive behavior therapy; CHF, congestive heart failure; COPD, chronic obstructive pulmonary disease; CSA, central sleep apnea; CVD, cardiovascular disease; ESRD, end-stage renal disease; MET, motivational enhancement therapy; MMSE, Minimental State Examination; PSG, polysomnogram; RDI, respiratory disturbance index.

Table 2
Overview of studies showing the impact of telemedicine on continuous positive airway pressure adherence for the treatment of obstructive sleep apnea

Study/Year	Study Design	Age (y)	BMI (kg/m²)	ESS	AHI/RDI (Events/h)	Intervention	Inclusion/Exclusion Criteria	Usual Care Adherence (h/Night)	Intervention Adherence (h/Night)
Stepnowsky et al,[44] 2007	Parallel, 2-arm RCT; Duration 2 mo; N = 45; Completed study: Intervention = 20; Usual care = 20	59 ± 14.3	32.8 ± 5.7	12.6 ± 5.8	39 ± 16.8	The intervention consisted of telemonitored compliance and efficacy that was then acted on collaboratively with the patient	Inclusion: ≥18 y/o, AHI ≥ 15, CPAP naive, stable sleep environment. Exclusion: sensitivity to CPAP mask material, supplemental oxygen, significant comorbid medical conditions that would interfere with daily CPAP use	2.8 ± 2.2	4.1 ± 1.8
Sparrow et al,[45] 2010	Parallel, 2-arm RCT; Duration 12 mo; N = 250; Completed study: Intervention = 112; Usual care = 122	Intervention 56.0 (48.0–63.0); Usual care 54.0 (45.0–62.0)	Intervention 34.4 (30.1–40.1); Usual care 35.9 (31.9–42.1)	Intervention 10.0 (6.0–15.0); Usual care 11.0 (8.0–15.0)	Intervention 36.0 (22.0–63.0); Usual care 40.5 (21.0–64.0)	Intervention included motivational interviewing implemented through up to 15 phone calls that used digitized voice responses	Inclusion: age 18–80 y/o, AHI ≥ 10, undergoing initial setup of fixed CPAP or bilevel PAP	0.99	2.98
Fox et al,[46] 2012	Parallel, 2-arm RCT; Duration 3 mo; N = 75; Completed study: Intervention = 28; Usual care = 26	Intervention 52 ± 10.8; Usual care 55.2 ± 11.5	Intervention 31.9 ± 5.0; Usual care 32.6 ± 16.2	Intervention 9.9 ± 5.0; Usual care 9.7 ± 4.7	Intervention 44.3 ± 24.8; Usual care 39.5 ± 19.6	Regular (every weekday) telemonitoring of adherence and efficacy data with corresponding clinical care and adjustments	Inclusion: ≥19 y/o, AHI ≥ 15, willing to initiate CPAP therapy. Exclusion: active cardiopulmonary or psychiatric disease, previously treated for OSA, did not have telephone line in their bedroom	1.75 ± 1.97	3.18 ± 2.45

(continued on next page)

Table 2
(continued)

Study/Year	Study Design	Age (y)	BMI (kg/m²)	ESS	AHI/RDI (Events/h)	Intervention	Inclusion/Exclusion Criteria	Usual Care Adherence (h/Night)	Intervention Adherence (h/Night)
Kuna et al,[47] 2015	Parallel, 3-arm RCT Duration 3 mo N = 138 Completed study: Web-based access = 40 Web-based access and financial incentive = 39 Usual care = 43	50.9 ± 12.1	36.7 ± 8.7	10.0 ± 4.4	37.8 ± 26.7	(1) Web-based access to PAP usage (2) Web-based access to PAP usage and a financial incentive ($30/d in the first week for objective PAP use ≥4 h/d) (3) Usual care	Inclusion: ≥18 y/o, AHI ≥ 10, newly diagnosed, 2 mo of stable medical history, daily access to phone and Internet Exclusion: other sleep disorders, previous OSA treatment, supplemental oxygen or bilevel PAP, rotating or night shift work	3.8 ± 3.3	Web access to PAP usage 5.0 ± 3.2 Web access to PAP usage and financial incentive 4.8 ± 3.0
Munafo et al,[48] 2016	Parallel, 2-arm RCT Duration 3 mo N = 122 Completed study: Intervention = 58 Usual care = 64	Intervention 52.3 ± 10.6 Usual care 50.0 ± 11.7	Intervention 33.5 ± 8.2 Usual care 32.9 ± 7.1	Intervention 10.9 ± 4.7 Usual care 10.2 ± 5.7	Intervention 33.4 ± 24.5 Usual care 27.4 ± 18.0	Intervention participants received automated series of text messages and/or emails that were triggered by conditions based on telemonitoring of adherence and efficacy data	Inclusion: 18–80 y/o, CPAP naive, AHI 5–70, text messaging email access/usability Exclusion: prominent CSA (≥20%), claustrophobia, use of other OSA therapy	4.7 ± 2.1	5.1 ± 1.9
Hostler et al,[49] 2017	Parallel, 2-arm nonrandomized Duration 11 wk N = 61 Completed study: Intervention = 30 Usual care = 31	Intervention 44.5 ± 11.3 Usual care 42.1 ± 6.8	—	Intervention 10.9 ± 6.8 Usual care 7.7 ± 6.0	Intervention 19.3 (10.1–25.3) Usual care 18.1 (10.3–29.5)	Intervention used SleepMapper, a mobile, Web-based system that allows patients to self-monitor PAP therapy and provides real-time positive feedback and education	Inclusion: initiating CPAP for the first time, AHI ≥ 5 along with symptoms of OSA Exclusion: CSA	2.7 (1.7–3.9)	4.0 (2.4–4.8)

Study	Design					Intervention	Inclusion/Exclusion	Adherence
Turino et al,[50] 2017	Parallel, 2-arm RCT Duration 3 mo N = 100 Completed study: Intervention = 52 Usual care = 48	Intervention 56 ± 13 Usual care 54 ± 12	Intervention 35 ± 7 Usual care 35 ± 7	Intervention 9 ± 5 Usual care 10 ± 4	Intervention 52 ± 25 Usual care 53 ± 26	Intervention included telemonitoring program that collected information regarding compliance, air leaks, and residual respiratory symptoms on a daily basis and then contacted patient to resolve issues	Inclusion: ≥18 y/o, newly diagnosed OSA, AHI ≥ 15 Exclusion: impaired lung function, severe heart failure, psychiatric disorders, pregnancy, other sleep disorders, previous CPAP treatment	4.9 ± 2.2 5.1 ± 2.1
Hwang et al,[51] 2018	Parallel, 4-arm RCT Duration 3 mo N = 1455 Completed study: Telemedicine education = 164 Telemonitoring = 125 Both telemedicine education and telemonitoring = 138 Usual care = 129	49.1 ± 12.5	34.0 ± 7.9	9.1 ± 5.4	22.7 ± 23.9	Telemedicine education of OSA and CPAP Telemonitoring of CPAP with automated feedback Both telemedicine education and CPAP telemonitoring feedback	Inclusion: 18 y/o, AHI ≥ 5, eligible for home sleep test, no prior sleep testing or OSA therapy Exclusion: at risk for other sleep disorders, significant cardiopulmonary disease, English is not first language	3.8 ± 2.5 Telemedicine education 4.0 ± 2.4 Telemonitoring 4.4 ± 2.2 Both telemedicine education and telemonitoring 4.8 ± 2.3
Pépin et al,[52] 2019	Parallel, 2-arm RCT Duration 6 mo N = 306 Completed study: Intervention = 117 Usual care = 122	Intervention 60.8 (53.8–66.0) Usual care 61.8 (54.7–66.1)	Intervention 32.4 (29.6–36.5) Usual care 31.4 (28.1–35.2)	Intervention 9 (5–13) Usual care 9 (5–14)	Intervention 47 (35.0–60.5) Usual care 45 (35.4–61.2)	Intervention used multimodal telemonitoring, which collected information regarding blood pressure, symptoms, CPAP side effects, and physical activity that triggered home care providers to use prespecified protocoled actions	Inclusion: 18–75 y/o, AHI ≥ 30, at least 1 cardiovascular disease or >5% 10-y cardiovascular risk Exclusion: central sleep apnea or ejection fraction <40%	4.75 ± 2.5 5.28 ± 2.23

Only includes prospective trials that assessed the impact of telemedicine on CPAP adherence.
Values represent means ± standard deviation, or median (25th–75th percentile range).
Abbreviation: y/o, years old.

Table 3
Summary of studies assessing the impact of continuous positive airway pressure versus noninvasive ventilation on adherence and Epworth Sleepiness Scale for the treatment of obesity hypoventilation syndrome

Study/ Year	Study Design	Age (y)	BMI (kg/m²)	ESS at Baseline	Average AHI/RDI (Events/h)	Inclusion/ Exclusion Criteria	CPAP Adherence (h/Night)	NIV Adherence (h/Night)	ESS at End of Trial
Piper et al,[20] 2008	Parallel, 2-arm RCT Intervention: NIV (bilevel PAP spontaneous mode) vs CPAP Duration 3 mo N = 36 Completed study: NIV = 18 CPAP = 18	NIV 47 ± 13 CPAP 52 ± 17	NIV 54 ± 9 CPAP 52 ± 7	NIV 14 (12–19) CPAP 15 (8–17)	NIV: NREM RDI 70 (19–97) and REM RDI 48 (30–68) CPAP: NREM RDI 93 (59–112) and REM RDI 61 (57–91)	Inclusion: BMI>30, compensated respiratory failure with $Paco_2$>45 and pH>7.34, not currently on PAP Exclusion: patients with persistent severe nocturnal hypoxemia (Spo_2 <80% for >10 min) or CO_2 retention despite optimal CPAP; significant respiratory, neuromuscular, or other disorder that could account for hypercapnia, FEV1/FVC<70, major psychiatric illness	5.8 ± 2.4	6.1 ± 2.1	CPAP change – 6 ± 8 NIV change – 9 ± 5

Study	Design/Intervention	Age	BMI			Inclusion/Exclusion			
Howard et al,[22] 2017	Parallel, 2-arm RCT Intervention: NIV (bilevel PAP spontaneous/timed mode) vs CPAP Duration 3 mo N = 60 Completed study: NIV = 27 CPAP = 30	NIV 53.2 ± 10.7 CPAP 52.9 ± 10	NIV 55.3 ± 12.9 CPAP 54.5 ± 11.0	NIV 12.10 (standard error 1.16) CPAP 11.52 (standard error 1.12)	—	Inclusion: OHS (BMI>30 and daytime >45 mm Hg), prior ventilatory support (bilevel PAP or CPAP) was permitted provided the duration was <1 mo in the last 3 mo before enrollment, arterial pH in the normal range (7.35–7.45 mm Hg) at randomization, PSG was not required but undertaken if clinically required Exclusion: other conditions that contribute to hypoventilation, including neuromuscular disease, chest wall abnormalities, respiratory depressant medications, COPD, or FEV1/FVC ratio <70% after bronchodilators	5.0 ± 2.4	5.3 ± 2.6	NIV 7.60 (standard error 1.22) CPAP 7.26 (standard error 1.15)
Masa et al,[19] 2019	Parallel, 2-arm RCT Intervention: NIV (volume-targeted pressure support) vs CPAP Duration: Median follow-up of 5.44 y NIV 5.37 (4.36–6.32) y CPAP 5.55 (4.53–6.50) y N = 221 Completed study: NIV = 97 CPAP = 107	NIV 65 (56.5–71.5) CPAP 60.0 (49.0–71.0)	NIV 42.9 (38.1–47.6) CPAP 42.7 (38.2–48.8)	NIV 11.4 ± 4.96 CPAP 10.6 ± 5.19	NIV 68.7 (48.5–97.1) CPAP 68.2 (41.6–92.4)	Inclusion: 15–80 y/o, AHI>30, BMI>30, Paco2>45 mm Hg, pH>7.35 and no clinical exacerbation during the previous 2 mo Exclusion: COPD, other causes of hypoventilation, narcolepsy, and RLS	6.0 (3.0–7.0)	6.0 (1.3–7.2)	At 3 y NIV 4.94 ± 3.74 CPAP 4.60 ± 3.66

(continued on next page)

Table 3
(continued)

Study/Year	Study Design	Age (y)	BMI (kg/m²)	ESS at Baseline	Average AHI/RDI (Events/h)	Inclusion/Exclusion Criteria	CPAP Adherence (h/Night)	NIV Adherence (h/Night)	ESS at End of Trial
Murphy et al,[53] 2012	Parallel, 2-arm RCT Intervention: AVAPS vs bilevel PAP spontaneous/timed mode Duration 3 mo N = 50 Completed study AVAPS = 23 Bilevel PAP spontaneous/timed = 23	AVAPS 53 ± 9 Bilevel PAP spontaneous/timed 56 ± 11	AVAPS50 ± 8 Bilevel PAP spontaneous/timed 52 ± 8	AVAPS 11 ± 5 Bilevel PAP spontaneous/timed 13 ± 6	—	Inclusion: recent acute decompensated respiratory failure caused by OHS, BMI>40, $PaCO_2$ >6 kPa, and pH>7.35, absence of another identifiable cause of hypoventilation; FEV1/FVC>70, and FVC<70% predicted	—	AVAPS 4.18 ± 2.89 Bilevel PAP spontaneous/timed 5.13 ± 3.67	AVAPS 6 ± 5 Bilevel PAP spontaneous/timed 7 ± 5
Bouloukaki et a,[25] 2018	Prospective observational study NIV = bilevel PAP spontaneous mode Intervention: NIV (bilevel PAP spontaneous mode) vs CPAP Duration 2 y minimum; median 30 mo (24–52 mo) N = 252 Completed study: CPAP = 84 NIV = 141	63 (48–69)	43.3 (39–50)	14 (11–16)	58 (36–86)	Inclusion: newly diagnosed OHS with $PaCO_2$>45 mm Hg at rest and BMI>30 in the absence of other causes of hypoventilation, such as neuromuscular, chest wall disorders, and COPD; clinically stable for 4 wk before enrollment; higher than elementary school education Exclusion: CSA severe cardiomyopathy, significant CKD, untreated hypothyroidism, family or personal history of mental illness, drug or alcohol abuse, sedative use, severe cognitive impairment, oncological disease, narcolepsy or RLS	5.6 ± 1.6	6.3 ± 1.7	7 (4–9)

Only prospective studies in which all patients received PAP modalities in both arms were included.

Abbreviations: AVAPS, average volume-assured pressure support; CKD, chronic kidney disease; FEV1, forced expiratory volume at 1 second; FVC, forced vital capacity; NREM, non-rapid eye movement sleep; REM, rapid eye movement; RLS, restless legs syndrome.

the average of all 562 subjects across these 5 trials at 5.9 h/night. As shown in **Fig. 1**, patients with OHS enrolled in clinical trials show higher adherence to either CPAP or NIV therapy compared with patients with eucapnic moderate to severe OSA enrolled in clinical trials designed to improve CPAP adherence by either telehealth or behavioral interventions. Note that these patients with OHS were not undergoing any intervention to enhance or improve PAP adherence. To the best of our knowledge, thus far there have not been any studies designed to improve PAP adherence in patients with OHS.

The data summarized in **Tables 1–3** also show that patients with OHS have more severe sleepiness than patients with eucapnic OSA. The mean plus or minus standard deviation baseline ESS for patients with OSA in the behavioral intervention trials was 10.4 ± 1.4 and similarly the mean ESS for patients before randomization in the telemedicine trials was 9.6 ± 0.9 (see **Tables 1** and **2**). This value is considerably lower than the average baseline ESS calculated from OHS trials, which was 12.6 ± 1.5 (see **Table 3**). The higher adherence to PAP therapy in patients with OHS may reflect that they are more symptomatic than patients with eucapnic OSA. In addition, 58% of patients with OHS report dyspnea with a minimal amount of physical activity (eg, hurrying on level ground or walking up a slight hill) before initiating PAP therapy.[19] The great burden of symptoms at baseline plus the significant improvement in sleepiness and dyspnea after successful PAP therapy in patients with OHS is the likely reason that adherence to PAP therapy is higher than in patients with OSA.

In conclusion, adherence to long-term treatment with CPAP and NIV in patients with OHS leads to reduced burden of OHS-related symptoms, decreased rate of ICU and hospital admissions, and reduced overall morbidity and mortality. There is no significant difference in adherence between CPAP and NIV. However, patients with OHS tend to be more adherent to PAP therapy compared with patients with moderate to severe eucapnic OSA, which may in part be because they are more symptomatic.

DISCLOSURE

The authors have no conflicts of interest to declare.

REFERENCES

1. Burwell CS, Robin ED, Whaley RD, et al. Extreme obesity associated with alveolar hypoventilation: a Pickwickian syndrome. Am J Med 1956;21:811–8.

2. Mokhlesi B. Obesity hypoventilation syndrome: a state-of-the-art review. Respir Care 2010;55: 1347–62 [discussion 1363–45].

3. Berry RB, Budhiraja R, Gottlieb DJ, et al. Rules for scoring respiratory events in sleep: update of the 2007 AASM manual for the scoring of sleep and associated events. Deliberations of the sleep apnea definitions task force of the American academy of sleep medicine. J Clin Sleep Med 2012;8: 597–619.

4. Hales CM, Carroll MD, Fryar CD, et al. Prevalence of obesity and severe obesity among adults: United States, 2017–2018. NCHS Data Brief 2020;360:1–8.

5. Littleton SW, Mokhlesi B. The Pickwickian syndrome-obesity hypoventilation syndrome. Clin Chest Med 2009;30:467–478, vii-viii.

6. Balachandran JS, Masa JF, Mokhlesi B. Obesity hypoventilation syndrome: epidemiology and diagnosis. Sleep Med Clin 2014;9:341–7.

7. Mokhlesi B, Kryger MH, Grunstein RR. Assessment and management of patients with obesity hypoventilation syndrome. Proc Am Thorac Soc 2008;5: 218–25.

8. Hida W. Quality of life in obesity hypoventilation syndrome. Sleep Breath 2003;7:1–2.

9. Berg G, Delaive K, Manfreda J, et al. The use of health-care resources in obesity-hypoventilation syndrome. Chest 2001;120:377–83.

10. Masa JF, Mokhlesi B, Benitez I, et al, Spanish Sleep Network. Echocardiographic changes with positive airway pressure therapy in obesity hypoventilation syndrome. long-term pickwick randomized controlled clinical trial. Am J Respir Crit Care Med 2020;201:586–97.

11. Masa JF, Corral J, Romero A, et al, Spanish Sleep Network. Protective cardiovascular effect of sleep apnea severity in obesity hypoventilation syndrome. Chest 2016;150:68–79.

12. Castro-Anon O, Perez de Llano LA, De la Fuente Sanchez S, et al. Obesity-hypoventilation syndrome: increased risk of death over sleep apnea syndrome. PLoS One 2015;10:e0117808.

13. Masa JF, Pepin JL, Borel JC, et al. Obesity hypoventilation syndrome. Eur Respir Rev 2019;28:1–14.

14. Kakazu MT, Soghier I, Afshar M, et al. Weight loss interventions as treatment of obesity hypoventilation syndrome: a systematic review. Ann Am Thorac Soc 2020;17:492–502.

15. Mokhlesi B, Masa JF, Brozek JL, et al. Evaluation and management of obesity hypoventilation syndrome. An official American thoracic society clinical practice guideline. Am J Respir Crit Care Med 2019; 200:e6–24.

16. Mandal S, Suh ES, Harding R, et al. Nutrition and exercise rehabilitation in obesity hypoventilation syndrome (NERO): a pilot randomised controlled trial. Thorax 2018;73:62–9.

17. Heinemann F, Budweiser S, Dobroschke J, et al. Non-invasive positive pressure ventilation improves lung volumes in the obesity hypoventilation syndrome. Respir Med 2007;101:1229–35.

18. Afshar M, Brozek JL, Soghier I, et al. The role of positive airway pressure therapy in adults with obesity hypoventilation syndrome. A systematic review and meta-analysis. Ann Am Thorac Soc 2020;17:344–60.

19. Masa JF, Mokhlesi B, Benitez I, et al, Spanish Sleep Network. Long-term clinical effectiveness of continuous positive airway pressure therapy versus noninvasive ventilation therapy in patients with obesity hypoventilation syndrome: a multicentre, open-label, randomised controlled trial. Lancet 2019; 393:1721–32.

20. Piper AJ, Wang D, Yee BJ, et al. Randomised trial of CPAP vs bilevel support in the treatment of obesity hypoventilation syndrome without severe nocturnal desaturation. Thorax 2008;63:395–401.

21. Masa JF, Corral J, Alonso ML, et al. Efficacy of different treatment alternatives for obesity hypoventilation syndrome. Pickwick Study. Am J Respir Crit Care Med 2015;192:86–95.

22. Howard ME, Piper AJ, Stevens B, et al. A randomised controlled trial of CPAP versus noninvasive ventilation for initial treatment of obesity hypoventilation syndrome. Thorax 2017;72:437–44.

23. Soghier I, Brozek JL, Afshar M, et al. Noninvasive ventilation versus CPAP as initial treatment of obesity hypoventilation syndrome. Ann Am Thorac Soc 2019;16:1295–303.

24. Steier J, Jolley CJ, Seymour J, et al. Neural respiratory drive in obesity. Thorax 2009;64:719–25.

25. Bouloukaki I, Mermigkis C, Michelakis S, et al. The association between adherence to positive airway pressure therapy and long-term outcomes in patients with obesity hypoventilation syndrome: a prospective observational study. J Clin Sleep Med 2018;14:1539–50.

26. Basoglu OK, Tasbakan MS. Comparison of clinical characteristics in patients with obesity hypoventilation syndrome and obese obstructive sleep apnea syndrome: a case-control study. Clin Respir J 2014;8:167–74.

27. Priou P, Hamel JF, Person C, et al. Long-term outcome of noninvasive positive pressure ventilation for obesity hypoventilation syndrome. Chest 2010; 138:84–90.

28. Jennum P, Kjellberg J. Health, social and economical consequences of sleep-disordered breathing: a controlled national study. Thorax 2011;66:560–6.

29. Jennum P, Ibsen R, Kjellberg J. Social consequences of sleep disordered breathing on patients and their partners: a controlled national study. Eur Respir J 2014;43:134–44.

30. Masa JF, Mokhlesi B, Benítez I, et al. Cost-effectiveness of positive airway pressure modalities in obesity hypoventilation syndrome with severe obstructive sleep apnoea. Thorax 2020;75:459–67.

31. Nowbar S, Burkart KM, Gonzales R, et al. Obesity-associated hypoventilation in hospitalized patients: prevalence, effects, and outcome. Am J Med 2004;116:1–7.

32. Carrillo A, Ferrer M, Gonzalez-Diaz G, et al. Noninvasive ventilation in acute hypercapnic respiratory failure caused by obesity hypoventilation syndrome and chronic obstructive pulmonary disease. Am J Respir Crit Care Med 2012;186:1279–85.

33. Marik PE, Chen C. The clinical characteristics and hospital and post-hospital survival of patients with the obesity hypoventilation syndrome: analysis of a large cohort. Obes Sci Pract 2016;2:40–7.

34. Mokhlesi B, Masa JF, Afshar M, et al. The effect of hospital discharge with empiric noninvasive ventilation on mortality in hospitalized patients with obesity hypoventilation syndrome: an individual patient data meta-analysis. Ann Am Thorac Soc 2020; 17:627–37.

35. Budweiser S, Riedl SG, Jorres RA, et al. Mortality and prognostic factors in patients with obesity-hypoventilation syndrome undergoing noninvasive ventilation. J Intern Med 2007;261:375–83.

36. Mokhlesi B, Tulaimat A, Evans AT, et al. Impact of adherence with positive airway pressure therapy on hypercapnia in obstructive sleep apnea. J Clin Sleep Med 2006;2:57–62.

37. Aloia MS, Di Dio L, Ilniczky N, et al. Improving compliance with nasal CPAP and vigilance in older adults with OAHS. Sleep Breath 2001;5:13–21.

38. Richards D, Bartlett DJ, Wong K, et al. Increased adherence to CPAP with a group cognitive behavioral treatment intervention: a randomized trial. Sleep 2007;30:635–40.

39. Olsen S, Smith SS, Oei TP, et al. Motivational interviewing (MINT) improves continuous positive airway pressure (CPAP) acceptance and adherence: a randomized controlled trial. J Consult Clin Psychol 2012;80:151–63.

40. Aloia MS, Arnedt JT, Strand M, et al. Motivational enhancement to improve adherence to positive airway pressure in patients with obstructive sleep apnea: a randomized controlled trial. Sleep 2013; 36:1655–62.

41. Parthasarathy S, Wendel C, Haynes PL, et al. A pilot study of CPAP adherence promotion by peer buddies with sleep apnea. J Clin Sleep Med 2013; 9:543–50.

42. Lai AYK, Fong DYT, Lam JCM, et al. The efficacy of a brief motivational enhancement education program on CPAP adherence in OSA: a randomized controlled trial. Chest 2014;146:600–10.

43. Bakker JP, Wang R, Weng J, et al. Motivational enhancement for increasing adherence to CPAP: a randomized controlled trial. Chest 2016;150:337–45.

44. Stepnowsky CJ, Palau JJ, Marler MR, et al. Pilot randomized trial of the effect of wireless telemonitoring on compliance and treatment efficacy in obstructive sleep apnea. J Med Internet Res 2007;9:e14.

45. Sparrow D, Aloia M, Demolles DA, et al. A telemedicine intervention to improve adherence to continuous positive airway pressure: a randomised controlled trial. Thorax 2010;65:1061–6.

46. Fox N, Hirsch-Allen AJ, Goodfellow E, et al. The impact of a telemedicine monitoring system on positive airway pressure adherence in patients with obstructive sleep apnea: a randomized controlled trial. Sleep 2012;35:477–81.

47. Kuna ST, Shuttleworth D, Chi L, et al. Web-based access to positive airway pressure usage with or without an initial financial incentive improves treatment use in patients with obstructive sleep apnea. Sleep 2015;38:1229–36.

48. Munafo D, Hevener W, Crocker M, et al. A telehealth program for CPAP adherence reduces labor and yields similar adherence and efficacy when compared to standard of care. Sleep Breath 2016; 20:777–85.

49. Hostler JM, Sheikh KL, Andrada TF, et al. A mobile, web-based system can improve positive airway pressure adherence. J Sleep Res 2017;26:139–46.

50. Turino C, de Batlle J, Woehrle H, et al. Management of continuous positive airway pressure treatment compliance using telemonitoring in obstructive sleep apnoea. Eur Respir J 2017; 49:1601128.

51. Hwang D, Chang JW, Benjafield AV, et al. Effect of telemedicine education and telemonitoring on continuous positive airway pressure adherence. The Tele-OSA randomized trial. Am J Respir Crit Care Med 2018;197:117–26.

52. Pepin JL, Jullian-Desayes I, Sapene M, et al. Multimodal remote monitoring of high cardiovascular risk patients with OSA initiating CPAP: a randomized trial. Chest 2019;155:730–9.

53. Murphy PB, Davidson C, Hind MD, et al. Volume targeted versus pressure support non-invasive ventilation in patients with super obesity and chronic respiratory failure: a randomised controlled trial. Thorax 2012;67:727–34.

Alternative Care Pathways for Obstructive Sleep Apnea and the Impact on Positive Airway Pressure Adherence

Unraveling the Puzzle of Adherence

Martha E. Billings, MD, MSc[a],[*], Sachin R. Pendharkar, MD, MSc[b]

KEYWORDS

- Obstructive sleep apnea • Ambulatory care • Delivery of health care
- Treatment adherence and compliance

KEY POINTS

- Obstructive sleep apnea (OSA) is a common disorder that is underdiagnosed because of an insufficient supply of sleep physicians and limited access to polysomnography.
- Compared with laboratory-based models of OSA diagnosis and treatment, ambulatory management of OSA in properly selected patients results in similar positive airway pressure adherence while improving access and reducing costs.
- The use of nonphysicians, such as specialist nurses, respiratory therapists, or sleep technicians, is a promising option for the management of uncomplicated OSA within a sleep clinic setting.
- Given the unmet burden of disease, primary care delivery models for OSA may improve access and satisfy patient preference for care within the medical home.
- Models incorporating these innovations must align expertise with patient complexity and require validation outside of a research setting.

INTRODUCTION

Obstructive sleep apnea (OSA) is common, with an estimated population prevalence ranging from 3% to 50% depending on age, sex, definition of disease, and body mass index.[1,2] Globally, it estimated that 936 million individuals have OSA,[3] and most remain undiagnosed.[4,5] Untreated OSA in adults may have significant medical consequences, including increased risk of hypertension, atrial fibrillation, stroke, and cognitive impairment.[6–8] Furthermore, daytime symptoms from OSA, such as sleepiness, may contribute to depression, poor quality of life, decreased workplace productivity, and a higher risk of motor vehicle collisions and occupational injury.[9–15] Individuals with OSA make greater and more costly use of the health care system compared with the general population.[16,17] Overall, the downstream

Funding Source: M.E. Billings has no commercial or financial conflicts of interest. S.R. Pendharkar has no commercial or financial conflicts of interest.

[a] Division of Pulmonary, Critical Care and Sleep Medicine, University of Washington School of Medicine, UW Medicine Sleep Center at Harborview Medical Center, Box 359803, 325 Ninth Avenue, Seattle, WA 98104, USA;
[b] Departments of Medicine and Community Health Sciences, Cumming School of Medicine, University of Calgary, TRW Building, Room 3E23, 3280 Hospital Drive Northwest, Calgary, Alberta T2N 4Z6, Canada
* Corresponding author.
E-mail address: mebillin@uw.edu

Sleep Med Clin 16 (2021) 61–74
https://doi.org/10.1016/j.jsmc.2020.10.005
1556-407X/21/Crown Copyright © 2020 Published by Elsevier Inc. All rights reserved.

sequelae of OSA contribute to significant costs for health and society.[18–20] Treatment of OSA with positive airway pressure (PAP) improves clinical outcomes and is cost-effective.[21–27]

However, the limited availability of laboratory-based sleep testing coupled with an inadequate supply of sleep specialists has led to reduced access, delays to diagnosis, and undertreatment of OSA with insufficient follow-up to support PAP adherence.[28–32] These challenges are exacerbated in rural and remote communities, where access to services may be more limited compared with urban centers.[31,33] Insufficient OSA care has prompted a demand for innovative diagnostic and treatment strategies, such as the use of home sleep apnea testing or management of OSA by nonsleep specialists. These strategies and others have been integrated into novel care delivery models that have been proposed as potential solutions to mitigate the supply-demand imbalance that limits access to OSA care. However, before implementing such innovations in clinical practice, it is important to assess if new models of care impact PAP adherence and other OSA clinical outcomes.

This review summarizes current research on alternative care delivery models for OSA, presenting key findings, limitations, and practical considerations for implementation. Through this discussion, important knowledge gaps are highlighted as directions for future research.

AMBULATORY CARE PATHWAYS

System pressures arising from constrained health care resources, combined with advances in technology, have led to a shift from laboratory-based care, using polysomnography (PSG) for OSA diagnosis with an additional in-laboratory PAP titration for treatment initiation, to home-focused care. Home-based testing and therapy initiation can be accomplished through a home sleep apnea test (HSAT) and subsequent use of automatic positive airway pressure (APAP) devices, bypassing the laboratory for most patients. This pathway has emerged as the more dominant form of care in much of the world, in part because of payer preference, as it is overall less costly.[34–37] In 2008, the US Centers for Medicare and Medicaid Services (CMS) approved HSAT testing to qualify for PAP coverage, resulting in a marked shift away from laboratory testing. Since then, many commercial payers have instituted policies requiring a home-based pathway unless certain clinical conditions are met, leading to a restriction in the use of PSG.[38] In many integrated health care systems, this approach has been used to expedite initiation

of appropriate therapy for uncomplicated adults with OSA, reducing wait times for studies and improving patient satisfaction.[39,40] The home-based pathway has also been adapted as a cost-saving mode in resource-limited settings, requiring far fewer trained personnel and less dedicated physical space than a traditional sleep laboratory.

Several studies have confirmed that a home-based pathway is equally efficacious in properly selected patients, those *with* a high probability of OSA based on clinical history, examination, and *without* significant cardiopulmonary comorbidities, such as heart failure, underlying lung disease, neuromuscular disease, or use of opioids, who may have sleep-related hypoventilation, severe hypoxemia, or central sleep apnea. The American Academy of Sleep Medicine (AASM) clinical practice guidelines for the diagnosis of OSA recommends HSAT or PSG in medically uncomplicated adults with signs and symptoms consistent with moderate to severe OSA.[41] Home sleep apnea testing methods vary; many include cardiopulmonary monitoring with oximetry, nasal pressure transducer, effort bands, and position sensor (level III device), whereas another widely adopted device measures primarily peripheral artery tone with oximetry (WatchPAT, Itamar Medical Ltd, Israel). All HSATs have lower sensitivity than the gold-standard in-laboratory PSG, especially in certain populations (comorbid insomnia, milder desaturation, difficulty self-administering the test because of cognitive impairment).[41] Newer updates to technology include auto-scoring,[42] assessment of central apneas and Cheyne-Stokes breathing, and validation in patients with underlying lung disease.[43,44] The AASM task force completed a systemic review and metaanalysis of clinical trials comparing HSAT and PSG pathways when developing their guidelines; the metaanalysis revealed that PAP adherence was slightly but nonsignificantly higher in those who underwent home testing.[45]

In uncomplicated adults with OSA, initiating APAP instead of performing an in-laboratory PAP titration study is equally efficacious in reducing Apnea Hypopnea Index (AHI) and in improving both sleepiness and quality of life.[46–49] Most relevant, the home pathway compared with in-laboratory titration had similar to better overall adherence.[46,49–52] The most recent AASM clinical practice guidelines for PAP therapy initiation added a strong recommendation for home-based APAP as an equivalent alternative to an in-laboratory titration pathway in adults with OSA and no significant comorbidities, citing no clinically significant difference in patient-reported outcomes or adherence between the home and laboratory-based pathways.[45,53] Consideration of patient preferences, costs, access to testing, and clinician judgment should weigh into selection of the most appropriate pathway.

Another consideration would be empiric APAP therapy without diagnostic testing in those with a very high probability of OSA. This approach may bypass the monetary, time, and opportunity costs of confirming a diagnosis and has been shown in a randomized trial to result in quicker treatment initiation and more rapid improvement in daytime sleepiness.[54] However, treatment with empiric APAP could potentially lead to inappropriate use of therapy in patients who do not actually have OSA. Furthermore, patients with comorbid hypoxemia or hypoventilation that is missed in the absence of diagnostic testing may receive incomplete therapy, although no adverse effects were reported in the trial by the study investigators.[54] Use of device downloads may confirm OSA diagnosis as well as the efficacy of therapy based on residual AHI, mask interface leak, hours of use, and mean and maximum pressure titration. This approach may work in integrated health care systems looking to reduce overall costs and improve patient well-being but is unlikely to be accepted in traditional fee-for-service models of care. In addition, patients may be less eager to accept or adhere to therapy without a proven OSA diagnosis. It is possible that without a diagnostic testing rubric, the patients may require distinct education, support, and follow-up to achieve treatment success, with associated costs that may obviate the savings from bypassing testing. However, a small trial using empiric APAP without diagnostic testing during stroke rehabilitation showed reasonable 3-month adherence of 4.7 hours per night.[55]

USE OF NONPHYSICIAN PROVIDERS

In addition to ambulatory diagnostic pathways, several studies have explored strategies incorporating nonphysician providers (nurses or respiratory therapists) to improve access at various points in the clinical pathway. The underlying premise for using these providers is to offload demand from a limited supply of sleep physicians, particularly for follow-up of patients with an established diagnosis or management of those with uncomplicated OSA. Health system decision makers may also perceive nonphysician providers to be a less costly alternative to traditional physician-led care.

A study based in England, by Palmer and colleagues,[56] randomized 174 established CPAP users to annual clinical review by a hospital-based physician consultant or by a specialist nurse in the patient's home. The primary outcome of sleepiness, depression, and anxiety scores or quality of life did not differ by between the consultant clinic and nurse home visit arms at 3 months, nor did CPAP adherence (5.93 vs 5.64 hours, respectively, $P = .54$). Of note, patients had used CPAP for almost 3 years, which may explain nightly adherence much higher than has been reported in other studies and the lack of difference between groups. Similar results were found in a randomized trial evaluating a home ambulatory diagnostic pathway, in which follow-up was compared between hospital-based physicians and home follow-up by a specialist nurse. In this study of 65 patients, there were no significant differences in CPAP adherence, sleepiness, or daily function.[57]

Nonphysician providers have also been used in the initial diagnosis and management of OSA. In one of the first studies evaluating a nurse-led clinical service, 150 patients underwent ambulatory diagnostic sleep testing and initiation of CPAP by a specialist nurse in the home. Most patients (138/150) accepted CPAP, and at 3 months mean adherence was 5.2 hours among 118 patients still using therapy. Sleepiness also improved significantly and was strongly predictive of CPAP adherence.[58] However, there was no comparison group. Antic and colleagues[59] randomized 195 patients with a clinical presentation and overnight oximetry that were highly suggestive of OSA to a simplified nurse-led model of care or traditional care led by a sleep physician and using PSG. Nurses followed a predefined clinical protocol and could solicit advice from sleep specialists when necessary. Based on a clinically relevant difference of -2 points on the Epworth Sleepiness Scale (ESS), the nurse-led model was noninferior to physician-led care. Adherence to CPAP was slightly lower in the nurse-led care arm (4.11 vs 4.56 hours), but this did not achieve statistical significance. Furthermore, 15 patients (15%) in the nurse-led care arm were discussed with physicians, leading to 12 physician visits, of which nine were due to nonadherence to therapy. Patients expressed greater satisfaction with nurse-led care, primarily because of the shorter waiting time for care, longer time spent with the provider, and explanations of OSA and treatment options in the nurse-led group compared with physicians who had greater time constraints.

Respiratory therapists have also been used to provide OSA follow-up care in place of physicians in an effort to provide more timely access. A study evaluated clinical outcomes of patients with physician-diagnosed OSA when CPAP follow-up was provided by a sleep-trained respiratory therapist. Out of 746 patients who initiated CPAP, adherence data were available for 456 who attended follow-up visits; mean nightly CPAP use was 5.4 hours. Although an association between adherence and the number of follow-up visits with a respiratory therapist was seen on univariate analysis, the relationship was not robust to multivariate adjustment.[60] A subsequent study by the same investigators examined the role of sleep-trained respiratory therapists in the management of patients with severe sleep-disordered breathing (severe OSA with or without cardiopulmonary co-morbidity or hypoventilation). In this noninferiority study, 156 patients were randomized to usual care by a sleep physician or a model in which initial assessment was performed by respiratory therapists under physician supervision. A small nonsignificant difference in PAP adherence between groups (4 vs 3.5 hours, $P = .16$) led to an indeterminate result with respect to the noninferiority design; however, patients in the respiratory therapy arm had greater improvements in sleepiness and, although not statistically significant, tended to have better quality of life and satisfaction scores at 3 months.[61] Similar to Antic's study, respiratory therapists could consult sleep physicians if required, although this was rare (0.16 visits/patient).

Nonphysician providers have also been used in targeted interventions to improve PAP adherence. In a study evaluating an intensive support strategy to improve CPAP adherence, 80 patients with a new diagnosis of OSA were randomized to standard support that included 2 scheduled telephone calls and additional as-needed telephone support from a clinic nurse, or intensive support in which clinic nurses provided home-based education and made several home visits. Adherence to CPAP at 6 months was higher in the intensive support group (5.4 vs 3.8 hours, $P = .003$), but differences in patient-reported outcomes were not consistently observed.[62] A larger randomized study demonstrated that intensive home-based CPAP support with clinic nurses was associated with higher adherence at 24 months (6.9 vs 5.2 hours, $P<.001$). Daytime sleepiness, depressive symptoms, and quality of life all improved to a greater extent in the intensive support group.[63] In Australia, pharmacists are members of the sleep apnea management pathway as providers of PAP devices and equipment. Qualitative research and survey studies have explored how community pharmacists are integrated into OSA care delivery,[64,65] but to date there have been no outcome studies on PAP adherence.

Economic analyses of models incorporating nonphysicians have consistently demonstrated potential cost savings, including studies in which patients received more intensive care than standard practice[56,57,59,63]; these economic benefits may be underestimated, as studies primarily assessed direct costs of care and did not incorporate clinical benefits or downstream cost-savings into an analysis of cost-effectiveness. However, cost-saving may be mitigated by additional costs of provider training requirements. Nonphysician providers in all of these studies had additional training and expertise in sleep medicine. In contrast, a survey of 271 sleep centers in the United States revealed that although 109 (40%) centers employed advanced practice registered nurses or physician assistants to provide new or follow-up clinical care of patients with sleep-disordered breathing, only 1 provider had specialty training in sleep medicine. Thus, the findings of the above studies may not translate to current models that incorporate nonphysician providers.

PRIMARY CARE MANAGEMENT OF OBSTRUCTIVE SLEEP APNEA

Epidemiologic studies suggest that OSA prevalence is comparable or exceeds that of other common chronic diseases, such as hypertension, diabetes, asthma, or chronic obstructive pulmonary disease. These conditions are frequently managed in a primary care setting, with specialist referral reserved for more complex cases. Such a model for care delivery ostensibly allows patients with uncomplicated disease to obtain care without having to navigate a complex specialty care system or wait for specialist appointment and aligns strongly with patient preference for care delivery within their medical home.[66–68] Moreover, under a chronic disease management paradigm, comprehensive management of OSA and related comorbidities (eg, metabolic syndrome) may be best managed in a primary care setting.[69]

Several randomized, controlled trials have explored the role of primary care providers (PCPs) in the management of patients with uncomplicated OSA. In a noninferiority study conducted by Chai-Coetzer and colleagues,[70] 155 patients were randomized to receive management by PCPs and a community-based nurse or by a sleep specialist. Patients were included if results from a 4-item screening questionnaire indicated high likelihood of OSA and overnight oximetry was consistent with moderate to severe OSA. All PCPs participated in a 6-hour educational program on OSA management before the study. The results confirmed noninferiority of primary care management of OSA at 6 months with respect to the primary outcome of ESS score. Adherence to PAP was not statistically different by group (5.4 [standard deviation, SD 2.1] in the PCP arm versus 4.8 [SD 0.3] hours in the sleep specialist arm, $P = .11$) nor were other patient-reported outcomes. Of note, PCPs could request support or consultation from sleep specialists during the study, although this was only used for 3 patients (4%).

Three subsequent randomized noninferiority trials from Spain have demonstrated similar results using slightly different primary care delivery models for OSA management. The first evaluated CPAP adherence in 210 patients with severe OSA (AHI >30), daytime hypersomnolence, or high cardiovascular risk. Patients received a diagnosis of OSA in a sleep unit and were then randomized to follow-up care by a nurse in the sleep unit or by PCPs that had participated in a 6-hour education session on OSA. A nonsignificant difference in adherence was observed (5.23 vs 4.94 hours in the sleep unit and primary care arms, respectively), with noninferiority established based on the prespecified noninferiority margin of 1 hour of CPAP use. Improvements in sleepiness and patient satisfaction favored the sleep unit arm.[71] A subsequent study randomized 302 patients with suspected OSA to primary care versus sleep unit management, but expanded decision making by PCPs to include selection of testing in at-risk individuals and recommendations for treatment. The main outcomes, change in ESS and quality of life at 6 months, were not significantly different between groups. Adherence to CPAP was also similar at 5.3 hours, although less than 50% of patients were treated with CPAP, which was lower than in most other studies of primary care OSA management.[72] Finally, a third study compared a model of OSA management by PCPs, using portable sleep monitoring and an algorithm for therapeutic decision making, to management by sleep specialists using PSG. Overall, 307 patients were randomized, and no significant differences were noted in the primary outcome of change in ESS or several secondary outcomes related to quality of life, patient satisfaction, cardiometabolic risk, or health care utilization. Approximately 70% of patients were treated with CPAP, and adherence was comparable between study arms (4.3 hours in each arm).[73]

All of the above studies demonstrated significant cost savings associated with primary care management of OSA.[70–73] Although these data are encouraging, it is important to acknowledge that each study protocol included initial training of PCPs on OSA management, regular follow-up with nurses, and options to consult a sleep specialist, highlighting the importance of appropriate education, staffing, and infrastructure for such models to succeed. Moreover, differences in PAP adherence favoring sleep specialist care were noted in 2 studies; although these differences were not statistically significant, they approached or exceeded the minimal clinically important difference in PAP adherence of 30 minutes.[41] These considerations are important in implementing such models outside of a research setting.

In contrast to trial data, observational studies have explored potential benefits of care by sleep specialists compared with primary care. Pamidi and colleagues[74] reviewed the charts of 403 patients who underwent polysomnographic CPAP titration at the University of Chicago Sleep Laboratory, of whom 26% had undergone a consultation by a board-certified sleep specialist before PSG and the remainder of whom had been referred by nonsleep physicians. Adherence at 30 days was higher in the sleep specialist group (4.7 vs 3.7 hours, $P = .005$), and 13% more patients met the CMS adherence threshold of 4 or more hours of CPAP use per night on 70% of days ($P = .01$).[75] However, after adjustment for differences in the demographics of each group, the benefits of sleep specialist consultation were no longer significant. Adherence in this study was assessed at 30 days; although this time window is relatively short for drawing conclusions about clinical outcomes, it is highly likely to predict longer-term adherence to therapy.[76,77] Studies exploring the role of accreditation on patient outcomes demonstrated that physician certification in sleep medicine and sleep center accreditation were both independently associated with greater adherence to PAP. Improved education and perception of OSA risk were identified as possible mediators of this relationship, highlighting the importance of appropriate support for patients to facilitate treatment success.[78,79] These findings suggest that, in real-world settings, PCPs may not be able to meet the diagnostic and follow-up needs of their OSA patients without adequate infrastructural support.

NEWER MODELS OF CARE

Ambulatory pathways may be used to manage uncomplicated adults with OSA but are not appropriate for all sleep apnea patients. Thus, newer models need to incorporate assessment of when specialist-led diagnosis and PAP titration using PSG are warranted. Integration of specialists, advanced practice providers, and PCPs within a geographic area or health organization, a so-called hub-and-spoke model,[80] has been used to improve access to opioid use disorder treatment and in acute stroke care.[81,82] The term "hub" was notarized by the airline industry and in health care reflects the center with more highly trained subspecialists and facilities for procedures, whereas "spokes" reflect the outreach to community centers with more limited services.[80] Applying this model to sleep medicine, the hub is the site for complex care with a sleep laboratory, technicians, and specialty sleep physicians, and the spokes represent community-based primary care centers for routine OSA diagnosis and follow-up of OSA therapy.[83] A hub-and-spoke model has been proposed as a possible solution to the anticipated shortage of sleep specialists[84]; moreover, it would extend the reach of sleep care beyond traditional specialist-centred models to improve timely access as well as convenience for patients.

In addition, this hub-and-spoke model can better serve rural communities, geographically remote areas, and resource-limited settings.[83] A group in New Zealand has implemented this model with a community-based sleep assessment service. This integrated health care service allows for provision of sleep care through a multidisciplinary meeting between primary and specialty care providers. The goal of this model is to expedite treatment to those in need of urgent therapy (severely sleepy, risk of car accidents), appropriately triage those with more complex sleep apnea, and keep the bulk for community evaluation by PCPs.[85] A similar model has also been used in the integrated Veterans Affairs (VA) health system with the high burden of OSA within the veteran population and few sleep laboratories and specialists. By providing tele-education about OSA to PCPs, more providers will be able to perform routine OSA evaluation and PAP care in the community VA clinics.[86] Such models fit in well with the notion of the patient-centered medical home by keeping the patient in a familiar primary care setting.[35] The hub and spoke may also result in more cost-effective, efficient care[35] with appropriate utilization of more intensive resources limited to the medically complex. However, the system impacts, costs, and outcomes of a hub-and-spoke model for OSA care have not been evaluated.

Other Innovative Patient-Centered Models

There has been recent interest in different models of service delivery to improve adherence and other OSA outcomes. SMART DOCS is a randomized trial comparing a patient-centered care management strategy to conventional sleep care.[87] In this study, PCPs are integrated with the sleep center for diagnosis and treatment of sleep disorders, supported by a Web-based interactive portal to facilitate communication and sharing of data between providers. However, PAP adherence is not an outcome of interest; rather, the focus is on improving patient-reported outcomes and experience.

Peer-support models

A randomized trial comparing a peer-driven intervention to improve PAP adherence to standard care was conducted in veterans in Arizona. In the intervention arm, subjects newly prescribed CPAP for OSA were paired with experienced, adherent, and trained CPAP users ("peer buddy"); partners met in person initially and then through telephone calls for 3 months. Patients in the intervention arm had higher adherence and rated the program highly.[88] This pilot study was small (n = 39), however, and has not yet been verified in larger trials. It also required substantial administrative effort to coordinate the training sessions and peer-buddy meetings and telephone calls. However, the use of peer expertise, support, and guidance is a promising strategy to improve adherence.

Online OSA peer-support forums have emerged organically in the modern technological era. Users of PAP can connect in Facebook groups (some with >35,000 members) to share tips and tricks and form a virtual community. Other on-line peer-support groups are hosted by device manufacturers and suppliers (such as CPAPtalk.com). Nonprofit patient organizations also host patient support platforms; examples include the American Sleep Apnea Association AWAKE (Alert, Well, And Keeping Energetic) program (https://talk.sleepapnea.org/) and MyApnea.org, which is a consortium of sleep patients, researchers, and physicians (https://myapnea.org/forum).[89] Patient-developed educational platforms are also popular resources, such as the Apnea Board (http://www.apneaboard.com/). These tools facilitate patient engagement and motivation within online communities[90]; anecdotally, these sites are very useful to patients, empowering them to solve issues with their PAP and learn from more experienced users. However, objective data evaluating if these forums improve adherence and sleep health outcomes are not yet available.

Multidisciplinary care

A model offered as a potential way to improve sleep outcomes and specifically PAP adherence is the multidisciplinary sleep center with a team-based approach to patient care. This model incorporates multiple specialties into the sleep center to treat the OSA patient's needs more comprehensively. An example would be an embedded psychologist to attend to comorbid insomnia or manage claustrophobia or PAP desensitization.[91] Simultaneously addressing these issues may improve PAP acceptance and adherence in more challenging patients.[92] Similarly, office-based interventions to reduce nasal congestion by an otolaryngologist included in the sleep team may also facilitate PAP use. Such an approach has been used by the Tripler Army Medical Center; their sleep clinic includes an oral surgeon, dental sleep medicine specialist, and speech pathologist in their team-based approach to treating sleep apnea.[93] Although evaluation frameworks including PAP adherence have been proposed, there are as yet no published data on the effectiveness of such models.

DISCUSSION

Alternative pathways for OSA care may help to mitigate the imbalances between the high burden of disease and limited supply of sleep specialists and sleep laboratories, as well as enable more holistic approaches to patient care. Studies of such models have demonstrated promising results with respect to PAP adherence and other clinical outcomes. Home-based pathways for OSA diagnosis and initiation of PAP therapy have the most support from clinical trials, leading to endorsement by the AASM in recent clinical practice guidelines[41,53] and adoption as a standard of care in many parts of the world. With the marked decrease in laboratory-based evaluation of uncomplicated OSA, ambulatory models are hardly an "alternative" any longer and have now become the norm.

An important but underappreciated consequence of home-based OSA care is the increase in the complexity and morbidity of patients seen in the sleep laboratory.[94] More medically complex patients often require more intensive monitoring and lower ratios of PSG technicians per patient, substantially raising the per-person cost of studies for the facility, skill of the technicians, and time of study interpretation. In integrated health care systems, however, increases in per-person costs for more complex patients will likely be offset by reduced costs for most patients shifted to home testing, leading to overall cost savings with home-based pathways.

Appropriate selection of patients for home-based pathways is key, to avoid scenarios in which HSAT is likely to be nondiagnostic or where clinical factors necessitate more comprehensive testing with PSG. In addition to the increased total costs with 2 tests, the additional burden on patients (cost, time, inconvenience) may lead them to forego the additional testing and subsequent OSA care.[41] Home-based pathways in which HSAT is outsourced to third-party vendors risk compromising patient support and follow-up.[34] Potential consequences of such a model include acceptance of false negatives with a nondiagnostic HSAT leading to undertreatment, or use of HSAT outside of established clinical indications resulting in overtreatment of individuals without symptoms or comorbidity. Although difficult to capture, these are important considerations for a comprehensive economic evaluation of home-based OSA care.

Alternative pathways that incorporate nonphysician providers, while encouraging, lack robust real-world data. Models using respiratory therapists or nurses have proven effective in small, structured trials,[59,61] and observational studies of pharmacists and trained nurse specialists describe some success but also note challenges. Common to all of these pathways is a requirement for extra training in sleep medicine as well as time, resources, and infrastructure to embed nonphysician providers within sleep specialty care models. In addition, many of these providers may need to operate within an accredited sleep center after obtaining additional certification, or under sleep physician oversight to prevent untrained and unsupported practitioners from delivering potentially harmful or inappropriate care. These limitations will need to be addressed in large-scale implementation studies in order to determine clinical and economic feasibility in real-world health care settings.

Management of OSA by PCPs has been validated in randomized trials, but there are several potential implementation barriers that must be considered. First, knowledge about pathophysiology, clinical presentation, and management of OSA among PCPs is variable. Exposure to sleep medicine during medical training is minimal: a multinational survey of 106 medical schools revealed a median of 90 (range 0–300) minutes of sleep education. PCPs have limited exposure during internal and family medicine residency as well.[95] Unsurprisingly, studies have consistently revealed that nonsleep specialist physicians rate their knowledge of OSA as poor,[96,97] lack confidence in managing the disease, and have objective knowledge gaps.[96,98–102] Encouraging results from more recent studies indicate that knowledge of OSA among PCPs may be improving, and there has been recent interest in quality improvement interventions to increase awareness about OSA and OSA management.[103-106]

Second, time constraints faced by PCPs are also real barriers to OSA management. PCPs are tasked with managing multiple chronic illnesses, often in the same patient, in addition to meeting guidelines for cancer screening, vaccinations, and other preventative health care. Adding to this burden of chronic disease management, particularly with a disease that requires obtaining and reviewing treatment downloads and making adjustments to specialized and continually evolving equipment, technology, and rapidly changing interfaces, may be untenable to PCPs without additional infrastructure support (such as respiratory therapists, Web portals, and sleep technicians). Integrated models of care that partner sleep specialists with PCPs may address knowledge gaps and support the management of uncomplicated OSA within the medical home.[107,108] Such models could promote more holistic, patient-centered care in treating problems such as insomnia and depression that frequently coexist with sleep apnea,[9,109] perhaps yielding greater success in all therapies, including PAP adherence.

However, essential elements of success for such integrated care delivery models, such as effective communication between providers and clarity of provider roles, have been reported as lacking in systems of OSA care.[97,110] A recent Australian observational study showed that although PCPs were increasingly involved in the management of patients with sleep disordered breathing, more than 50% of patients were still referred to sleep specialists, indicating that barriers such as these continue to foster a reliance on specialty care.[111] Thoughtful design of an integrated model must account for these factors and others; for example, patient and system factors affecting PAP use may differ in primary and specialty care settings, suggesting that different strategies may be required to promote PAP adherence.[112]

Finally, the optimal OSA care pathway should be tailored to the patient's OSA clinical phenotype, as 1 approach will not fit all patients. Using metrics such as AHI or oxygen desaturation index without consideration of symptoms clusters of insomnia, sleepiness, or being asymptomatic[113] may contribute to poorer outcomes because of differences in diagnosis, experiences with PAP, and comorbid challenges. Sleep apnea phenotypes have been shown to predict PAP adherence and benefit.[114] Furthermore, complex comorbidity (such as cardiopulmonary disease) may warrant specialty care for advanced sleep testing and treatment as well

as for follow-up to ensure adequate PAP adherence.

Many enticing, innovative models described here, such as the hub and spoke, multidisciplinary team, or patient-centered care models, are more conceptual descriptions of local practices without multicenter trials, implementation studies, or outcome data to support widespread adoption. Although many of these proposed models seem to confer cost savings by avoiding overuse of sleep specialists and laboratory testing, these findings are difficult to verify without real-world application to diverse health care systems. Further implementation research is needed to validate these proposed models in different health care systems, assess patient outcomes within these models, and evaluate economic impacts on OSA care. Fortunately, such studies are underway by researchers in Australia (https://www.ncshsr.com) and Spain.[115]

SUMMARY

The looming shortage of sleep physicians and sleep laboratory beds, high burden of unmet sleep apnea care needs, and notoriously poor PAP adherence call for the development of novel, patient-centered models of OSA care. These models may encompass features of the medical home by integrating PCPs into the sleep team through hub-and-spoke models and may also integrate nonphysician providers, such as sleep-trained nurses and respiratory therapists, to support patients to improve adherence. Technological advancements in OSA care, ambulatory testing, remote monitoring, and adjustments of PAP therapy, may facilitate the implementation of new models with the ability to incorporate telehealth. Telemedicine is well suited to support these alternative models, allowing virtual patient assessment, follow-up, and communication among providers at a distance. Any pathway should begin with an assessment of unique patient needs, including symptoms, competing illnesses, and psychosocial demands, in order to align care delivery with patient preferences and clinically appropriate care. Comparative effectiveness studies and implementation interventions should thus use patient-partnerships and include all stakeholders to inform design of sustainable models of care.

Importantly, the design and implementation of cost-effective models of OSA care must retain a broader view of health care quality. Market-driven or payer-driven OSA care that may emerge without thoughtful consideration of patient or system consequences may lead to insufficient

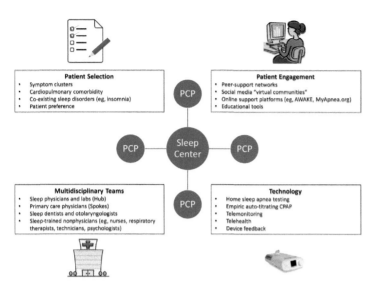

Fig. 1. Features of a comprehensive model of OSA care. AWAKE, Alert, Well, And Keeping Energetic; CPAP, continuous positive airway pressure. (*Adapted from* Pepin J-L, Baillieul S, Tamisier R. Reshaping Sleep Apnea Care: Time for Value-based Strategies. *Ann Am Thorac Soc.* 2019;16(12):1501-1503; with permission.)

support to foster PAP adherence and potentially deterioration of treatment effectiveness. Although a comprehensive framework of quality indicators for OSA care has been developed,[116] measurement is inconsistent among sleep centers.[117] A proposed model for comprehensive OSA care has been illustrated by Pepin and colleagues.[118] Incorporating different testing strategies, providers, and patients in a service delivery model to improve PAP adherence is a complex endeavor with several clinical and logistical considerations (**Fig. 1**). Although there is evidence to support individual "alternative" features of the comprehensive care model for OSA, integration into a cohesive, cost-effective model that accounts for unique patient and system needs is required. Optimally integrating these features may yield high-quality, accessible OSA care at lower cost and promote high adherence to PAP.

CLINICS CARE POINTS

- Multidisciplinary teams comprising sleep specialist, primary care physicians and non-physician providers may enable more diagnosis and testing of OSA.
- Expanding use of telemonitoring with patient engagement may facilitate better PAP adherence.
- Integration of comprehensive care into health care systems may improve cost-effectiveness but implementation studies are needed.
- Home-based pathways of diagnosis are effective and may improve access when incorporated into delivery models.

REFERENCES

1. Peppard PE, Young T, Barnet JH, et al. Increased prevalence of sleep-disordered breathing in adults. Am J Epidemiol 2013;177(9):1006–14.
2. Heinzer R, Vat S, Marques-Vidal P, et al. Prevalence of sleep-disordered breathing in the general population: the HypnoLaus study. Lancet Respir Med 2015;3(4):310–8.
3. Benjafield AV, Ayas NT, Eastwood PR, et al. Estimation of the global prevalence and burden of obstructive sleep apnoea: a literature-based analysis. Lancet Respir Med 2019;7(8):687–98.
4. Kapur V, Iber C. Underdiagnosis of sleep apnea syndrome in U.S. communities. Sleep Breath 2002;6(2):49–54.
5. Costa LE, Uchôa CHG, Harmon RR, et al. Potential underdiagnosis of obstructive sleep apnoea in the cardiology outpatient setting. Heart 2015;101(16):1288–92.
6. Hla KM, Young T, Hagen EW, et al. Coronary heart disease incidence in sleep disordered breathing: the Wisconsin Sleep Cohort Study. Sleep 2015;38(5):677–84.
7. Redline S, Yenokyan G, Gottlieb DJ, et al. Obstructive sleep apnea-hypopnea and incident stroke: the Sleep Heart Health Study. Am J Respir Crit Care Med 2010;182(2):269–77.
8. Dzierzewski JM, Dautovich N, Ravyts S. Sleep and cognition in older adults. Sleep Med Clin 2018;13(1):93–106.
9. Lang CJ, Appleton SL, Vakulin A, et al. Associations of undiagnosed obstructive sleep apnea and excessive daytime sleepiness with depression: an Australian population study. J Clin Sleep Med 2017;13(4):8.

10. Moyer CA, Sonnad SS, Garetz SL, et al. Quality of life in obstructive sleep apnea: a systematic review of the literature. Sleep Med 2001;2(6):477–91.

11. Tregear S. Obstructive sleep apnea and risk of motor vehicle crash: systematic review and meta-analysis. J Clin Sleep Med 2009;6:19.

12. Karimi M, Hedner J, Häbel H, et al. Sleep apnea related risk of motor vehicle accidents is reduced by continuous positive airway pressure: Swedish traffic accident registry data. Sleep 2015;38(3):341–9.

13. Garbarino S, Guglielmi O, Sanna A, et al. Risk of occupational accidents in workers with obstructive sleep apnea: systematic review and meta-analysis. Sleep 2016;39(06):1211–8.

14. Povitz M, Bansback N, Fenton M, et al. Workplace and driving consequences of sleepiness in Canadians with obstructive sleep apnea: results of a market research Survey. Abstract presented at the: World Sleep 2019 Congress; 2019; Vancouver, BC, September 21-25, 2019.

15. Walia HK, Thompson NR, Pascoe M, et al. Effect of positive airway pressure therapy on drowsy driving in a large clinic-based obstructive sleep apnea cohort. J Clin Sleep Med 2019;15(11):1613–20.

16. Banno K, Ramsey C, Walld R, et al. Expenditure on health care in obese women with and without sleep apnea. Sleep 2009;32(2):247–52.

17. Albarrak M, Banno K, Sabbagh AA, et al. Utilization of healthcare resources in obstructive sleep apnea syndrome: a 5-year follow-up study in men using CPAP. Sleep 2005;28(10):1306–11.

18. Hillman D, Mitchell S, Streatfeild J, et al. The economic cost of inadequate sleep. Sleep 2018; 41(8). https://doi.org/10.1093/sleep/zsy083.

19. Tarasiuk A, Reuveni H. The economic impact of obstructive sleep apnea. Curr Opin Pulm Med 2013;19(6):639–44.

20. Watson NF. Health care savings: the economic value of diagnostic and therapeutic care for obstructive sleep apnea. J Clin Sleep Med 2016; 12(08):1075–7.

21. Jennum P, Kjellberg J. Health, social and economical consequences of sleep-disordered breathing: a controlled national study. Thorax 2011;66(7):560–6.

22. Marin JM, Agusti A, Villar I, et al. Association between treated and untreated obstructive sleep apnea and risk of hypertension. JAMA 2012;307(20):2169–76.

23. Bratton DJ, Gaisl T, Wons AM, et al. CPAP vs mandibular advancement devices and blood pressure in patients with obstructive sleep apnea: a systematic review and meta-analysis. JAMA 2015; 314(21):2280–93.

24. Rizzi CF, Ferraz MB, Poyares D, et al. Quality-adjusted life-years gain and health status in patients with OSAS after one year of continuous positive airway pressure use. Sleep 2014;37(12):1963–8.

25. Campos-Rodriguez F, Queipo-Corona C, Carmona-Bernal C, et al. Continuous positive airway pressure improves quality of life in women with obstructive sleep apnea. A randomized controlled trial. Am J Respir Crit Care Med 2016;194(10):1286–94.

26. AlGhanim N, Comondore VR, Fleetham J, et al. The economic impact of obstructive sleep apnea. Lung 2008;186(1):7–12.

27. Kim J, Tran K, Seal K, et al. Interventions for the treatment of obstructive sleep apnea in adults: a health technology assessment. Ottawa: CADTH; 2017. CADTH optimal use report; vol.6, no.1b.

28. Rotenberg B, George C, Sullivan K, et al. Wait times for sleep apnea care in Ontario: a multidisciplinary assessment. Can Respir J 2010;17(4):170–4.

29. Flemons WW, Douglas NJ, Kuna ST, et al. Access to diagnosis and treatment of patients with suspected sleep apnea. Am J Respir Crit Care Med 2004;169(6):668–72.

30. Pendharkar SR, Bischak DP, Rogers P. Evaluating Healthcare Systems with Insufficient Capacity to Meet Demand. In: Laroque C, Himmelspach J, Pasupathy R, et al, editors. Proceedings of the 2012 Winter Simulation Conference. Piscataway: Institute for Electrical and Electronics Engineers; 2012. p. 859–71.

31. Povitz M, Jenkyn KB, Kendzerska T, et al. Clinical pathways and wait times for OSA care in Ontario, Canada: A population cohort study. Canadian Journal of Respiratory, Critical Care, and Sleep Medicine 2019;3(2):91–9.

32. Phillips B, Gozal D, Malhotra A. What is the future of sleep medicine in the United States? Am J Respir Crit Care Med 2015;192(8):915–7.

33. Allen AJMH, Amram O, Tavakoli H, et al. Relationship between travel time from home to a regional sleep apnea clinic in British Columbia, Canada, and the severity of obstructive sleep apnea. Ann Am Thorac Soc 2016;13(5):719–23.

34. Kim RD, Kapur VK, Redline-Bruch J, et al. An economic evaluation of home versus laboratory-based diagnosis of obstructive sleep apnea. Sleep 2015; 38(7):1027–37.

35. Kundel V, Shah N. Impact of portable sleep testing. Sleep Med Clin 2017;12(1):137–47.

36. Hui DS, Ng SS, Tam WWS. Home-based approach noninferior to hospital-based approach in managing patients with suspected obstructive sleep apnea syndrome. Am J Respir Crit Care Med 2018; 197(9):1233–4.

37. Stewart SA, Penz E, Fenton M, et al. Investigating cost implications of incorporating level III at-home

testing into a polysomnography based sleep medicine program using administrative data. Can Respir J 2017;2017:1–7.

38. Parish JM, Freedman NS, Manaker S. Evolution in reimbursement for sleep studies and sleep centers. Chest 2015;147(3):600–6.

39. Safadi A, Etzioni T, Fliss D, et al. The effect of the transition to home monitoring for the diagnosis of OSAS on test availability, waiting time, patients' satisfaction, and outcome in a large health provider system. Sleep Disord 2014;2014:1–6.

40. Stewart SA, Skomro R, Reid J, et al. Improvement in obstructive sleep apnea diagnosis and management wait times: a retrospective analysis of home management pathway for obstructive sleep apnea. Can Respir J 2015;22(3):167–70.

41. Kapur VK, Auckley DH, Chowdhuri S, et al. Clinical practice guideline for diagnostic testing for adult obstructive sleep apnea: an American Academy of Sleep Medicine Clinical Practice Guideline. J Clin Sleep Med 2017;13(3):479–504.

42. Topor ZL, Remmers JE, Grosse J, et al. Validation of a new unattended sleep apnea monitor using two methods for the identification of hypopneas. J Clin Sleep Med 2020. https://doi.org/10.5664/jcsm.8324.

43. Pillar G, Berall M, Berry R, et al. Detecting central sleep apnea in adult patients using WatchPAT—a multicenter validation study. Sleep Breath 2019. https://doi.org/10.1007/s11325-019-01904-5.

44. Chang Y, Xu L, Han F, et al. Validation of the Nox-T3 portable monitor for diagnosis of obstructive sleep apnea in patients with chronic obstructive pulmonary disease. J Clin Sleep Med 2019;15(04):587–96.

45. Patil SP, Ayappa IA, Caples SM, et al. Treatment of adult obstructive sleep apnea with positive airway pressure: an American Academy of Sleep Medicine systematic review, meta-analysis, and GRADE assessment. J Clin Sleep Med 2019;15(02):301–34.

46. Rosen CL, Auckley D, Benca R, et al. A multisite randomized trial of portable sleep studies and positive airway pressure autotitration versus laboratory-based polysomnography for the diagnosis and treatment of obstructive sleep apnea: the HomePAP study. Sleep 2012;35(6):757–67.

47. Kuna ST, Gurubhagavatula I, Maislin G, et al. Non-inferiority of functional outcome in ambulatory management of obstructive sleep apnea. Am J Respir Crit Care Med 2011;183(9):1238–44.

48. Chai-Coetzer CL, Antic NA, Hamilton GS, et al. Physician decision making and clinical outcomes with laboratory polysomnography or limited-channel sleep studies for obstructive sleep apnea: a randomized trial. Ann Intern Med 2017;166:332–40.

49. Berry RB, Sriram P. Auto-adjusting positive airway pressure treatment for sleep apnea diagnosed by home sleep testing. J Clin Sleep Med 2014;10(12):1269–75.

50. Berry RB, Hill G, Thompson L, et al. Portable monitoring and autotitration versus polysomnography for the diagnosis and treatment of sleep apnea. Sleep 2008;31(10):1423–31.

51. Skomro RP, Gjevre J, Reid J, et al. Outcomes of home-based diagnosis and treatment of obstructive sleep apnea. Chest 2010;138(2):257–63.

52. Lettieri CF, Lettieri CJ, Carter K. Does home sleep testing impair continuous positive airway pressure adherence in patients with obstructive sleep apnea? Chest 2011;139(4):849–54.

53. Patil SP, Ayappa IA, Caples SM, et al. Treatment of adult obstructive sleep apnea with positive airway pressure: an American Academy of Sleep Medicine Clinical Practice Guideline. J Clin Sleep Med 2019;15(02):335–43.

54. Drummond F, Doelken P, Ahmed QA, et al. Empiric auto-titrating CPAP in people with suspected obstructive sleep apnea. J Clin Sleep Med 2010;06(02):140–5.

55. Khot S, Barnett H, Davis A, et al. Intensive continuous positive airway pressure adherence program during stroke rehabilitation. Stroke 2019;50(7):1895–7.

56. Palmer S, Selvaraj S, Dunn C, et al. Annual review of patients with sleep apnea/hypopnea syndrome—a pragmatic randomised trial of nurse home visit versus consultant clinic review. Sleep Med 2004;5:61–5.

57. Andreu AL, Chiner E, Sancho-Chust JN, et al. Effect of an ambulatory diagnostic and treatment programme in patients with sleep apnoea. Eur Respir J 2012;39(2):305–12.

58. Tomlinson M, John Gibson G. Obstructive sleep apnoea syndrome: a nurse-led domiciliary service. J Adv Nurs 2006;55(3):391–7.

59. Antic NA, Buchan C, Esterman A, et al. A randomized controlled trial of nurse-led care for symptomatic moderate–severe obstructive sleep apnea. Am J Respir Crit Care Med 2009;179(6):501–8.

60. Pendharkar SR, Dechant A, Bischak DP, et al. An observational study of the effectiveness of alternative care providers in the management of obstructive sleep apnea. J Sleep Res 2016;25(2):234–40.

61. Pendharkar SR, Tsai WH, Penz ED, et al. A randomized controlled trial of an alternative care provider clinic for severe sleep-disordered breathing. Ann Am Thorac Soc 2019;16(12):1558–66.

62. Hoy CJ, Vennelle M, Kingshott RN, et al. Can intensive support improve continuous positive airway

pressure use in patients with the sleep apnea/hypopnea syndrome? Am J Respir Crit Care Med 1999;159(4):1096–100.

63. Bouloukaki I, Giannadaki K, Mermigkis C, et al. Intensive versus standard follow-up to improve continuous positive airway pressure compliance. Eur Respir J 2014;44(5):1262–74.

64. Hanes CA, Wong KKH, Saini B. Consolidating innovative practice models: the case for obstructive sleep apnea services in Australian pharmacies. Res Soc Adm Pharm 2015;11(3):412–27.

65. Hanes CA, Wong KKH, Saini B. An overview of service quality of continuous positive airway pressure services in Australian pharmacies: CPAP service quality in pharmacies. Respirology 2014;19(1):85–91.

66. Grumbach K, Selby JV, Damberg C, et al. Resolving the gatekeeper conundrum: what patients value in primary care and referrals to specialists. J Am Med Assoc 1999;282(3):261–6.

67. Jackson GL, Powers BJ, Chatterjee R, et al. Improving patient care. The patient centered medical home. A systematic review. Ann Intern Med 2013;158(3):169–78.

68. Sampson R, Cooper J, Barbour R, et al. Patients' perspectives on the medical primary-secondary care interface: systematic review and synthesis of qualitative research. BMJ Open 2015;5(10): e008708.

69. Heatley EM, Harris M, Battersby M, et al. Obstructive sleep apnoea in adults: a common chronic condition in need of a comprehensive chronic condition management approach. Sleep Med Rev 2013;17(5):349–55.

70. Chai-Coetzer CL, Antic NA, Rowland LS, et al. Primary care vs specialist sleep center management of obstructive sleep apnea and daytime sleepiness and quality of life: a randomized trial. J Am Med Assoc 2013;309:997–1004.

71. Sánchez-de-la-Torre M, Nadal N, Cortijo A, et al. Role of primary care in the follow-up of patients with obstructive sleep apnoea undergoing CPAP treatment: a randomised controlled trial. Thorax 2015;70(4):346–52.

72. Tarraubella N, Sánchez-de-la-Torre M, Nadal N, et al. Management of obstructive sleep apnoea in a primary care vs sleep unit setting: a randomised controlled trial. Thorax 2018. https://doi.org/10.1136/thoraxjnl-2017-211237.

73. Sánchez-Quiroga MÁ, Corral J, Gómez-de-Terreros FJ, et al. Primary care physicians can comprehensively manage patients with sleep apnea. a noninferiority randomized controlled trial. Am J Respir Crit Care Med 2018;198(5):648–56.

74. Pamidi S, Knutson KL, Ghods F, et al. The impact of sleep consultation prior to a diagnostic polysomnogram on continuous positive airway pressure adherence. Chest 2012;141(1):51–7.

75. Kribbs NB, Pack AI, Kline LR, et al. Objective measurement of patterns of nasal CPAP use by patients with obstructive sleep apnea. Am Rev Respir Dis 1993;147(4):887–95.

76. McArdle N, Devereux G, Heidarnejad H, et al. Long-term use of CPAP therapy for sleep apnea/hypopnea syndrome. Am J Respir Crit Care Med 1999;159(4 Pt 1):1108–14.

77. Van Ryswyk E, Anderson CS, Antic NA, et al. Predictors of long-term adherence to continuous positive airway pressure in patients with obstructive sleep apnea and cardiovascular disease. Sleep 2019;42(10):zsz152.

78. Parthasarathy S. A national survey of the effect of sleep medicine specialists and American Academy of Sleep Medicine Accreditation on management of obstructive sleep apnea. J Clin Sleep Med 2006;2(2):133–42.

79. Parthasarathy S, Subramanian S, Quan SF. A multicenter prospective comparative effectiveness study of the effect of physician certification and center accreditation on patient-centered outcomes in obstructive sleep apnea. J Clin Sleep Med 2014;10(3):243–9.

80. Elrod JK, Fortenberry JL. The hub-and-spoke organization design: an avenue for serving patients well. BMC Health Serv Res 2017;17(S1):457.

81. Reif S, Brolin MF, Stewart MT, et al. The Washington State Hub and Spoke Model to increase access to medication treatment for opioid use disorders. J Subst Abuse Treat 2020;108:33–9.

82. Hunter RM, Davie C, Rudd A, et al. Impact on clinical and cost outcomes of a centralized approach to acute stroke care in london: a comparative effectiveness before and after model. PLoS One 2013; 8(8):e70420.

83. Donovan LM, Shah A, Chai-Coetzer CL, et al. Redesigning care for obstructive sleep apnea. Chest 2019. https://doi.org/10.1016/j.chest.2019.10.002. S0012369219340243.

84. Watson NF, Rosen IM, Chervin RD. The past is prologue: the future of sleep medicine. J Clin Sleep Med 2017;13(01):127–35.

85. Epton MJ, Kelly PT, Shand BI, et al. Development and outcomes of a primary care-based sleep assessment service in Canterbury, New Zealand. NPJ Prim Care Respir Med 2017;27(1):26.

86. Parsons EC, Mattox EA, Beste LA, et al. Development of a sleep telementorship program for rural Department of Veterans Affairs primary care providers: sleep Veterans Affairs extension for community healthcare outcomes. Ann Am Thorac Soc 2017;14(2):267–74.

87. Kushida CA, Nichols DA, Holmes TH, et al. SMART DOCS: a new patient-centered outcomes and coordinated-care management approach for the future practice of sleep medicine. Sleep 2015;38(2):315–26.

88. Parthasarathy S, Wendel C, Haynes PL, et al. A pilot study of CPAP adherence promotion by peer buddies with sleep apnea. J Clin Sleep Med 2013;9(6):543–50.

89. Redline S, Baker-Goodwin S, Bakker JP, et al. Patient partnerships transforming sleep medicine research and clinical care: perspectives from the sleep apnea patient-centered outcomes network. J Clin Sleep Med 2020;12(7):1053–8.

90. Hwang D. Monitoring progress and adherence with positive airway pressure therapy for obstructive sleep apnea. Sleep Med Clin 2016;11:161–71.

91. Shelgikar AV, Durmer JS, Joynt KE, et al. Multidisciplinary sleep centers: strategies to improve care of sleep disorders patients. J Clin Sleep Med 2014; 10(06):693–7.

92. Sweetman A, Lack L, Catcheside PG, et al. Cognitive and behavioral therapy for insomnia increases the use of continuous positive airway pressure therapy in obstructive sleep apnea participants with comorbid insomnia: a randomized clinical trial. Sleep 2019;42(12):zsz178.

93. Camacho M, Ryhn MJ, Fukui CS, et al. Multidisciplinary sleep clinic: a patient-centered approach. Cranio 2017;35(2):129.

94. Colaco B, Herold D, Johnson M, et al. Analyses of the complexity of patients undergoing attended polysomnography in the era of home sleep apnea tests. J Clin Sleep Med 2018;14(04):631–9.

95. Mindell JA, Bartle A, Wahab NA, et al. Sleep education in medical school curriculum: a glimpse across countries. Sleep Med 2011;12(9): 928–31.

96. Papp KK, Penrod CE, Strohl KP. Knowledge and attitudes of primary care physicians toward sleep and sleep disorders. Sleep Breath 2002;6(3): 103–9.

97. Hayes SM, Murray S, Castriotta RJ, et al. (Mis)perceptions and interactions of sleep specialists and generalists: obstacles to referrals to sleep specialists and the multidisciplinary team management of sleep disorders. J Clin Sleep Med 2012;8(6): 633–42.

98. Chung SA, Hussain MRG, Shapiro CM, et al. Knowledge of sleep apnea in a sample grouping of primary care physicians. Sleep Breath 2001; 5(3):115–21.

99. Ozoh OB, Iwuala SO, Desalu OO, et al. An assessment of the knowledge and attitudes of graduating medical students in Lagos, Nigeria, regarding obstructive sleep apnea. Ann Am Thorac Soc 2015;12(9):1358–63.

100. Ozoh OB, Ojo OO, Iwuala SO, et al. Is the knowledge and attitude of physicians in Nigeria adequate for the diagnosis and management of obstructive sleep apnea? Sleep Breath 2017; 21(2):521–7.

101. Cherrez Ojeda I, Jeffe DB, Guerrero T, et al. Attitudes and knowledge about obstructive sleep apnea among Latin American primary care physicians. Sleep Med 2013;14(10):973–7.

102. Chérrez-Ojeda I, Calderón JC, Fernández García A, et al. Obstructive sleep apnea knowledge and attitudes among recent medical graduates training in Ecuador. Multidiscip Respir Med 2018;13(1):5.

103. Chang J-WR, Akemokwe FM, Marangu DM, et al. Obstructive sleep apnea awareness among primary care physicians in Africa. Ann Am Thorac Soc 2020;17(1):98–106.

104. Showalter L, O'Keefe C. Implementation of an obstructive sleep apnea screening tool with hypertensive patients in the primary care clinic. J Am Assoc Nurse Pract 2019;31(3):184–8.

105. Ononye T, Nguyen K, Brewer E. Implementing protocol for obstructive sleep apnea screening in the primary care setting. Appl Nurs Res 2019;46: 67–71.

106. Bakhai SY, Nigam M, Saeed M, et al. Improving OSA screening and diagnosis in patients with hypertension in an academic safety net primary care clinic: quality improvement project. BMJ Open Qual 2017;6:1–7.

107. Strollo PJ, Badr MS, Coppola MP, et al. The future of sleep medicine. Sleep 2011. https://doi.org/10.5665/sleep.1410.

108. Badr MS. The future is here. J Clin Sleep Med 2013;09(09):841–3.

109. Sweetman AM, Lack LC, Catcheside PG, et al. Developing a successful treatment for co-morbid insomnia and sleep apnoea. Sleep Med Rev 2017;33:28–38.

110. Pendharkar SR, Blades KG, Kelly JE, et al. Perspectives on primary care management of obstructive sleep apnea: a qualitative study of patients and healthcare providers. J Clin Sleep Med 2020. https://doi.org/10.5664/jcsm.8814.

111. Cross NE, Harrison CM, Yee BJ, et al. Management of snoring and sleep apnea in Australian primary care: the BEACH study (2000-2014). J Clin Sleep Med 2016;12(8):1167–73.

112. Nadal N, de Batlle J, Barbé F, et al. Predictors of CPAP compliance in different clinical settings: primary care versus sleep unit. Sleep Breath 2018; 22(1):157–63.

113. Ye L, Pien GW, Ratcliffe SJ, et al. The different clinical faces of obstructive sleep apnoea: a cluster analysis. Eur Respir J 2014;44(6):1600–7.

114. Gagnadoux F, Le Vaillant M, Paris A, et al. Relationship between OSA clinical phenotypes and CPAP treatment outcomes. Chest 2016;149(1):288–90.

115. Mayos M, Peñacoba P, Pijoan AMP, et al. Coordinated program between primary care and sleep unit for the management of obstructive

sleep apnea. Npj Prim Care Respir Med 2019; 29(1):39.

116. Aurora RN, Collop NA, Jacobowitz O, et al. Quality measures for the care of adult patients with obstructive sleep apnea. J Clin Sleep Med 2015; 11(3):357–83.

117. Liang A, Santana MJ, Perry S, et al. A survey of quality measurement in Canadian sleep centers. Can J Respir Crit Care Sleep Med 2020;1–7. https://doi.org/10.1080/24745332.2019.1699478.

118. Pepin J-L, Baillieul S, Tamisier R. Reshaping sleep apnea care: time for value-based strategies. Ann Am Thorac Soc 2019;16(12):1501–3.

The Impact of Device Modifications and Pressure Delivery on Adherence

Roo Killick, MBBS, FRACP, PhD[a], Nathaniel S. Marshall, PhD[a,b],*

KEYWORDS

• CPAP • Humidification • APAP • Expiratory pressure relief • Bilevel • C-Flex • Ramp • OSA

KEY POINTS

• No positive airway pressure (PAP) device modification has been shown by robust evidence to improve objective adherence to therapy meaningfully.
• A small increase in adherence has been seen using automatically titrating PAP over fixed-pressure continuous PAP, but whether this is clinically significant is doubtful.
• The decision to purchase a device with any of these optional modifications may come down to patient choice and cost.

INTRODUCTION

Obstructive sleep apnea (OSA) is a chronic condition affecting at least 24% of middle-aged men and 9% of women,[1] with some more reports suggesting the prevalence is higher still.[2,3] Repetitive upper airway obstruction occurs during sleep, leading to sleep fragmentation and several associated comorbidities, including daytime sleepiness, increased mortality, cardiovascular disease, and possibly cancer morbidity.[4,5] It is a major global health burden, and, with obesity a major risk factor for OSA and as globally obesity rates increase, prevalence of OSA is certain to increase accordingly. Finding a tolerable effective therapy for patients, therefore, is critical.

Continuous positive airway pressure (CPAP) is the gold standard treatment of moderate to severe OSA syndrome. When used regularly, it is an effective treatment; however, adherence, as with many medical interventions, often is limited due to various factors, both physical and psychological.[6,7] Acceptable adherence of therapy often is described in the research literature with an arbitrary cutoff of 4 h/night usage, which is far from

optimal considering normal sleep duration is considered 7 h/night to 8 h/night; however, this also is reflective of how many individuals find the therapy hard to use. Whether therapy is going to be tolerated often is determined within the first few days on treatment.[6] From a clinician's perspective, it is important that the patient is monitored closely after starting PAP and, if appropriate, adjustments to therapy are made, prior to the patient potentially abandoning PAP and being lost to follow-up.

Since the initial development of CPAP in Sydney in 1981,[8] there have been a variety of engineering modifications made to the initial rather cumbersome apparatus, with the aim of ameliorating patient comfort and, therefore, increasing adherence to therapy. This review provides an overview of the various PAP device modifications that are widely accessible globally to patients and discusses the evidence that exists regarding their use. With the advance of engineering and software associated with device production in recent years, there now are many extra options for patients to choose between prior to purchasing a device, some in

a Woolcock Institute of Medical Research, The University of Sydney, 431 Glebe Pt Road, Glebe, Sydney, New South Wales 2037, Australia; b Faculty of Medicine and Health, The University of Sydney, Sydney, New South Wales, Australia
* Corresponding author.
E-mail address: nathaniel.marshall@sydney.edu.au

Sleep Med Clin 16 (2021) 75–84
https://doi.org/10.1016/j.jsmc.2020.10.008
1556-407X/21/© 2020 Elsevier Inc. All rights reserved.

conjunction with their prescribing sleep physician; but, more often than not, these can become a personal choice at the time of purchasing. It can prove to be a confusing and overwhelming consumer experience for individuals; hence, it is important to review the evidence examining whether these modifications are worthwhile and whether they provide subjective and/or objective improvements in symptoms and outcomes to justify the extra cost to the patient. The authors are indebted to the investigators of a recent Cochrane systematic review and meta-analysis on this exact topic (search date up to October 2018), which pooled 64 studies of 3922 adults with OSA and have based this review substantially on their robust work.[9]

CONTINUOUS POSITIVE AIRWAY PRESSURE—THE BASICS

CPAP therapy essentially delivers pressurized air through a closed circuit to a patient to prevent airway collapse and maintain a patent airway during sleep.[8] The circuit consists of an electrical pump and a hose, which connect to a mask on the patient's face. The face masks are used most often either as a nasal mask covering the nose only or a full-face mask covering nose and mouth. Many different options of masks exist, however, and mask selection is a critical point in establishing an early successful relationship between the patient and the PAP device.[10] Nasal pillow masks are popular with patients and have been shown to be as effective as full nasal masks in terms of adherence, pressure delivery, and other outcomes.[11]

A majority of side effects experienced by patients relate to the level of pressure being delivered to the airway. Minimizing the pressure required tends to alleviate many of these symptoms and improve adherence. PAP can cause nasal dryness and stuffiness. Nasal obstruction often results in higher PAP pressures being required, hence making sure nasal patency is as optimum as possible is important to minimizing the pressure delivered. Pressurized air can be very dry and also is dependent on the ambient temperature and humidity of the environment. Dryness can be alleviated by humidifying the air delivered, to enhance the humidifying natural function of the nose. This is achieved by a separate water heater chamber within the PAP machine and can be controlled by the patient.[12,13]

Despite all efforts, at least 1 analysis has shown that CPAP adherence reported in clinical research does not seem to have improved in the past 20 years.[14]

CONTINUOUS POSITIVE AIRWAY PRESSURE ADHERENCE—FACTORS TO CONSIDER

The commonsense assumption behind all device modifications to PAP is that less pressure equals greater patient comfort, which in turn produces greater adherence with therapy. Case series describing patients' experiences with CPAP sometimes have reported that patients who have been prescribed high pressures often have problems with adherence and there is a correlation between pressure and adherence.[15,16] The problem with this generally sensible idea and everyday observation is that in the authors' analysis of 3 clinical trials where patients received both real CPAP and sham CPAP (with close to zero pressure), there was a strong correlation (r = 0.73) between adherence with real CPAP and adherence with sham CPAP.[17] The average amount of use of CPAP per night in intention-to-treat analyses in those trials combined was 4.3 h/night compared with the use of sham per night of 3.6 h/night. Because of these effects, there naturally is a correlation between adherence with sham CPAP and the prescribed pressure on the unrelated CPAP arm (reported in 1 trial as r = 0.42[18] [**Fig. 1**]), indicating that there is something about patients who require higher pressure that explains some of their CPAP adherence (**Fig. 2**).[19] Patients who end up needing higher pressures to control their OSA tend to have greater problems with adherence. What the authors have learned from these rare sham CPAP crossover trials is that pressure delivered has little to do with adherence with PAP. So machines that make minor adjustments to the amount or timing of pressure of PAP should not be assumed to have major effects on adherence (see **Figs. 1** and **2**).[17,19]

The major limitation of reliance on any of the existing clinical trials when thinking about long-term routine clinical use of PAP is that all of them are relatively short term—often between 3 weeks and 12 weeks, and mostly studied patients who are therapy-naïve and commencing PAP for the first time. In clinical practice, OSA is a chronic disease and ongoing patient adherence over years rather than weeks is more clinically relevant to sleep physicians and to patients; however, these longer-term outcomes often are not recorded. The European guidelines[20] also make the point that the adherence trials have been conducted on naïve patients and not on what should perhaps be the real target population—patients who are failing to be able to use standard CPAP. Another one of the authors' clinical trials recruited subjects who had tried, but given up, CPAP therapy and, as part of the screening procedure, 27 of 74 patients

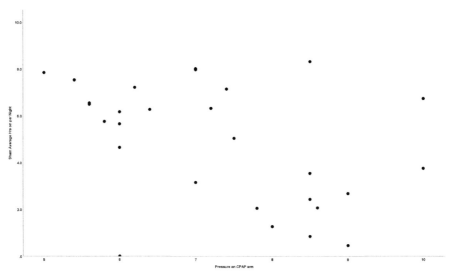

Fig. 1. Scattergram showing the negative correlation between adherence with sham CPAP in hours per night and the pressure in cm H_2O prescribed on the unrelated full-pressure CPAP arm. (*Data from* Marshall NS, Neill AM, Campbell AJ, Sheppard DS. Randomised controlled crossover trial of humidified continuous positive airway pressure in mild obstructive sleep apnoea. *Thorax.* 2005;60(5):427-432.)

screened were successfully reestablished on to CPAP therapy by the authors' clinical service.[21]

CONTINUOUS POSITIVE AIRWAY PRESSURE MODIFICATIONS

CPAP machines have a variety of functionalities added by the manufacturers to improve the patient experience. Many have now become standard

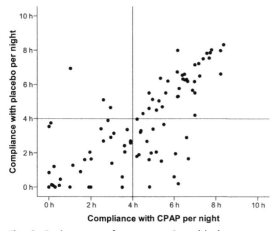

Fig. 2. Patient use of treatment is stable between a real CPAP device and a placebo version of the same device ($r^2 = 0.53$; $P<.001$). X and Y axes are in units of average hours per night of use. (*From* Crawford MR, Bartlett DJ, Coughlin SR, et al. The effect of continuous positive airway pressure usage on sleepiness in obstructive sleep apnoea: real effects or expectation of benefit? *Thorax.* 2012;67(10):920-924; with permission.)

additions to most devices (eg, ramp function and humidification) and others are manufacturer specific (eg, C-Flex [Phillips Respironics, Philadelphia, USA] or SensAwake [Fisher & Paykel, Auckland, New Zealand]). With so many brands available in the marketplace globally, with differing marketing strategies for similar features, it can be a confusing experience for patients. Despite the equivocal empiric or theoretic evidence for improving patient comfort, however, some of the choice about whether to pay extra for these modifications has now gone, because they have become built into many of the standard PAP devices on the market.

This section discusses each modification individually. A summary of the findings adapted from the Cochrane review[9] is shown in **Table 1**.

Ramp Function

The ramp function gradually increases pressure from a predetermined low pressure (usually 4 cm H_2O) up to the prescribed therapeutic pressure over a period of time (often between 5 minutes and 45 minutes) after the device is turned on. This allows the patient time to fall asleep with a lower pressure, with the aim of the patient fully asleep once the higher therapeutic pressure is delivered. Patients find this useful especially in the first few weeks of treatment as they are acclimatizing to the device. They often continue to use this feature routinely, but in many cases once acclimatized they opt to turn the function to the minimum time duration, or turn it off, so that the full therapeutic pressure is delivered as soon

Table 1
Summary of the effects of device modifications on adherence with continuous positive airway pressure as reported by the Cochrane review

Modality	Studies (no.)	Patients (no.)	Duration of Follow-up (wk)	Comparator: Fixed-Pressure Continuous Positive Airway Pressure Adherence (h/Night)	Mean Difference (h/Night) over Fixed Continuous Positive Airway Pressure (CI)	Certainty of the Evidence (Grade)
APAP	31	1452	Median: 6	5	0.21 (13 min) (0.11 longer to 0.31 longer)	Moderate
Bilevel	4	268	Range: 4–52	5.5	0.14 (8 min) (0.17 shorter to 0.45 longer)	Low
EPR using CPAP	9	609	Range: 2–24	5.1	0.14 (8 min) (0.07 shorter to 0.35 longer)	Low
Humidification using CPAP	6	277	Range: 3–12	5	0.37 (22 min) (0.1 shorter to 0.64 longer)	Low

Adapted from Kennedy B, Lasserson TJ, Wozniak DR, Smith I. Pressure modification or humidification for improving usage of continuous positive airway pressure machines in adults with obstructive sleep apnoea. Cochrane Database Syst Rev 2019;12:CD003531; with permission.

as the device is turned on. This tends to occur when patients are on higher pressures for more severe OSA. It also can be restarted by patients, for instance, if they wake during the night. As far as the authors are aware, there are no randomized trials looking at whether the ramp function improves patients sleep or their adherence with PAP. But it is used routinely in clinical practice with positive feedback from patients. Hypothetically, there could be greater residual OSA if the ramp function is utilized, in particular on a longer setting or repeatedly used during the night, and this could affect compliance and patient perception of therapy, but the authors were unable to find any research to validate this theory.

Humidification

Most PAP machines have either built-in humidification chambers or the ability to attach a separate chamber as an addition. This warms the air delivered and aims at reducing airway dryness that often is experienced. They are popular with patients, and all PAP therapists and sleep physicians have a substantial number of patients who prefer to use humidification routinely. The amount of humidification generated can be controlled by the patient, and heated hoses also are available to assist with temperature control. Humidification might work well in climates with relatively low humidity, in more temperate climates, or in societies where bedroom temperatures are lower.[22]

A recent meta-analysis of 9 studies[23] looked at outcomes, including hours of usage and subjective sleepiness by Epworth Sleepiness Scale (ESS) score, and also broke down the groups using CPAP versus Automatically titrating PAP (APAP) and those with or without upper airway symptoms prior to PAP therapy. They found that there were no improvements in any of the measures when using humidification versus not. In the recent Cochrane review, there was low-grade to very-low-grade evidence in measured outcomes in studies using heated humidification or not in fixed-pressure CPAP devices (see **Table 1**).[9] In studies reporting hours of usage, a small increase of 0.37 h/patient/night was seen across 6 studies (n = 277), with a range of follow-up of 3 weeks to 12 weeks. There was no significant change seen in symptoms scores (ESS/Functional Outcomes of Sleepiness Questionnaire [FOSQ]) or apnea/hypopnea index (AHI) (however, these outcomes were only examined in 1 study of 44 patients), and only 1 study reported patient preference[22] showing no difference. Adverse events as measured by symptoms of blocked nose were lower in the humidification group (2 randomized controlled trials [RCTs]; n = 147; odds ratio [OR] 0.32 [0.16–0.63]).

Automatically Titrating Positive Airway Pressure

One of the most studied options in device choice is whether a patient uses a fixed-pressure CPAP or an automatically titrating (APAP) device. Machines that can deliver APAP also can be switched to deliver fixed pressure; however, the reverse is not the case. Furthermore, the cost of an APAP device is significantly higher than CPAP. Often, APAP machines initially are used by sleep clinics to determine the appropriate pressure required, if an in-laboratory titration study is not performed, and then the patient can go onto purchase a fixed-pressure device in the longer term. In those areas where home APAP therapy trials are the mainstay of initiating treatment, however, arguably the additional cost of an APAP device by a sleep service may end up being cost effective if the expense of an in-laboratory attended titration polysomnogram is avoided. The HomePAP study, which compared the pathways of diagnosis and initiating therapy in the laboratory versus home settings, found 1 h/night better compliance at 3 months in those who completed a home diagnostic test followed by a 1-week APAP trial and then switched onto fixed-pressure PAP compared with those who were diagnosed and commenced on CPAP in the laboratory setting after a diagnostic and in-laboratory PAP titration studies.[24]

Consumers often associate increased cost with better outcomes and the question of whether an APAP device is better therapy probably is the most frequent conversation sleep physicians have with their patients concerning decisions pertaining to cost. The Cochrane review[9] examined 36 studies involving 2135 participants, looking specifically at APAP versus CPAP. It concluded that APAP increased therapy usage overall on average by only 13 minutes per night (CPAP, 5 hours, vs APAP, 5 hours and 13 minutes; 31 RCTs; n = 1452) after 6 weeks' duration (see **Table 1**), with a modest improvement in ESS (<0.5 points). There was a significant improvement in ESS in both types of therapy, however, so this difference unlikely is of clinical relevance. The proportion of participants who withdrew from therapy in the APAP arm of studies was not significantly superior (CPAP 11% vs APAP 10%; OR 0.90 [0.64–1.27]; 13 RCTs; n = 1275). Only 2 studies examined whether APAP increased the proportion of patients using therapy for greater than 4 h/night, and this was not enough to be conclusive, although a weak positive trend existed (CPAP 60.1% vs APAP 63.6%; OR 1.16 [0.75–1.81]; 2 RCTs, n = 346). Quality of life measured by FOSQ was similar between therapies (although only measured in 3 studies; n = 352).

Two older meta-analyses published in 2012[25,26] also showed similar changes in adherence between APAP and CPAP (improvement in 11 min/night with APAP in 24 studies,[25] and by 14 minutes in 19 studies[26]). ESS scores improved by 0.5 points in 1 report,[25] but no significant change in the second.[26]

Looking at objective treatment outcomes, APAP pressure utilized was on average between 1 cm H_2O and 3 cm H_2O lower than CPAP, and CPAP showed a greater improvement in treated AHI compared with APAP (by 0.48 events/h; 26 studies; n = 1256).[9] One of the meta-analyses also reported that CPAP improved minimum oxygen saturation by 1.3% over APAP.[23] CPAP demonstrated a better improvement in diastolic blood pressure (by <3 mm Hg) in the Cochrane review, although with low certainty evidence (and only 2 trials reporting) but with no significant difference in systolic blood pressure (moderate certainty).[9] Fixed-pressure CPAP also has been associated with an attenuation in decline in renal function compared with APAP in a large clinical cohort of the European Sleep Apnoea Database.[27] Such variance, therefore, requires more consistent approaches to measuring physiologic outcomes, such as blood pressure, during such trials because a few studies' results can significantly influence pooled analyses.

It is difficult to argue that the 13-minute advantage is clinically significant. It might be a slight placebo effect driven by the less than optimal blinding in these studies (see Cochrane report[9]). Overall, therefore, there is no high-quality convincing evidence showing improvement in adherence or outcomes to justify recommending a significant increase in expenditure in purchasing APAP over fixed-pressure CPAP. If an individual has no cost restrictions and subjectively prefers the device, then arguably there also is no evidence of increased adverse effects using APAP over CPAP. Ultimately it comes down to patient choice.

Bilevel

Bilevel ventilation is not first-line therapy for OSA and is used predominantly in patients requiring more complex respiratory support. It essentially provides the ability to alter the inspiratory and expiratory pressures separately in addition to more complex features. The machines are significantly more expensive than CPAP/APAP devices because their functionality is more advanced. Some patients with OSA who struggle to acclimatize to CPAP, however, can be offered a trial of bilevel to see if the differing pressures applied in inspiration and expiration offer a more comfortable therapy.

The 4 trials in the Cochrane meta-analysis[9] examined adherence of bilevel versus CPAP. The investigators concluded there was insufficient evidence to show a significant difference between therapies (only 8 min/night improvement in adherence; CI, −0.17–0.45 minutes; range of follow-up

4–52 weeks; n = 268 [see **Table 1**]). A small reduction in ESS score with bilevel was seen (−0.49 points), but once again that and other symptom scores outcomes did not have enough combined data to either rule in or out a potentially clinically relevant effect.

Expiratory Pressure Relief

Patients with OSA often describe finding it difficult to breathe out against positive pressure airflow. Because pressure is not actually needed to control OSA during at least the initial phase of exhalation, the ability to drop the pressure during expiration was added to many CPAP machines, without compromising the therapeutic effect on breathing parameters[28] or work of breathing[29,30] (**Fig. 3**).[19] This has been variously branded as, for example, expiratory pressure relief (EPR; ResMed, Sydney, Australia), C-Flex, C-Flex+, A-Flex, Bi-Flex, P-Flex (Phillips Respironics, Philadelphia, USA), and SoftPAP (Löwenstein, Bad Ems, Germany), with some of these features being available in APAP and bilevel machines.

The initial (nonrandomized) study raised hopes that this might be an effective modification, reporting 1.7 h/night greater adherence on C-Flex.[31] The Cochrane review[9] found 9 randomized trials of 609 participants over 2 weeks' to 24 weeks' duration, comparing fixed-pressure CPAP with and without this feature, and ascertained it provided only a modest increase in 0.14 h/night (see **Table 1**). There were little differences in symptom or quality of life scores, with little or no difference in residual AHI

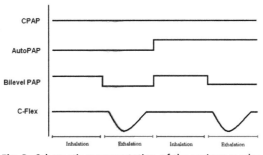

Fig. 3. Schematic representation of the various modes of pressure delivery. Pressure deviations not necessarily are to scale and the magnitude of change not necessarily is comparable between PAP types. Pressure traces indicate the direction and immediacy of pressure shift only. APAPs also can change pressure down. APAPs also tend to change pressure in response to upper airway resistance/blockage rather than strictly at the start of inhalation. (*From* Marshall NS. Positive airway pressure for obstructive sleep apnoea: systematic evaluation versus clinical and technological drift. Massey University, Sleep/Wake Research Centre, Wellington, New Zealand; 2005; with permission.)

or treatment pressure levels. This concurs with 1 of the authors' earlier meta-analyses of 10 trials showing no significant improvement in adherence with this method of delivery[32] and no change in objective measures of sleepiness, including ESS score, residual AHI, maintenance of wakefulness testing, or psychomotor vigilance testing. One study[33] looked specifically at bilevel with EPR (Bi-Flex) versus CPAP in 104 participants and found an increase in adherence of 3.7 h/night versus 2.9 h/night usage. The participants, however, were previously poorly tolerant to fixed CPAP despite standard CPAP clinical interventions. This is a patient population that requires further evaluation compared with therapy-naïve individuals.

In conclusion, although the concept sounds plausible, there is no evidence to suggest that EPR is a modification that significantly improves adherence or objective outcomes in standard CPAP therapy initiation. It is not recommended as a first-line therapy in the European guidelines,[20] although it may be worth trialing in patients who already have started CPAP but are struggling. I does not appear, however, to result in worse patient outcomes, so patients should not be concerned if their CPAP machine does or does not support the feature.

Wake-Sensing Continuous Positive Airway Pressure—SensAwake

Specific to 1 PAP manufacturer is a modification, called SensAwake, which acts to reduce CPAP pressure on detection of changes in respiration consistent with wakefulness. The device seemed to successfully reduce mean pressure applied through the night, while maintaining clinically effective control of sleep apnea in the authors' single-night trial, which was too short to have adherence data.[34] A subsequent longer crossover trial was conducted in 65 participants (with and without SensAwake activated) and found no differences in adherence after 4 weeks; however, they did report decreased amounts of leak.[35] Another recent randomized crossover trial, published too recently to be included in the Cochrane review, examined SensAwake use in patients with OSA and comorbid PTSD in 85 participants, and found improvements in adherence at 4 weeks but only after adjustment for ESS scores at baseline.[36] Another study looking at OSA and insomnia sufferers utilizing the SensAwake feature has yet to be reported and the authors look forward to seeing their results (ClincalTrials.gov registration no. NCT02721329).[37] More data are required on this modification to be able to assess its effect on adherence; however, the feature has been available and incorporated into devices for a decade and the feature can be turned on or off by patients.

CHANGE OF PRESSURE DELIVERY MODE IN THOSE WHO HAVE INITIALLY FAILED CONTINUOUS POSITIVE AIRWAY PRESSURE

Arguably, those patients who previously have failed PAP may be a subgroup who does better with some form of device modification than during their first failed attempt at therapy. Several studies have explored this further with differing protocols and results. One pilot RCT found a statistically non-significant 30 minute difference in compliance at 90 days between continuing PAP versus switching to automatically titrating bilevel therapy (n=51),[38] and in a similar sized cohort[39] (n = 66), no difference between groups was seen at 6 months either between CPAP and automatic titrating bilevel. A study of n = 204 non-compliant PAP users first were all given standard help to improve adherence, after which 24% became compliant.[33] The remaining agreeable cohort of 104 patients then were randomized to either PAP or flexible bilevel (using a modification that allows small pressure reductions in late inspiration and early expiration, marketed as Bi-Flex), and a significant improvement in the proportion who then were deemed compliant was seen at 90 days in the bilevel group (28% vs 49%, respectively; $P = .03$, and 2.9 h/night vs 3.7 h/night, respectively; $P<.05$). It can be technically difficult or impossible to blind these sorts of trials. This may cause a bias whereby patients are using the newer or more expensive favored treatment more than they would without that knowledge.

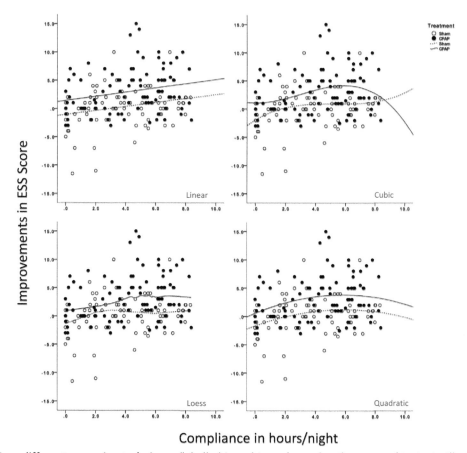

Fig. 4. Four different regression techniques (labelled in red in each quadrant) were used to try to illustrate the shape of the dose-response curve between the amount of time that CPAP is used per night and symptomatic relief as measured by the ESS. Raw data also are plotted to show how weak these correlations are and how uncertain the authors are about what the true shape of the dose-response curve (line) really is. (*From* Crawford MR, Bartlett DJ, Coughlin SR, et al. The effect of continuous positive airway pressure usage on sleepiness in obstructive sleep apnoea: real effects or expectation of benefit? *Thorax.* 2012;67(10):920-924; with permission.)

IS MARGINALLY IMPROVING CONTINUOUS POSITIVE AIRWAY PRESSURE ADHERENCE GOING TO DRIVE PATIENT-CENTERED OUTCOME IMPROVEMENTS?

The effects of improving CPAP adherence from generally suboptimal usage (for instance 2 h/night sporadic use) to a regular 6 h/night probably are genuine and have clinically meaningful benefits.[17,40,41] There is no evidence, however, that any device modification improves adherence by that much—the effects are touted as much more marginal.

But what actually happens in RCTs? For instance, the Cochrane review[9] reported that APAP increased adherence from approximately 5 h/night by approximately 13 minutes longer per night. But does that translate into a meaningful clinical effect for patient quality of life? The authors' analyses of sham-controlled trials indicate that it probably does not—particularly where adherence already is over 4 h/night to 5 h/night. This is because the effects of adherence on outcomes might not be linear but rather asymptotic.[17,40] Other groups do not necessarily find this shaped association, although because the relationship sometimes is reported as linear (more is better), and the shape can be dramatically different, depending on the outcome selected.[41] The typical shape of the effect could be different on ESS scores between patient groups and it could be different even among the various measures of quality of life. The authors' analyses of sham-controlled data indicate at least some of this dose-response shape is due to patients' knowledge that they are using the device, because sometimes there is a dose-response relationship between higher sham CPAP use and patients reported outcomes improving (**Fig. 4**).[9]

POSSIBLE NEGATIVE EFFECTS OF INCREASED CONTINUOUS POSITIVE AIRWAY PRESSURE ADHERENCE ON OBESITY

A recent hot topic in OSA treatment has been that CPAP has a recently described side effect that was not expected (although may have been reported some time ago).[42] Although there were some hopes that high CPAP adherence might drive weight loss,[43] it seems instead that high levels of adherence with CPAP cause a very small increase in weight.[44–46] In a separate analysis of sham CPAP controlled clinical trials the authors conducted, they were not able to tell whether this weight gain was fat, water, or muscle mass. They also did not find an adverse effect on lipids or glucose markers. Although the authors currently believe that this weight gain effect is real, they also think it is subtle and not clinically significant.[47] There are some plausible mechanisms for this weight gain effect, because OSA patients seem to burn more energy during normal sleeping hours than controls and treating their sleep apnea may be reducing this nocturnal energy use caused by their restless sleep.[48] How this fascinating effects plays out over the longer term certainly warrants further investigation.

SUMMARY

In conclusion, there have been a variety of device modifications available to OSA patients for several years, without robust clinical trial evidence that any of them actually improves adherence or patient outcomes, as assessed by several gold standard systematic reviews and meta-analyses.[9,25,26,32] The patients recruited in a majority of the clinical trials described within these thorough reviews had OSA in the moderate to severe categories, were treatment naïve, and were male. There is a developing clinical trial literature on those who previously failed CPAP and are being reintroduced to therapy with different equipment—arguably, this group of patients may do better with some form of device modification than on their first failed attempt. Evidence on this group of patients is worth watching for.

CLINICAL CARE POINTS

- APAP may improve adherence over fixed CPAP by a small amount (approximately 13 min/night) and produced a small improvement in ESS, but whether this is clinically meaningful is uncertain.
- Residual AHI may be better on CPAP than APAP and used on average higher pressures than APAP.
- Minimal long-term data are available for adherence with any device modifications, and longer-term studies should be planned (ie, years).
- Certain subgroups are under-represented in meta-analysis data, for instance, those who have initially failed to use CPAP.

DISCLOSURE

R. Killick has nothing to declare. N.S. Marshall previously has conducted a trial mentioned in this review, funded by Fisher & Paykel (SensAwake device). He has received in-kind support (investigational product supplied free of charge) from Respironics (now Phillips—the C-Flex modification) for another trial discussed in this review. He also has received in-kind support (investigational product) from Teva (formerly Cephalon) and Neurim for trials outside of the scope of this review, except for 1 trial supported by Teva, which is cited in this review in the context of reestablishing patients on PAP after they have abandoned it.

REFERENCES

1. Young T, Palta M, Dempsey J, et al. The occurrence of sleep-disordered breathing among middle-aged adults. N Engl J Med 1993;328(17):1230–5.
2. Heinzer R, Vat S, Marques-Vidal P, et al. Prevalence of sleep-disordered breathing in the general population: the HypnoLaus study. Lancet Respir Med 2015; 3(4):310–8.
3. Senaratna CV, Perret JL, Lodge CJ, et al. Prevalence of obstructive sleep apnea in the general population: a systematic review. Sleep Med Rev 2017;34: 70–81.
4. Young T, Finn L, Peppard PE, et al. Sleep disordered breathing and mortality: eighteen-year follow-up of the Wisconsin sleep cohort. Sleep 2008;31(8): 1071–8.
5. Marshall NS, Wong KK, Cullen SR, et al. Sleep apnea and 20-year follow-up for all-cause mortality, stroke, and cancer incidence and mortality in the busselton health study cohort. J Clin Sleep Med 2014;10(4):355–62.
6. Weaver TE, Grunstein RR. Adherence to continuous positive airway pressure therapy: the challenge to effective treatment. Proc Am Thorac Soc 2008;5(2): 173–8.
7. Cayanan EA, Bartlett DJ, Chapman JL, et al. A review of psychosocial factors and personality in the treatment of obstructive sleep apnoea. Eur Respir Rev 2019;28(152).
8. Sullivan CE, Issa FG, Berthon-Jones M, et al. Reversal of obstructive sleep apnoea by continuous positive airway pressure applied through the nares. Lancet 1981;1(8225):862–5.
9. Kennedy B, Lasserson TJ, Wozniak DR, et al. Pressure modification or humidification for improving usage of continuous positive airway pressure machines in adults with obstructive sleep apnoea. Cochrane Database Syst Rev 2019;12:CD003531.
10. Rowland S, Aiyappan V, Hennessy C, et al. Comparing the efficacy, mask leak, patient adherence, and patient preference of three different CPAP interfaces to treat moderate-severe obstructive sleep apnea. J Clin Sleep Med 2018;14(1): 101–8.
11. Lanza A, Mariani S, Sommariva M, et al. Continuous positive airway pressure treatment with nasal pillows in obstructive sleep apnea: long-term effectiveness and adherence. Sleep Med 2018;41:94–9.
12. Freedman N. Positive airway pressure treatment for obstructive sleep. In: Kryger M, Thomas Roth T, Dement WC, editors. Principles and practice of sleep medicine. 6th edition. Philadelphia: Elsevier; 2017. p. 1125–37.e6.
13. Greenberg H, Lakticova V, Scharf SM. Obstructive sleep apnea: clinical features, evaluation, and principles of management. In: Kryger M, Thomas Roth T, Dement WC, editors. Principles and practice of sleep medicine. 6th edition. Philadelphia: Elsevier; 2017. p. 1110–24.e6.
14. Rotenberg BW, Murariu D, Pang KP. Trends in CPAP adherence over twenty years of data collection: a flattened curve. J Otolaryngol Head Neck Surg 2016;45(1):43.
15. Wild MR, Engleman HM, Douglas NJ, et al. Can psychological factors help us to determine adherence to CPAP? A prospective study. Eur Respir J 2004; 24(3):461–5.
16. Shapiro GK, Shapiro CM. Factors that influence CPAP adherence: an overview. Sleep Breath 2010; 14(4):323–35.
17. Crawford MR, Bartlett DJ, Coughlin SR, et al. The effect of continuous positive airway pressure usage on sleepiness in obstructive sleep apnoea: real effects or expectation of benefit? Thorax 2012;67(10): 920–4.
18. Marshall NS, Neill AM, Campbell AJ, et al. Randomised controlled crossover trial of humidified continuous positive airway pressure in mild obstructive sleep apnoea. Thorax 2005;60(5):427–32.
19. Marshall NS. Positive airway pressure for obstructive sleep apnoea: systematic evaluation versus clinical and technological drift. Wellington (New Zealand): Massey University, Sleep/Wake Research Centre; 2005.
20. Fischer J, Dogas Z, Bassetti CL, et al. Standard procedures for adults in accredited sleep medicine centres in Europe. J Sleep Res 2012;21(4):357–68.
21. Chapman JL, Cayanan EA, Hoyos CM, et al. Does armodafinil improve driving task performance and weight loss in sleep apnea? A randomized trial. Am J Respir Crit Care Med 2018;198(7):941–50.
22. Neill AM, Wai HS, Bannan SP, et al. Humidified nasal continuous positive airway pressure in obstructive sleep apnoea. Eur Respir J 2003;22(2):258–62.
23. Zhu D, Wu M, Cao Y, et al. Heated humidification did not improve compliance of positive airway pressure and subjective daytime sleepiness in obstructive sleep apnea syndrome: a meta-analysis. PLoS One 2018;13(12):e0207994.
24. Rosen CL, Auckley D, Benca R, et al. A multisite randomized trial of portable sleep studies and positive

airway pressure autotitration versus laboratory-based polysomnography for the diagnosis and treatment of obstructive sleep apnea: the HomePAP study. Sleep 2012;35(6):757–67.

25. Ip S, D'Ambrosio C, Patel K, et al. Auto-titrating versus fixed continuous positive airway pressure for the treatment of obstructive sleep apnea: a systematic review with meta-analyses. Syst Rev 2012; 1:20.

26. Xu T, Li T, Wei D, et al. Effect of automatic versus fixed continuous positive airway pressure for the treatment of obstructive sleep apnea: an up-to-date meta-analysis. Sleep Breath 2012;16(4): 1017–26.

27. Marrone O, Cibella F, Pepin JL, et al. Fixed but not autoadjusting positive airway pressure attenuates the time-dependent decline in glomerular filtration rate in patients with OSA. Chest 2018;154(2): 326–34.

28. Canisius S, Kesper K, Jerrentrup L, et al. C-flex technology: effects on breathing parameters and inspiratory flow limitation. Respiration 2009;78(2):168–76.

29. Jerrentrup L, Canisius S, Wilhelm S, et al. Work of breathing in fixed and pressure relief continuous positive airway pressure (C-Flex): a post hoc analysis. Respiration 2017;93(1):23–31.

30. Ruhle KH, Domanski U, Happel A, et al. Analysis of expiratory pressure reduction (C-Flex method) during CPAP therapy. Pneumologie 2007;61(2):86–9.

31. Aloia MS, Stanchina M, Arnedt JT, et al. Treatment adherence and outcomes in flexible vs standard continuous positive airway pressure therapy. Chest 2005;127(6):2085–93.

32. Bakker JP, Marshall NS. Flexible pressure delivery modification of continuous positive airway pressure for obstructive sleep apnea does not improve compliance with therapy: systematic review and meta-analysis. Chest 2011;139(6):1322–30.

33. Ballard RD, Gay PC, Strollo PJ. Interventions to improve compliance in sleep apnea patients previously non-compliant with continuous positive airway pressure. J Clin Sleep Med 2007;3(7):706–12.

34. Dungan GC 2nd, Marshall NS, Hoyos CM, et al. A randomized crossover trial of the effect of a novel method of pressure control (SensAwake) in automatic continuous positive airway pressure therapy to treat sleep disordered breathing. J Clin Sleep Med 2011;7(3):261–7.

35. Bogan RK, Wells C. A randomized crossover trial of a pressure relief technology (sensawake) in continuous positive airway pressure to treat obstructive sleep apnea. Sleep Disord 2017;2017:3978073.

36. Holley A, Shaha D, Costan-Toth C, et al. A randomized, placebo-controlled trial using a novel PAP delivery platform to treat patients with OSA and comorbid PTSD. Sleep Breath 2019. https://doi.org/10.1007/s11325-019-01936-x.

37. Pepin JL, Gagnadoux F, Foote A, et al. Combination of obstructive sleep apnoea and insomnia treated by continuous positive airway pressure with the SensAwake pressure relief technology to assist sleep: a randomised cross-over trial protocol. BMJ Open 2017;7(10):e015836.

38. Powell ED, Gay PC, Ojile JM, et al. A pilot study assessing adherence to auto-bilevel following a poor initial encounter with CPAP. J Clin Sleep Med 2012; 8(1):43–7.

39. Carlucci A, Ceriana P, Mancini M, et al. Efficacy of bilevel-auto treatment in patients with obstructive sleep apnea not responsive to or intolerant of continuous positive airway pressure ventilation. J Clin Sleep Med 2015;11(9):981–5.

40. Weaver TE, Maislin G, Dinges DF, et al. Relationship between hours of CPAP use and achieving normal levels of sleepiness and daily functioning. Sleep 2007;30(6):711–9.

41. Antic NA, Catcheside P, Buchan C, et al. The effect of CPAP in normalizing daytime sleepiness, quality of life, and neurocognitive function in patients with moderate to severe OSA. Sleep 2011;34(1):111–9.

42. Redenius R, Murphy C, O'Neill E, et al. Does CPAP lead to change in BMI? J Clin Sleep Med 2008; 4(3):205–9.

43. Ong JC, Crisostomo MI. The more the merrier? Working towards multidisciplinary management of obstructive sleep apnea and comorbid insomnia. J Clin Psychol 2013;69(10):1066–77.

44. Quan SF, Budhiraja R, Clarke DP, et al. Impact of treatment with continuous positive airway pressure (CPAP) on weight in obstructive sleep apnea. J Clin Sleep Med 2013;9(10):989–93.

45. Drager LF, Brunoni AR, Jenner R, et al. Effects of CPAP on body weight in patients with obstructive sleep apnoea: a meta-analysis of randomised trials. Thorax 2015;70(3):258–64.

46. Ou Q, Chen B, Loffler KA, et al. The effects of long-term CPAP on weight change in patients with comorbid OSA and cardiovascular disease: data from the SAVE trial. Chest 2019;155(4):720–9.

47. Hoyos CM, Murugan SM, Melehan KL, et al. Dose-dependent effects of continuous positive airway pressure for sleep apnea on weight or metabolic function: individual patient-level clinical trial meta-analysis. J Sleep Res 2019;28(5):e12788.

48. Stenlof K, Grunstein R, Hedner J, et al. Energy expenditure in obstructive sleep apnea: effects of treatment with continuous positive airway pressure. Am J Phys 1996;271(6 Pt 1):E1036–43.

Using the Remote Monitoring Framework to Promote Adherence to Continuous Positive Airway Pressure

Brendan T. Keenan, MS[a], Richard J. Schwab, MD[b],*

KEYWORDS

- Continuous positive airway pressure • Treatment adherence • Telemedicine • Remote monitoring

KEY POINTS

- The ability to remotely, reliably, and objectively monitor data from positive airway pressure devices, the first-line therapy for obstructive sleep apnea, allows real-time interventions and modifications to maximize efficacy and adherence.
- Research shows telemedicine approaches incorporating remote monitoring can improve shorter-term adherence and efficiency, but results in more limited improvements in patient-reported outcomes.
- Remote monitoring should be further incorporated into other treatment enhancement techniques, including support and education, behavioral therapy, behavioral economics, and gamification, to improve scalability and, potentially, adherence and outcomes.
- Development and evaluation of interventions that can sustain and increase longer-term positive airway pressure treatment adherence and efficacy is an important next step.
- Combining data from remote monitoring in real-world patients with increasingly available clinical information in their electronic medical record would create a powerful future resource for sleep medicine practice and research.

INTRODUCTION

Obstructive sleep apnea (OSA) is a complex and common sleep disorder associated with a number of adverse outcomes,[1,2] from excessive daytime sleepiness[3,4] and reduced quality of life[5] to cardiovascular disease,[6,7] cognitive decline,[8] and cancer.[9] Thus, OSA carries a large public health burden. Fortunately, positive airway pressure (PAP) therapy, the first-line treatment for OSA, is highly efficacious at eliminating the nightly respiratory events characteristic of the disorder.[10] However, establishing and maintaining adherence to PAP therapy is a consistent concern that ultimately can limit overall treatment effectiveness.[10–12] Using the standard accepted Centers for Medicare and Medicaid Services (CMS) criteria of more than 4 hours of PAP use per night, adherence rates vary from 50% to 80% across studies.[13] A comprehensive systematic literature review of 66 clinical studies from 1994 to 2015 estimated a

[a] Biostatistics Core, Division of Sleep Medicine, Department of Medicine, University of Pennsylvania, Translational Research Laboratories, 125 South 31st Street, Suite 2100, Office 2121, Philadelphia, PA 19104, USA;
[b] Division of Sleep Medicine, Department of Medicine, University of Pennsylvania, University of Pennsylvania Medical Center, 3624 Market Street, Suite 205, Philadelphia, PA 19104, USA
* Corresponding author.
E-mail address: rschwab@pennmedicine.upenn.edu

Sleep Med Clin 16 (2021) 85–99
https://doi.org/10.1016/j.jsmc.2020.11.001
1556-407X/21/© 2020 Elsevier Inc. All rights reserved.

weighted mean nightly PAP usage of 4.46 hours per night and an adherence rate of 63.7% (based on an estimated time of 7 hours in bed per night).[14] Interestingly, despite the advancements in PAP technology over the 20-year review period and a number of attempted adherence intervention programs, nonadherence rates remained relatively consistent.[14] Thus, nonadherence persists in clinical trials including patients closely monitored for research purposes. As these trials typically include less-severe patients, generalizability to real-world patients remains in question. Toward this end, a large-scale analysis of real-world data in 2.62 million patients estimated 90-day adherence to be 74.6%, with median usage of 5.54 hours per night.[15] Although this level of adherence is more impressive, a clear limitation recognized by the authors is the lack of data on patients who were prescribed PAP and either never obtained it or never turned it on, which may represent as many as 24% of patients.[15,16] Moreover, given the heterogeneity of OSA and its outcomes, it is likely that more refined definitions of adherence are required to fully optimize therapy.

A number of techniques to improve PAP adherence have been evaluated and show promise when compared with usual care.[10–12,17–19] Approaches include clinical support and patient education, behavioral therapies (including motivational enhancement therapy, cognitive behavioral therapy [CBT], and social support), behavioral economics, and both hands-on and automated telemedicine approaches. Each of these techniques could likely be further strengthened by leveraging the ongoing technological advances of sleep medicine and PAP devices, including remote monitoring of usage, residual disease severity, and mask leak via cloud-based systems, and enhanced telemedicine.[12,20] Telemonitoring interventions, in particular, are already leveraging these remote monitoring resources. Ultimately, these data can be automatically returned to patients, closely monitored by practitioners, and combined with readily available electronic health record resources to improve patient adherence and outcomes (**Fig. 1**). Moreover, systems to effectively provide patients access to data on use and efficacy are rapidly developing.[11,12,20] The effectiveness of and opportunities for leveraging remote monitoring to promote adherence to PAP and improve patient outcomes are the focus of this review.

WHAT IS AVAILABLE THROUGH REMOTE MONITORING?

OSA clinical medicine is in the advantageous position of having the ability to remotely and reliably monitor objective adherence to the first-line therapy: PAP.[20,21] As such, real-time interventions and modifications can be applied to maximize treatment efficacy, and, ideally, improve overall adherence. As discussed in this official American Thoracic Society statement on PAP adherence tracking systems,[20] specific and reliable metrics of adherence and efficacy exist (**Box 1**), and technologies for monitoring these measures are evolving. Readily available summaries of usage derived from PAP machines include specific dates used, total and percentage of nights using PAP, and average hours per night on nights used and all nights. Importantly, these measures are more accurate and more easily obtainable than self-reported adherence and surrogates such as refills.[10] In addition to measures of adherence, measures of efficacy, including residual apnea-hypopnea index (AHI) (eg, disease severity while using the device), mask leak, and device pressure are routinely tracked. Although less standardized across devices than mask-on time, these metrics offer additional opportunity to intervene to improve treatment efficacy, particularly early in the treatment initiation process or in patients who meet acceptable adherence criteria based on usage duration.[20] Importantly, despite specific differences in the quantification, extremely high or low values of these measures likely have clinical implications. Standardizing metrics and reporting across devices would enhance the utility of these data, while also decreasing the effort required to incorporate data into the electronic health record (EHR). This integration between the EHR and PAP tracking systems, which has been accomplished by some institutions (eg, through HL7 interfacing at the University of Pennsylvania), will further improve the ability to evaluate the impact of treatment on relevant outcomes. For example, although standard practice uses a binary classification of adherent or nonadherent (eg, using CMS criteria of $\geq$4 hours per night on $\geq$70% of nights during a consecutive 30-day period during the first 90 days), data have shown that increased hours of use is associated with improved sleepiness, quality of life, and health outcomes.[22,23] Combining remotely collected data from PAP machines with outcomes in the EHR would allow enhancement of adherence definitions, ultimately improving understanding of individual differences in adherence requirements. See **Fig. 1** for an illustration of the potential interplay between remote monitoring resources and both patient-based and provider-based interventions, as well as the role of the EHR.

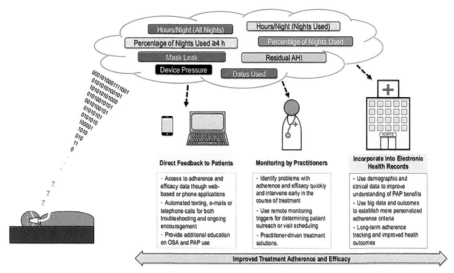

Fig. 1. Approaches for using remote PAP monitoring to improve adherence, patient care, and outcomes.

WHAT ARE THE TECHNIQUES AVAILABLE FOR IMPROVING ADHERENCE TO POSITIVE AIRWAY PRESSURE?

Numerous interventions for improving adherence rates and hours of PAP usage have been investigated, with a number showing benefits for patients.[10–12,17–19] The primary focus of this review is on telemedicine-based approaches that leverage remote monitoring capabilities of modern PAP machines.[17] We then briefly describe other approaches, including how they may be enhanced by incorporating remote monitoring technology (**Box 2**).

Telemedicine and Telemonitoring Approaches Using Remote Monitoring

The field of sleep medicine has increasingly used telehealth and telemedicine approaches to diagnose patients with OSA (via home-based sleep studies) and monitor treatment adherence and efficacy.[21] With respect to enhancing PAP adherence, telemonitoring approaches range from hands-on interventions by trained medical staff to patient-facing applications developed by companies such as ResMed and Philips Respironics that automatically deliver summaries of nightly adherence (**Table 1**).

Smaller randomized studies evaluating telemedicine approaches

A number of small, randomized studies have evaluated the benefits of telemonitoring interventions that are based on data obtained from remote monitoring.[24–28] In general, most studies show either enhanced PAP adherence in telemedicine arms, or similar adherence to usual care, but obvious cost benefits. In 2007, Stepnowsky and colleagues[24] randomized 45 patients to either standard care or telemonitored clinical care based on a clinical pathway defined by wireless tracking of PAP adherence and efficacy. In this small sample, the telemonitored group demonstrated 1.3 hours per night more PAP usage and an 18% increase in the number of nights with any PAP use, although neither reached statistical significance. The benefit of telemonitoring was confirmed by these same investigators in a larger

---

> **Box 1**
> **Variables routinely available from remote monitoring of PAP machines**
>
> Metrics of Treatment Adherence
> - Dates of usage
> - Mask-on time
> - Usage (hours per night) on days used
> - Usage (hours per night) on all days
> - Total and proportion of nights used
> - Total and proportion of nights used ≥4 hours
>
> Metrics of Treatment Efficacy
> - Residual apnea-hypopnea index
> - Mask leak measurements
>   - Average mask leak
>   - Percentiles
>   - Time with large mask leak
> - Device pressure settings

Box 2
Treatment enhancement approaches and how remote monitoring could be incorporated into designs

Technique	Description	Opportunity for Using Remote Monitoring Data
Telemedicine and telemonitoring	The delivery of health care services, where distance is a critical factor, by all health care professionals using information and communication technologies for the exchange of valid information for diagnosis, treatment, and prevention of disease and injuries, research and evaluation, and for the continuing education of health care providers, all in the interests of advancing the health of individuals and their communities.[17,21,43]	Currently using remote monitoring data on PAP adherence and efficacy to provide summary data to patients and trigger automated feedback or practitioner-initiated contact with patient. Could be further enhanced with more complex and longer-term automated interactions.
Physician support and education	Providing patients with information on OSA and PAP benefits and proper use, with different sources of delivery (eg, providing materials, nurse or physician-led clinical support, or telemedicine and Web-based education).[10–12,19]	Support and education could be further incorporated into telemedicine platforms that use remote monitoring.
Behavioral therapy	Multiple approaches focused on self-efficacy, motivating patients and improving attitudes toward therapy and adherence. Approaches include motivational enhancement therapy, cognitive behavioral therapy, and social support and encouragement.[10–12,19]	Using Web-based delivery techniques for these approaches (eg, through Web-based video content) or incorporating therapies into the automated telemonitoring responses based on remote monitoring of data may further enhance telemedicine approaches, while also increasing efficiency of behavioral therapy techniques.
Behavioral economics	The broad concept of leveraging knowledge from economics, marketing. and psychology to improve individuals' choices and health behaviors.[37]	Create different financial incentives (short/long-term, positive/negative) and lottery-based interventions based on amount of adherence captured through remote monitoring.
Gamification	Using gaming elements to motivate and engage people in nongame contexts to promote health behaviors.[38–41]	Incorporate usage data from remote monitoring among patients into supportive, collaborative, or competitive gamification techniques.

Table 1
Overview of selected telemedicine-based studies using remote monitoring

Study	Design	Sample Size	Sample Characteristics[a]	Intervention	Summary of Main Conclusions
Stepnowsky et al,[24] 2007	Randomized pilot study	N = 45	Age: 59 y BMI: 33 kg/m^2 Male: 98% ESS: 12.6 points	Telemonitored clinical care pathway with wireless tracking of PAP data	Nonsignificant, but trending increase in usage (1.3 hours per night) and adherence (18% more) in the intervention compared with standard care.
Fox et al,[26] 2012	Randomized study	N = 75	Age: 54 y BMI: 32 kg/m^2 Male: 80% ESS: 9.8 points	Telemedicine-based remote monitoring with telephone contact to resolve issues	Increased usage in intervention arm (3.18 h/d) compared with standard care (1.75 h/d), as well as 1.1 h more time spent with intervention arm over the 90-d period.
Stepnowsky et al,[25] 2013	Randomized study	N = 241	Age: 52 y BMI: 32.5 kg/m^2 Male: n/a ESS: 10.6 points	Wireless, Internet-based telemonitoring of PAP data (MyCPAP)	Significantly increased usage in the MyCPAP arm compared with usual care at 2-mo (4.1 vs 3.4 hours per night) and 4-mo (3.9 vs 3.2 hours per night) follow-up, but no difference in patient-reported outcomes.
Hardy et al,[29] 2014	Retrospective analysis	N = 15,242	Age: 53 y BMI: n/a Male: 64% ESS: n/a	Patient-facing, Web-based engagement platform (SleepMapper, Philips Respironics)	Higher adherence and hours per night of PAP usage in those with SleepMapper compared with standard care alone.

(continued on next page)

Table 1
(continued)

Study	Design	Sample Size	Sample Characteristics[a]	Intervention	Summary of Main Conclusions
Kuna et al,[34] 2015	Randomized, multi-arm study	N = 138	*Age:* 51 y *BMI:* 36.7 kg/m^2 *Male:* 61% *ESS:* 10.0 points	Web-based access to adherence data (1) with and (2) without a short-term financial incentive	Greater average daily PAP usage in the arms receiving Web-access to PAP data with (5.9 hours per night) and without (6.3 hours per night) financial incentive, compared with usual care (4.7 hours per night) No additional benefit of financial incentive and differences in patient-reported outcomes.
Hardy et al,[31] 2016	Retrospective analysis	N = 172,679	*Age:* 53 y *BMI:* n/a *Male:* 66% *ESS:* n/a	Patient-facing, web-based engagement platform (DreamMapper, Philips Respironics)	Higher adherence and hours per night of PAP usage in those with DreamMapper compared with standard care alone.
Munafo et al,[27] 2016	Randomized study	N = 122	*Age:* 51 y *BMI:* 33.2 kg/m^2 *Male:* 69% *ESS:* 10.6 points	Telehealth intervention with automated text/e-mail (U-Sleep, ResMed Corporation)	Nonsignificant trend toward increased adherence in the intervention arm compared with standard care with scheduled telephone contact. Fewer patient contacts and less labor time in the telehealth arm.
Hostler et al,[30] 2017	Randomized study	N = 61	*Age:* 43 y *BMI:* n/a *Male:* n/a *ESS:* 9.3 points	Patient-facing, web-based engagement platform (SleepMapper, Philips Respironics)	Greater percentage of nights with any use (78.0% vs 55.5%) and >4 h of use (54.0% vs 37.0%), and trend toward increase hours of use in group receiving SleepMapper compared with standard of care.

(continued on next page)

Table 1
(continued)

Study	Design	Sample Size	Sample Characteristics[a]	Intervention	Summary of Main Conclusions
Turino et al,[28] 2017	Randomized study	N = 100	*Age:* 55 y *BMI:* 35.0 kg/m² *Male:* 77% *ESS:* 9.5 points	Telemonitoring based on daily compliance and efficacy data, with contact by providers	No difference in hours of use (5.1 vs 4.9 hours per night) or patient-reported outcomes over 3 mo, but a 28% lower cost per patient in intervention compared to standard of care.
Hwang et al,[35] 2018	Randomized, multi-arm study	N = 1455[b]	*Age:* 49 y *BMI:* 34.0 kg/m² *Male:* 49% *ESS:* 9.1 points	Telemedicine interventions with (1) Web-based education (Tel-Ed), (2) PAP telemonitoring with automated feedback (Tel-TM), or (3) both (Tel-both)	Increased PAP usage in Tel-TM (4.4 h/d) and Tel-both (4.8 h/d) arms, but not the Tel-Ed (4.0 h/d), compared with usual care (3.8 h/d). Increased clinical attendance in education arm. Evidence of more sustained adherence at 1 y in group in which telemessaging was mistakenly left on.
Malhotra et al,[32] 2018	Retrospective study with propensity scores	N = 128,037	*Age:* 52 y *BMI:* n/a *Male:* n/a *ESS:* n/a	Patient-facing, Web-based engagement platform (myAir, ResMed Corporation)	Compared with AirView alone, patients also receiving active patient engagement with myAir had increased adherence (87.3% vs 70.4%) and higher nightly PAP usage (5.9 h vs 4.9 h).
Woehrle et al,[33] 2018	Retrospective study with propensity scores	N = 1000	*Age:* 56 y *BMI:* n/a *Male:* 88% *ESS:* n/a	Patient-facing, Web-based engagement platform (myAir, ResMed Corporation)	Group receiving both AirView and myAir showed increased proportion of nights with PAP usage ≥4 h (77% vs 63%), as well as higher average usage (6.2 hours per night vs 5.5 hours per night) compared with AirView alone.

(continued on next page)

Table 1
(continued)

Study	Design	Sample Size	Sample Characteristics[a]	Intervention	Summary of Main Conclusions
Pepin et al,[36] 2019	Randomized study	N = 306	*Age:* 61 y *BMI:* 31.9 kg/m² *Male:* 74% *ESS:* 9.0 points	Multimodal telemonitoring of blood pressure and activity using available devices, remote monitoring of PAP adherence and efficacy, and electronic questionnaires.	No differences in blood pressure or cardiometabolic risk factors between intervention and usual care, but improvements in PAP adherence (5.28 vs 4.75 hours per night) and patient-reported outcomes (ESS and quality of life) in the multimodal monitoring arm.

Abbreviations: BMI, body mass index; ESS, Epworth Sleepiness Scale; n/a, not available; PAP, positive airway pressure.
 [a] Average sample characteristics estimated based on summary data provided in each article, when available.
 [b] n = 556 of 1455 randomized patients received PAP therapy.

follow-up study.[25] In this study, 115 patients were randomized to usual care and 126 to wireless, Internet-based telemonitoring of continuous PAP (CPAP) data (labeled "MyCPAP"). Patients randomized to MyCPAP used their devices significantly more hours per night at both the 2-month (4.1 vs 3.4 hours per night) and 4-month (3.9 vs 3.2 hours per night) follow-up timepoints. As noted by the investigators,[25] there was an initial improvement in the telehealth arm in the first 14 days, which persisted during the course of the study. Beyond adherence, there was also evidence that patients randomized to MyPAP increased their use of the Internet to obtain information about OSA, suggesting a benefit in the ability to convey clinical education. However, although adherence to PAP was improved, no differences in patient-reported outcomes (eg, Epworth Sleepiness Scale [ESS], Sleep Apnea Quality of Life Scale, and Center for Epidemiologic Studies–Depression) were observed between the 2 groups, a recurring theme in a number of telemedicine studies.

In another small, randomized study, Fox and colleagues[26] compared patients receiving either standard care (n = 36) or telemedicine-based remote monitoring via modems (EncoreAnywhere; Philips Respironics, Murrysville, PA) with telephone contact to resolve issues (n = 39). Data in the intervention arm were reviewed by research coordinators every weekday morning (except holidays), and patients were contacted as a result of a large mask leak (>40 L/min for >30% of night), or

high residual AHI (>10 events/h) and/or pressure (90th percentile >16 cm H_2O), as well as 2 consecutive nights with less than 4 hours of use. An improvement in adherence of nearly 1.5 hours was seen in the telemonitoring arm (3.18 h/d) compared with standard care (1.75 h/d). Notably, in contrast to later studies, overall adherence in both study arms was generally low, with less than 2 hours per night usage in the control arm. As may be expected given the hands-on nature of the telemonitoring, study personnel spend more than 1 hour additional time, on average, with the telemonitoring arm (3.5 hours) than the standard care arm (2.4 hours) over the 90-day duration of the study.[26] This relatively small increase in time spent with the individual patients over the course of 3 months may be justifiable based on the improvement in average adherence. Moreover, automated telemonitoring methods could increase efficiency.

In this regard, randomized studies by Munafo and colleagues[27] and Turino and colleagues[28] emphasize the ability of automated telehealth programs to increase efficiency, although neither observed significantly improved adherence. Munafo and colleagues[27] randomized 122 patients to either standard of care with scheduled telephone contact on days 1, 7, 14, and 20 (n = 64) or a telehealth intervention with automated text/e-mail through the U-Sleep platform (ResMed Corporation, San Diego, CA) (n = 58). U-Sleep uses pre-set notification triggers to message the patient and/or provider based on remotely collected PAP adherence data, including no usage for 2 consecutive days, less than 4 hours per night for 3 nights, large leak or high AHI, or achieving Medicare criteria for adherence.[27] Overall, the telemedicine arm demonstrated trends toward improved adherence and usage, although differences were not statistically significant in this small sample and both the telemedicine and standard care arms had high adherence rates (83% and 73%, respectively). However, the telehealth arm required fewer resources, including fewer contacts with providers and less labor time (eg, total time spent attempting to contact patients, on telephone calls with patients, and at clinic visits). Thus, similar adherence was achieved more cost-effectively. Similarly, Turino and colleagues[28] conducted a small study of 100 patients with moderate-severe OSA randomized to either standard PAP management (n = 48) or telemedicine based on daily compliance and efficacy monitoring, with providers contacting patients to resolve issues in cases of high mask leak or less than 4 hours of use on 2 consecutive nights (n = 52). Overall, the study found no significant improvement in hours per night of use with telemonitoring (5.1 vs 4.9 hours per night) over 3 months, as well as no differences in patient-reported outcomes.[28] However, telemonitoring was again shown to be more cost-effective, with a 28% lower cost per patient in the telemonitoring group primarily due to lower costs related to follow-up visits, which were included in the standard care arm.

Larger-scale retrospective studies evaluating telemedicine approaches

In contrast to these smaller randomized studies, several recent large-scale, retrospective, industry-supported interrogations of patient-facing applications developed by Philips Respironics and ResMed and have suggested benefits and excellent CPAP adherence.[29–33] Although results in these large-scale databases are encouraging, there remains limited data available on patient demographics and other characteristics that may influence treatment adherence (eg, body mass index, disease severity, and symptoms), which likely biases results. Combining these large-scale, remote monitoring resources with the increasingly available clinical data from electronic medical records would help to greatly improve the causal inferences from these designs, and enhance confidence in the results.

Two white papers evaluating the Philips Respironics Web-based PAP monitoring systems, including SleepMapper[29] and, later, DreamMapper,[31] showed the benefit of interventions based on data from the cloud-based adherence monitoring system, EncoreAnywhere. First, in a large retrospective study of the EncoreAnywhere database, Hardy and colleagues[29] analyzed more than 15,000 records among patients who did (n = 7641) and did not (n = 7601) use SleepMapper. Among all patients, adherence was estimated to be 78% in the SleepMapper group, compared with only 56% in the standard care group (P < .0001), with 1.4 hours per night more average usage in the SleepMapper group. When restricting this analysis to those with available data over a full 90 days, adherence was 84% in the SleepMapper group, compared with 74% in the standard care group, with a 0.6 hour per night increase among those using SleepMapper.[29] This benefit of SleepMapper is also supported by a small study of 61 patients randomized to either SleepMapper plus standard education and follow-up versus standard of care alone.[30] In a subsequent retrospective analysis in more than 10 times as many patients (n = 172,679), Hardy and colleagues[31] similarly showed the benefit of the DreamMapper application. In particular, among all included patients, 90-day adherence was 78% in those using DreamMapper, compared with 63% among those receiving standard care. Thus, reports demonstrate the potential benefit of Web-based patient-facing applications that leverage remotely collected PAP data to improve adherence. However, there was limited ability to control for underlying covariates that may influence adherence.

In investigations using the AirView and myAir resources from the ResMed Corporation, Malhotra and colleagues[32] and Woehrle and colleagues[33] combined retrospective data with propensity score matching in an attempt to reduce bias in the nonrandomized comparisons. In a large-scale retrospective analysis, Malhotra and colleagues[32] leveraged the AirView and myAir cloud-based systems to evaluate the impact of active patient engagement technology versus usual care on PAP adherence. AirView alone was considered usual care, whereas patients who signed up for the myAir platform made up the active patient engagement cohort. Thus, both arms relied on remote monitoring of PAP adherence data, with the addition of patient engagement in the myAir arm, including messaging-related usage and efficacy, personalized messaging, and a myAir score based on usage hours, mask leak, residual AHI, and mask-on/off times.[32] Of nearly 1 million patients with available data, a 1:2 propensity score–matched cohort was created, including a total of 42,679 patients in the active patient engagement group and 85,358 in the usual care arm. Compared with usual care, patients in the active patient engagement arm demonstrated increased US Medicare adherence (87.3% vs 70.4%) and higher nightly PAP usage (5.9 hours vs 4.9 hours). Moreover, there were modest improvements in efficacy measurements, including average daily mask leak and residual AHI among those in the active patient engagement group. Although the high level of adherence is encouraging, this study also illustrates the notable limitations inherent in leveraging a large-scale data source focused only on remote monitoring of adherence. Most strikingly, although the investigators leverage propensity score matching to help reduce bias, included covariates are limited to a small number of variables available in the database, including age, device model/type, start date of PAP therapy, residual AHI on day 1, and mask leak on day 1.[32] Important clinical covariates, including sex, obesity, or disease severity at diagnosis, were unavailable, and thus may still confound the results. In addition, by relying on self-selected participant groups, those in the active patient engagement arm may have been more motivated or have increased health care education, compared with those who remained in standard care. In a similar investigation in Germany, Woehrle and colleagues[33] examined data from the ResMed Healthcare Germany database in 500 patients using telemedicine (AirView) and 500 patients using telemedicine and patient engagement (AirView and myAir). Propensity score matching was again limited to a model that included sex, age at start of therapy, first device type, first mask type, and private versus public insurance. Within this sample, the group receiving both telemedicine and patient engagement showed increased proportion of nights with PAP usage ≥ 4 hours (77% vs 63%), as well as higher average usage (6.2 hours per night vs 5.5 hours per night), and there was evidence of reduced leak in the patient engagement arm.[33]

Thus, data from these large-scale retrospective studies support high levels of adherence in real-world data and emphasize the potential utility of combining remote monitoring and technological advances. However, combining these remote monitoring resources with the increasingly available clinical data from electronic medical records would help to greatly improve causal inferences from propensity score designs, reducing bias and increasing confidence in the estimated effects. Although the results are supportive of a benefit of patient engagement in terms of adherence and efficacy, there remain a number of unaccounted for or unavailable covariates that may have influenced results.

Randomized studies evaluating multiple telemedicine approaches

In addition to the small randomized and larger-scale retrospective evaluations of telemonitoring approaches, several randomized studies have compared the benefits of multiple approaches, including telemedicine.[34–36] These interventions include the addition of a short-term financial incentive to providing Web access to adherence data,[34] comparisons of tele-education and telemonitoring alone and in combination,[35] and a multimodal telemonitoring intervention.[36]

In a 3-arm study by Kuna and colleagues,[34] patients were randomly assigned to 1 of 3 adherence-related arms: (1) usual care, (2) usual care with online access to their PAP data, or (3) usual care with online access to PAP data and a financial incentive during the first week of treatment. The Web portal was updated daily using wirelessly transmitted data from the patient's PAP machine. Participants in the Web-access arms were able to log onto the Web site at any time to view their daily mask-on time. The group also receiving a financial incentive could earn $30/d during the first week of treatment for logging onto the Web site and using their PAP for at least 4 hours in the prior day. The study observed higher average daily PAP usage in both arms receiving Web access to PAP data with (5.9 hours per night) and without (6.3 hours per night) financial incentive, compared with usual care (4.7 hours per night). Interestingly, there was no difference between the 2 arms receiving Web access, suggesting that a 1-week financial incentive does not further improve adherence beyond providing patients access to their remotely collected adherence data. Similar differences were observed across the entire 3-month follow-up period, although average hours per night decreased at similar rates in all groups, to an average of 4.8 and 5.0 hours per night in the groups with and without financial incentive, respectively, and 3.8 hours per night in the usual care group at 3 months. In addition to improved adherence among the study arms receiving Web access, there was some evidence of improved adherence among those with more logins to the Web portal (based on number of times patients completed a PAP survey). Despite the improvement in PAP adherence, Kuna and colleagues[34] observed no statistically significant differences in Functional Outcomes of Sleep Questionnaire-10, ESS, or 12-item Short Form Health Survey (SF-12) among study arms. Thus, the question of the clinical benefit of increased PAP adherence remains. Nonetheless, these data support the beneficial effect of leveraging remote monitoring capabilities of

PAP machines, combined with platforms to allow patients to visualize data, for enhancing adherence. Although this benefit was maintained over the 3-month course of the study, adherence steadily declined in all groups. Thus, additional interventions are required to maintain longer-term PAP adherence.

A study providing some insight into potential longer-term effects was a randomized study to evaluate the benefit of telemedicine approaches to enhance PAP adherence by Hwang and colleagues.[35] The study compared 4 management arms: (1) usual care alone, (2) usual care plus telemedicine Web-based education (Tel-Ed), (3) usual care plus PAP telemonitoring with automated feedback messaging based on usage data (Tel-TM), and (4) usual care plus both telemedicine-based interventions (Tel-both). Telemonitoring was performed using remote upload of PAP data through the U-sleep platform (ResMed Corporation). At the primary 90-day endpoint, data supported significant increases in average PAP usage within both the Tel-TM (4.4 h/d) and Tel-both (4.8 h/d) arms, but not the Tel-Ed (4.0 h/d), when compared with usual care (3.8 h/d). There was also evidence of increased proportion of days using PAP and higher adherence rates in the 2 telemedicine-based feedback arms. Although no effect of telemedicine-based education was observed on PAP adherence, there was increased clinical attendance in arms receiving education, suggesting some OSA-related benefit. In addition to PAP usage at 90 days, adherence trends over 1 year were evaluated.[35] As in other studies, PAP usage declined over time, albeit with some evidence of less decline within the arms receiving telemonitoring feedback. When examining more long-term adherence patterns, the investigators discovered a protocol deviation through which telemessaging had serendipitously been left on in nearly 30% of patients longer than the planned 90 days. Although those in whom messaging had been turned off returned to adherence levels seen in those not receiving telemonitoring, the group in which messaging had been mistakenly left on maintained an increased adherence rate similar to that seen in the initial 90 days. Thus, these data suggest that prolonged telemedicine interventions leveraging remote PAP monitoring data may have longer-term benefits. Importantly, automated telemonitoring has the potential for increased efficiency and scalability in these type of long-term interventions.

Finally, in a randomized trial examining the benefit of multimodal telemonitoring of patients with OSA on blood pressure (primary) and PAP compliance, symptoms and activity (secondary),

Pepin and colleagues[36] compared patients starting PAP randomized to usual care (n = 149) or multimodal telemonitoring (n = 157). The intervention arm included blood pressure and activity monitoring using wearable devices, remote monitoring of PAP adherence and efficacy, and electronic questionnaires. Automatic algorithms were used to respond to issues with PAP therapy, based on both remote monitoring and patient-reported sleepiness. Although no differences were observed in blood pressure or other cardiometabolic risk factors, improvements in PAP adherence (5.28 hours per night vs 4.75 hours per night) and patient-reported outcomes (ESS and quality of life) were observed in the multimodal monitoring arm. For exploratory patient-reported outcomes, there was evidence of substantial improvements in both arms, with larger improvements in ESS, SF-12 (physical), and Pichot fatigue scale in the telemonitoring arm ranging from 1.0 to 1.5 points. Thus, overall these data support the benefits of remote monitoring for increasing CPAP adherence and, possibly, improving patient-reported outcomes beyond usual care alone.

Other Approaches to Improving Positive Airway Pressure Adherence that Could Leverage Remote Monitoring

In addition to telemedicine-based approaches with remote monitoring, alternative approaches include clinical support and patient education, behavioral therapies (such as motivational enhancement therapy, CBT, and social support), and behavioral economics and gamification (see **Box 2**). These are briefly mentioned later in this article; we refer the reader to more in-depth reviews on these topics for additional information on these and other approaches.[10–12,17,19,37]

Education and support
Nearly all patients starting PAP therapy receive some amount of education on OSA and instruction on best practices. Different studies have evaluated both the content of OSA-related education (eg, standard or reinforced) and the delivery (eg, providing materials, nurse or physician-led clinical support, or telemedicine and Web-based education).[10–12,19] Overall, studies show a small benefit of educational interventions for increasing adherence, as well as with respect to attending clinic visits and accepting treatment.[11,19] However, these interventions are generally not sufficient for greatly improving PAP adherence, particularly compared with other approaches. As several studies have noted that telemedicine with remote monitoring approaches typically increase a

patient's Web-based activity and interaction,[25,34,35] additional studies on the benefit of incorporating educational materials into telehealth (potentially automatically triggered by observed issues with adherence or efficacy) are warranted.

Behavioral therapy

Interventions using behavioral therapy focused on motivating patients and improving attitudes toward therapy have perhaps shown the greatest impact on overall adherence.[10–12,19] In particular, a number of studies have demonstrated a benefit of motivational enhancement therapy: an approach based on motivational interviewing that aims to improve patients' attitude toward treatment and adherence through critical thought.[11] Other interventions targeting self-efficacy include CBT and social support and encouragement, both of which may rely on sharing patient experiences with PAP.[10–12] Although effective, these approaches generally rely on trained staff, and therefore increase utilization of health resources. Developing Web-based delivery techniques for these approaches (eg, through Web-based video content) or incorporating motivational enhancement therapy into the automated telemonitoring responses based on remote monitoring of data may further enhance telemedicine approaches, while also increasing efficiency of behavioral therapy techniques.

Behavioral economics and gamification

Both behavioral economics (the concept of leveraging knowledge from economics, marketing, and psychology to improve individual choices and behaviors)[37] and gamification (incorporating gaming elements to motivate and engage people in nongame contexts)[38–41] have shown promise in improving health behaviors. This broad set of techniques, which have not been systematically studied in the context of influencing PAP adherence, may represent new and novel interventions. Although the previously described study by Kuna and colleagues[34] suggested no benefit of a short-term, positive financial incentive based on remotely monitored adherence, a number of alternative approaches exist that should be evaluated.[37] With respect to gamification, a recently published study by Patel and colleagues[42] (the STEP UP Trial) used remote monitoring to compare 3 different gamification interventions (support, collaboration, and competition) with usual care with respect to increasing physical activity. Overall, the study showed a significant benefit of competitive gamification compared with all other arms, including evidence of better longer-term improvement. Whether this approach

could also work for improving PAP adherence remains to be determined. However, the quantitative and goal-oriented nature of remotely monitored adherence and efficacy data could be readily incorporated into these approaches.

FUTURE APPLICATIONS: WHAT COMES NEXT?

Although interventions leveraging remote monitoring of PAP data show promise with respect to improving adherence and increasing efficiency, a number of questions are left to be answered. Most importantly, it remains unclear (1) whether any interventions can maintain longer-term adherence, and (2) what level of increase in adherence is required to observe reproducible improvements in health and patient-reported outcomes.

A number of studies discussed in this review observed increased PAP adherence with the proposed interventions, but also described consistent and similar declines in adherence rates over time. In particular, although Kuna and colleagues[34] observed significant improvement among groups receiving Web access to their adherence data, the investigators noted relatively constant rates of decline in all groups over the 3-month intervention. Although the 2 Web-based arms demonstrated more than 6 hours per night of usage on average during the first week, compared with 4.7 hours in the usual care group, average usage in all 3 arms was less than 4 hours per night at 3 months.[34] Similarly, Hwang and colleagues[35] observed approximately 70% adherence at 90 days in arms receiving telemonitoring, compared with 53.5% among those receiving usual care. However, after 1 year, adherence rates declined to less than 60% in all groups, with the group that stopped telemonitoring at 90 days returning to the same level as controls.[35] Fortunately, this study may provide some insight into approaches to maintain longer-term adherence. Although adherence declined in all groups, a subset of patients in which telemessaging was mistakenly left on during follow-up demonstrated evidence of increased adherence at 1 year. Whether more intensive telemessaging over this period or alternative approaches geared toward engaging patients over the longer term would be beneficial is an important area of future research.

Future research using data obtained through remote monitoring would also be greatly enhanced if combined with in-depth clinical data available through electronic health records. Large-scale databases supported by industry partners such as ResMed and Philips Respironics have amassed PAP adherence data on millions of patients.

Although these data have been used to illustrate the potential benefit of patient-facing platforms (such as DreamMapper and myAir),[29–33] clinical information is limited to age, gender, and device-specific characteristics. The lack of critical information related to patient disease severity, obesity, and clinical outcomes ultimately limits the utility of these datasets. Incorporating adherence data into EHRs in a consistent and automated fashion would improve the ability of clinicians and researchers to understand individual differences in adherence and usage, evaluate the differential responses of clinical outcomes to varying levels of PAP adherence, and robustly study the benefits of PAP within real-world patient populations using causal analysis approaches, such as propensity score matching. Ultimately, knowledge gained from the combination of these 2 "big data" resources may prove to be invaluable to the future of clinical sleep medicine practice and clinical research.

SUMMARY

Remote monitoring of PAP data provides a unique opportunity for the field of sleep medicine to quickly and efficiently improve patient adherence. Studies of telemedicine approaches that respond to these PAP data show promise in increasing adherence or efficiency of care. Moreover, alternative techniques to promote PAP adherence may benefit from incorporating the remote monitoring data. Larger randomized studies incorporating multiple techniques and combining PAP adherence data with clinical information in electronic health records would greatly benefit the future of sleep medicine and clinical research. Ultimately, remote monitoring of PAP data can be used by individual patients, practitioners and care management teams, and the larger health system to enhance treatment adherence and to improve patient outcomes and care.

CLINICS CARE POINTS

- Data from remote monitoring of PAP machines includes mask-on time, hours used per night, total and proportion of nights used, residual AHI, and mask leak.
- Remote monitoring of PAP data provides a unique opportunity for the field of sleep medicine to quickly and efficiently improve patient adherence.
- Techniques for improving adherence to medical interventions include telemonitoring, support and education, behavioral therapy, behavioral economics, and gamification.

- Studies show that telemedicine and telemonitoring approaches can increase shorter-term PAP usage and improve efficiency of care.
- Results show more limited improvements in patient-reported outcomes (such as sleepiness and quality of life) with telemedicine interventions, as well as a decline in PAP adherence over time.
- Remote monitoring of PAP can benefit individual patients, practitioners, and care management teams, and should be incorporated into the larger electronic health system.

DISCLOSURE

Dr R.J. Schwab reports grant and research funding support from the National Institutes of Health, Inspire, CryOSA, and ResMed, including studies of obstructive and central sleep apnea and continuous positive airway pressure in hospitalized patients. Mr B.T. Keenan has no relevant conflicts to disclose.

REFERENCES

1. Lim DC, Pack AI. Obstructive sleep apnea: update and future. Annu Rev Med 2017;68:99–112.
2. Punjabi NM. The epidemiology of adult obstructive sleep apnea. Proc Am Thorac Soc 2008;5(2): 136–43.
3. Rakel RE. Clinical and societal consequences of obstructive sleep apnea and excessive daytime sleepiness. Postgrad Med 2009;121(1):86–95.
4. Bixler EO, Vgontzas AN, Lin HM, et al. Excessive daytime sleepiness in a general population sample: the role of sleep apnea, age, obesity, diabetes, and depression. J Clin Endocrinol Metab 2005;90(8): 4510–5.
5. Baldwin CM, Griffith KA, Nieto FJ, et al. The association of sleep-disordered breathing and sleep symptoms with quality of life in the sleep heart health study. Sleep 2001;24(1):96–105.
6. Shahar E, Whitney CW, Redline S, et al. Sleep-disordered breathing and cardiovascular disease: cross-sectional results of the sleep heart health study. Am J Respir Crit Care Med 2001;163(1):19–25.
7. Mazzotti DR, Keenan BT, Lim DC, et al. Symptom subtypes of obstructive sleep apnea predict incidence of cardiovascular outcomes. Am J Respir Crit Care Med 2019;200(4):493–506.
8. Olaithe M, Bucks RS, Hillman DR, et al. Cognitive deficits in obstructive sleep apnea: insights from a meta-review and comparison with deficits observed in COPD, insomnia, and sleep deprivation. Sleep Med Rev 2018;38:39–49.
9. Gozal D, Farre R, Nieto FJ. Obstructive sleep apnea and cancer: epidemiologic links and

theoretical biological constructs. Sleep Med Rev 2016;27:43–55.

10. Sawyer AM, Gooneratne NS, Marcus CL, et al. A systematic review of CPAP adherence across age groups: clinical and empiric insights for developing CPAP adherence interventions. Sleep Med Rev 2011;15(6):343–56.

11. Bakker JP, Weaver TE, Parthasarathy S, et al. Adherence to CPAP: what should we be aiming for, and how can we get there? Chest 2019; 155(6):1272–87.

12. Weaver TE. Novel aspects of CPAP treatment and interventions to improve CPAP adherence. J Clin Med 2019;8(12):2220.

13. Weaver TE, Grunstein RR. Adherence to continuous positive airway pressure therapy: the challenge to effective treatment. Proc Am Thorac Soc 2008;5(2): 173–8.

14. Rotenberg BW, Murariu D, Pang KP. Trends in CPAP adherence over twenty years of data collection: a flattened curve. J Otolaryngol Head Neck Surg 2016;45(1):43.

15. Cistulli PA, Armitstead J, Pepin JL, et al. Short-term CPAP adherence in obstructive sleep apnea: a big data analysis using real world data. Sleep Med 2019;59:114–6.

16. Lin HS, Zuliani G, Amjad EH, et al. Treatment compliance in patients lost to follow-up after polysomnography. Otolaryngol Head Neck Surg 2007;136(2): 236–40.

17. Pepin JL, Tamisier R, Hwang D, et al. Does remote monitoring change OSA management and CPAP adherence? Respirology 2017;22(8):1508–17.

18. Shaughnessy GF, Morgenthaler TI. The effect of patient-facing applications on positive airway pressure therapy adherence: a systematic review. J Clin Sleep Med 2019;15(5):769–77.

19. Askland K, Wright L, Wozniak DR, et al. Educational, supportive and behavioural interventions to improve usage of continuous positive airway pressure machines in adults with obstructive sleep apnoea. Cochrane Database Syst Rev 2020;4:CD007736.

20. Schwab RJ, Badr SM, Epstein LJ, et al. An official American thoracic society statement: continuous positive airway pressure adherence tracking systems. The optimal monitoring strategies and outcome measures in adults. Am J Respir Crit Care Med 2013;188(5):613–20.

21. Singh J, Badr MS, Diebert W, et al. American academy of sleep medicine (AASM) Position paper for the use of telemedicine for the diagnosis and treatment of sleep disorders. J Clin Sleep Med 2015; 11(10):1187–98.

22. Weaver TE, Maislin G, Dinges DF, et al. Relationship between hours of CPAP use and achieving normal levels of sleepiness and daily functioning. Sleep 2007;30(6):711–9.

23. Antic NA, Catcheside P, Buchan C, et al. The effect of CPAP in normalizing daytime sleepiness, quality of life, and neurocognitive function in patients with moderate to severe OSA. Sleep 2011;34(1):111–9.

24. Stepnowsky CJ, Palau JJ, Marler MR, et al. Pilot randomized trial of the effect of wireless telemonitoring on compliance and treatment efficacy in obstructive sleep apnea. J Med Internet Res 2007;9(2):e14.

25. Stepnowsky C, Edwards C, Zamora T, et al. Patient perspective on use of an interactive website for sleep apnea. Int J Telemed Appl 2013;2013:239382.

26. Fox N, Hirsch-Allen AJ, Goodfellow E, et al. The impact of a telemedicine monitoring system on positive airway pressure adherence in patients with obstructive sleep apnea: a randomized controlled trial. Sleep 2012;35(4):477–81.

27. Munafo D, Hevener W, Crocker M, et al. A telehealth program for CPAP adherence reduces labor and yields similar adherence and efficacy when compared to standard of care. Sleep Breath 2016; 20(2):777–85.

28. Turino C, de Batlle J, Woehrle H, et al. Management of continuous positive airway pressure treatment compliance using telemonitoring in obstructive sleep apnoea. Eur Respir J 2017;49(2):1601128.

29. Hardy W, Powers J, Jasko JG, et al. SleepMapper: a mobile application and website to engage sleep apnea patients in PAP therapy and improve adherence to treatment. Philips Respironics 2014. Available at: http://cdn.sleepreviewmag.com/sleeprev/2014/06/SleepMapper-Adherence-White-Paper.pdf. Accessed June 22, 2020.

30. Hostler JM, Sheikh KL, Andrada TF, et al. A mobile, web-based system can improve positive airway pressure adherence. J Sleep Res 2017;26(2): 139–46.

31. Hardy W, Powers J, Jasko JG, et al. A mobile application and website to engage sleep apnea patients in PAP therapy and improve adherence to treatment. Philips Respironics 2016. Available at: http://alliednlassets.s3.amazonaws.com/rt-mrkt/phlprp-dm-1611/PR_DreamMapperWhitePaperV2-Final.pdf. Accessed June 22, 2020.

32. Malhotra A, Crocker ME, Willes L, et al. Patient engagement using new technology to improve adherence to positive airway pressure therapy: a retrospective analysis. Chest 2018;153(4):843–50.

33. Woehrle H, Arzt M, Graml A, et al. Effect of a patient engagement tool on positive airway pressure adherence: analysis of a German healthcare provider database. Sleep Med 2018;41:20–6.

34. Kuna ST, Shuttleworth D, Chi L, et al. Web-based access to positive airway pressure usage with or without an initial financial incentive improves treatment use in patients with obstructive sleep apnea. Sleep 2015;38(8):1229–36.

35. Hwang D, Chang JW, Benjafield AV, et al. Effect of telemedicine education and telemonitoring on continuous positive airway pressure adherence. the tele-OSA randomized trial. Am J Respir Crit Care Med 2018;197(1):117–26.

36. Pepin JL, Jullian-Desayes I, Sapene M, et al. Multi-modal Remote monitoring of high cardiovascular risk patients with OSA initiating CPAP: a randomized trial. Chest 2019;155(4):730–9.

37. Stevens J. Behavioral economics strategies for promoting adherence to sleep interventions. Sleep Med Rev 2015;23:20–7.

38. King D, Greaves F, Exeter C, et al. 'Gamification': influencing health behaviours with games. J R Soc Med 2013;106(3):76–8.

39. Edwards EA, Lumsden J, Rivas C, et al. Gamification for health promotion: systematic review of behaviour change techniques in smartphone apps. BMJ open 2016;6(10):e012447.

40. Kawachi I. It's all in the game-the uses of gamification to motivate behavior change. JAMA Intern Med 2017;177(11):1593–4.

41. Sardi L, Idri A, Fernandez-Aleman JL. A systematic review of gamification in e-Health. J Biomed Inform 2017;71:31–48.

42. Patel MS, Small DS, Harrison JD, et al. Effectiveness of behaviorally designed gamification interventions with social incentives for increasing physical activity among overweight and obese adults across the United States: the STEP UP randomized clinical trial. JAMA Intern Med 2019;179:1–9.

43. WHO. Telemedicine: opportunities and developments in Member States: report on the second global survey on eHealth 2009. 2010. Available at: https://www.who.int/goe/publications/goe_telemedicine_2010.pdf.

Summary and Update on Behavioral Interventions for Improving Adherence with Positive Airway Pressure Treatment in Adults

Angela L. D'Rozario, PhD[a,b,c,]*, Yael Galgut, PGDip (ProfPsych)[b],
Megan R. Crawford, PhD[d], Delwyn J. Bartlett, PhD[b,c]

KEYWORDS

- Adherence • Compliance • Obstructive sleep apnea • Behavioral interventions • Psychoeducation
- Psychosocial factors • Cognitive behavioral therapy • Sleep-disordered breathing

KEY POINTS

- Despite initial uptake and adherence to positive airway pressure (PAP) treatment, ongoing use is generally not maintained by 3 to 6 months.
- Continued support (phone calls, booster sessions) are recommended for improved adherence outcomes. Positive messages around PAP that are repeated frequently and ease of access to health professionals are crucial.
- Approaches to identify the characteristics of those most at risk of nonadherence should be explored at the time of obstructive sleep apnea diagnosis and again at 1 to 2 weeks after initiating treatment.
- Individualized and tailored interventions can optimize adherence. The patient's perspective, feelings heard and concerns met, is an important consideration.

BACKGROUND

Prevalence and Burden of Obstructive Sleep Apnea

Obstructive sleep apnea (OSA) is a prevalent sleep disorder characterized by chronic fragmentation, and intermittent hypoxia resulting in considerable comorbidity and mortality.[1] Recent research estimated 1 billion men and women aged 30 to 69 years had OSA with and without symptoms, and in some countries there is a prevalence of up to 50%.[2] OSA is also prevalent in older adults,[3] with a burgeoning cost to health care systems.[4] Untreated OSA in older adults was associated with increased utilization of primary care visits and hospital admissions, occurring 5 to 10 years before the diagnosis of OSA.[4] With a rapidly aging population,[5] it is crucial to screen earlier for OSA and optimize current treatment approaches.[6]

[a] School of Psychology, Faculty of Science, Brain and Mind Centre and Charles Perkins Centre, The University of Sydney, Level 2, Building D17, Johns Hopkins Drive, Camperdown, New South Wales 2050, Australia; [b] Sleep and Circadian Research Group, Woolcock Institute of Medical Research, The University of Sydney, PO Box M77, Missenden Road, Camperdown, Sydney, New South Wales 2050, Australia; [c] Sydney Medical School, The University of Sydney; [d] The University of Strathclyde, Graham Hills Building, 50 George Street, Glasgow G1 1QE, UK

* Corresponding author. Sleep and Circadian Research Group, Woolcock Institute of Medical Research, The University of Sydney, PO Box M77, Missenden Road, New South Wales 2050, Australia.
E-mail address: angela.drozario@sydney.edu.au

Sleep Med Clin 16 (2021) 101–124
https://doi.org/10.1016/j.jsmc.2020.10.006
1556-407X/21/© 2020 Elsevier Inc. All rights reserved.

Effects of Positive Airway Pressure Treatment

Positive airway pressure (PAP) therapy stabilizes nocturnal oxygen saturation levels, normalizes sleep architecture, improves daily functioning, and reduces physical, psychological, and neurocognitive comorbidity when used effectively.[7,8] PAP treatment potentially reduces the risk for adverse cardiovascular events.[9] However, in the large SAVE trial (Sleep Apnea Cardiovascular Endpoints),[10] the low PAP usage of 3.3 hours per night was a factor in not reducing cardiovascular disease (CVD) mortality over 3.7 years. Moreover, the patients with CVD were possibly more concerned about their cardiac diagnosis compared with their OSA, as many were asymptomatic.[11] PAP treatment must be perceived by the individual as having physical and psychological benefits. Moreover, poor adherence in large clinical trials impedes the evaluation of PAP on comorbidities.[12]

Effective PAP use can reduce accidents in the workplace and on the road and improve neurocognitive function and mood.[13–16] However, not all cognitive deficits are reversed.[17] Despite these positive effects, 1 night of not using PAP can result in the return of apneas and hypopneas and associated impairments/risks.[12]

There is wide interindividual variability in the subjective and objective response to hours of PAP use. Improved subjective and objective sleepiness[18] and quality-of-life ratings occurred with more than 5 hours of PAP per night,[13] whereas 7 hours produced the most effective improvement in symptoms.[15] Four hours or more of PAP use can improve neurocognitive function,[13] and 6 hours can normalize memory.[15] However, improving neurocognitive function with PAP may be dependent on the presence of daytime sleepiness, which in turn influences adherence.[19] Even 1 hour of PAP is better than no PAP,[20] whereas using PAP across the night, every night has potentially beneficial health outcomes.

Challenges with Positive Airway Pressure Adherence

Despite considerable technological advances to equipment, including humidifiers and the availability of quieter and more portable machines, PAP adherence continues to be low. In the first week to 6 months, the dropout rate ranges from 5% to 50%,[21] with the first 3 days being critical.[22] Adherence thresholds to PAP usage[23–25] of 4.7 hours per night or 4.0 hours on 70% of the nights used is problematic for sustaining positive health outcomes when most individuals sleep for approximately 7 hours each night.

Factors that may determine the uptake and continuation of PAP therapy include race/ethnicity, socioeconomic and income status, education level, age, obesity, gender, and smoking, as well as nasal congestion and nasal function, that is, deviated septum; however, outcomes in terms of continuation of treatment are variable despite the presence of these factors within the individual.[26–28] Treatment intervention in asymptomatic patients is particularly challenging. Patients who are minimally symptomatic have a reduced likelihood of successful PAP treatment compared with those with persistent symptoms of being sleepy.[29,30]

Challenges Around Side Effects of Using Positive Airway Pressure

Mask-related difficulties with leakages, skin soreness, and overall mask discomfort often drive discontinuation. The type of mask selected at titration affects initial acceptance. Switching to a different mask was associated with a 7.2 odds ratio of giving up PAP treatment in the first year,[31] even with a 61% resolution of physical difficulties. Women were 1.2 times more likely to change masks, which may relate to most masks being originally designed for men. Other commonly reported side effects include nasal stuffiness, a dry mouth/throat and frequent awakenings, and claustrophobia, as well as the general inconvenience of using the device and maintaining/cleaning equipment.[21,32–36]

Technological improvements, such as trialing different mask interfaces[37–39] or enhancing device capability, such as heated humidification[40,41] and flexible pressure delivery,[42,43] are continually being tested. In a meta-analysis, auto-titrating PAP resulted in an extra 13 minutes per night at approximately 6 weeks than those using fixed-pressure PAP, and heated humidification resulted in an additional 0.37 hours of PAP use.[44] Craniofacial phenotyping[45] and engineering approaches for customizing mask interfaces to fit the individual[46] appear to be important future strategies for enhancing PAP adherence.

PATIENTS' PERSPECTIVE: QUALITATIVE RESEARCH IN POSITIVE AIRWAY PRESSURE USAGE

In their guidance document on complex interventions, the Medical Research Council alluded to the importance of considering qualitative methodologies for the development and evaluation of complex treatments.[47] PAP is a complex intervention, and several qualitative methodologies have been adopted to explore the barriers and facilitators of PAP use. PAP-naïve patients do not all start from the same baseline, and the need for more consideration of their perspective and willingness to undertake this difficult treatment is backed up by numerous cross-sectional and some longitudinal qualitative investigations. Some individuals struggle using their PAP machine, which they believe identifies them as ill, odd, or not able to take care of themselves,[48–51] or they experience side effects, which have repeatedly been voiced as a barrier to continued PAP use.[48,49,52–55] Social support can help many patients increase their PAP use and includes spousal support.[48,49,52–54,56,57] However, not all spousal input is the same, and partners who are too invasive can negatively affect PAP use.[56] Regular PAP users find themselves having to use internal means, such as willpower, positive attitudes, and self-efficacy,[52,53,58] and engage in a cost-benefit evaluation.[53,57] If advantages (especially the elimination of negative consequences of OSA and witnessing improvements in functioning) outweigh the disadvantages, this can lead to engagement in the treatment. From these qualitative studies, adherence to PAP is not a 1-stop decision in which patients either adhere or not, but a dynamic process.

In a qualitative study with 61 patients prescribed PAP, Zarhin and Oksenberg[51] explored the dynamic nature and found ambivalence toward PAP in both regular users and those who rejected PAP outright/after 1 night of use. There was evidence in both groups that the behavior (use PAP vs reject PAP) is not synonymous with specific beliefs about PAP. Those who accepted it sometimes doubted its use, and those who rejected it sometimes reevaluated their decision. Even 18 months after rejecting the PAP, individuals in the nonadherent group had doubts around rejecting the treatment and queried potential benefits. In the adherence group, patients reported not being satisfied with this nonaesthetic treatment. They were ashamed of using it in front of partners or grandchildren and frustrated that it was not a cure for OSA.

Many adherers reported intermittent interruptions in use either while traveling or during the night, that is, taking the mask off in the middle of the night after waking up. Often patients report taking off the mask after a few hours of use, to be "free"[51] of the machine and finally get a "proper sleep."[57] This mask-off behavior might be driven by the cutoff information of 4 hours, in the literature as a level of optimal use, despite evidence for continued improvement beyond this cutoff.[15] This behavior is witnessed clinically, yet it is rarely investigated quantitatively. In a recent commentary,[59] it was suggested how the decision to wear PAP to bed occurs during waking hours, whereas the middle of the night is a time in which decision-making is impaired. The decision to keep the mask on after waking up in the middle of the night may be impaired by sleep inertia, heightened emotions during our circadian night, or the sleep/bed context, that is, a sleeping partner who cannot offer support. In summary, PAP use is a dynamic process, and future research (quantitative and qualitative) requires more explicit investigation.

BEHAVIORAL TREATMENT INTERVENTIONS TO INCREASE ADHERENCE

This section provides a background of behavioral treatments used to increase adherence and includes psychosocial interventions, cognitive behavioral therapy (CBT), motivational enhancement, standard care and educational programs, and combined treatments.

A review of educational, supportive, and behavioral approaches showed that most studies used more than 1 intervention to address PAP adherence.[60] In treatment-naïve patients, behavioral therapy showed the largest effect of 1.44 hours of additional PAP usage and more patients using their machine for more than 4 hours per night, compared with supportive and educational interventions.[60]

Psychosocial Interventions

The work by Bandura[61,62] on social cognitive theory created another perspective on the impact of psychosocial factors that could be applied to PAP adherence. This perspective is based on self-efficacy and how an individual can stick with and maintain a treatment when faced with considerable difficulties. Risk perception of the disorder, outcome expectancies of the treatment process, and the coping mechanisms are key components of this model.[63–65] Components of self-efficacy can be explored using the Ways of Coping questionnaire[65] and the self-efficacy measure in sleep apnea (SEMSA).[66] Self-efficacy has been assessed at numerous time points of PAP treatment[63,64,67,68]; however, it is unclear whether it changes with PAP usage or is a baseline predictor of adherence.[69–71] However, an increase of 1 point higher on the self-efficacy scale did predict 1 more hour of PAP usage in the intervention group at 6 months,[69,70] and lower self-efficacy scores indicate the need for increased support.[67,72]

Cognitive Behavioral Therapy

CBT for PAP adherence was initially a combination of components that educated patients on their disease severity and efficacy of treatment, helped set goals, and discussed realistic treatment expectations.[73] No group adherence differences were found at 1 and 4 weeks; however, by 12 weeks the intervention group used their PAP for 3.2 hours longer compared with the control group.[73] Two brief behavioral therapies (education and motivational enhancement) decreased PAP dropouts compared with standard care at 3 months.[74] A group-based CBT approach increased PAP use by 2.9 hours per night and uptake at 1 month, compared with treatment as usual (TAU).[69]

Motivational Interviewing/Enhancement

The Health Belief Model explores the cues, for example, health, partner, or health professional cues, that enable individuals to initiate and continue to use PAP despite encountering difficulties.[75] Combining motivational interviewing around healthy lifestyles (diet/exercise) to increase positive expectations associated with change, that is, of using PAP, resulted in an additional 1.5 hours per night compared with the control group at 12 months.[76]

In a 3-arm randomized controlled trial (RCT) there was no difference in the rate of decline in PAP adherence across 12 months among educational, motivational enhancement, and standard care groups but usage decreased in all groups.[77] Retrospectively stratifying patients based on adherence in the first week, motivational enhancement appeared more effective in moderate users, high users responded more to the educational intervention, and low PAP users did not show benefits. Patient profiling at this early stage to tailor the best intervention for the individual may enhance adherence.[77,78]

A brief motivational enhancement education program plus standard care increased PAP usage by 2 hours per night with a fourfold increase in adherence compared with standard care at 3 months.[79] Self-efficacy was also increased in this intervention. In a health action process, self-efficacy, outcome expectations, and risk perception all improved PAP adherence at 3 months.[80] However, unequal time exposure for both control arms of these studies highlights the ongoing difficulties around what constitutes "standard care."

A proof-of-concept trial aimed to increase PAP in previously nonadherent patients.[81] Following an educational session, if there was less than a 25% improvement in adherence, patients were randomized to either motivational enhancement treatment or self-management treatment. Both additional interventions were effective (based on >4 hours per night), highlighting effective interventions for baseline nonadherent PAP.

Standard Care and Educational Programs

Standard patient education is difficult to assess, as the specific content, evaluation and effectiveness of the programs used is often lacking.[82] Educational strategies include slide presentations, videos, and general discussions/demonstrations. Timing of PAP education pre or post titration, and personal contact often determines PAP uptake and adherence. A 4-tiered intervention strategy with reinforced sessions (additional per need) compared with standard care, increased PAP usage to >5 hours per night from 3 to 12 months. High-rate PAP users could account for this finding[83]; however, the frequency of the booster sessions is a more likely long-term factor.

An early seminal multimodal intervention compared with standard care increased adherence by 1.6 hours per night at 6 months.[84] However, this program was labor intensive and expensive. A more recent but less intensive multimodal intervention of individual education and a slide presentation in a group setting enhanced PAP usage by >1 hour per night.[85]

Telehealth and Support-Based Approaches

Telephone counseling and peer support may provide feasible, cost-effective programs to improve PAP adherence.[86] In a parallel RCT of 379 patients with OSA, 5 sessions of telephone-based coaching (15–20 minutes) increased both the proportion of adherent users and PAP usage after 4 months of treatment.[87]

In a smaller parallel RCT of 40 patients with OSA, daily phone reinforcement messages from their sleep doctor, in the first week and at 1 month increased adherence. This outcome was not sustained at 1 year.[88] After using PAP for 1 month, 146 patients with OSA were randomly assigned to a 1-hour group-based education intervention or to no education resulting in no differences in adherence.[89] Early support in the initiation process, and ongoing support appears necessary to optimize ongoing adherence to PAP.[90]

In a study of 3100 patients with OSA, an intensive support program (physicians and nurses) significantly increased PAP adherence relative to usual care (6.9 vs 5.2 hours per night) after 2 years.[91] The program reduced sleepiness, improved mood and quality of life, and lowered CVD morbidity and mortality. Partners and family accompanied the patient during the follow-up care. In another similar study (predominantly nurse-led) positive outcomes were observed on

PAP adherence at 1 year, highlighting personal contact roles.[92]

A pilot study of "peer buddies" (experienced PAP users) was introduced to promote adherence in veteran patients with OSA.[93] The peer buddies shared their experiences and coping strategies, which improved usage at 3 months. Patient satisfaction of the peer buddy system was high and correlated with adherence.

The Role of Partners in Positive Airway Pressure Adherence

The presence of a partner increases PAP usage compared with no partner,[94,95] potentially improving the bedpartner's sleep.[96] In a review approaching spousal support from a dyad framework perspective, social support (ways of coping and response to stressors) and control were significant adherence factors.[97] A small study introducing a 1-day educational program including partners did not significantly increase adherence.[98] In a CBT study, social support was a significant factor in adherence but not partner participation.[69] Being unmarried and having more variation in bedtimes (>75 minutes) was associated with more nonadherence at 1 month.[99] Overall, the role of the immediate social environment and important close relationships appear to positively impact adherence.[67]

Updated Research: Behavioral Treatment Interventions to Increase Adherence

This section extends an earlier review of behavioral interventions to improve PAP adherence.[100] It focuses on new approaches that have emerged in the last 4 years and explores their impact and practicality.

METHODS

An electronic search was conducted using Scopus, Medline, PsychInfo, and Embase databases. The search terms included ('Sleep Apnea' OR 'Obstructive Sleep Apnea') AND ('CPAP Adherence' OR 'Continuous Positive Airway Pressure' OR 'Positive Airway Pressure') AND (behavio?r* intervention* OR 'Behavi?r* Therap*' OR 'behavio?r* treatment'). The search was limited to include full-text and English-language publications between January 1, 2016, and February 8, 2020, and included only articles that outlined a behavioral intervention to increase PAP adherence. All articles were reviewed for relevance by title, abstract, and, if necessary, full text. We excluded articles if they (1) did not focus on behavioral interventions, (2) did not outline an

RCT, (3) did not include a measure of PAP adherence as an outcome, and (4) did not include adult subjects.

RESULTS

The combined search produced 128 articles of which 44 were duplicates. After filtering the selection based on the exclusion criteria, 12 articles were selected for inclusion.[101-112] We serendipitously found 2 additional papers[113,114] from searching the references as we were reviewing potential articles for inclusion in review. Fourteen articles therefore met inclusion criteria and are outlined in **Table 1**. One[108] of the 14 articles did use an RCT design and was therefore selected for inclusion; however, the investigators did not statistically compare the effects of the intervention and control groups on adherence outcomes due to not reaching the required sample size, but instead reported effect sizes.

Psychosocial Interventions

A different modeling approach (CPAP-SAVER) was introduced to increase PAP adherence in 66 patients randomized to the intervention or usual care.[110] The Theory of Planned Behavior seeks to understand how personal, social, internal, and environmental factors influence what individuals intend to do and what they do. Attitude, social pressure, anxiety, self-efficacy, or perceived personal control were key components. Within the first week of using PAP, the risks and benefits were explored, with a video, education handouts, an adherence report card, and nurse-led telephone calls. At 1-month, adherence (4 hours on 70% of nights) was not different between the groups on weekly hours 154.1 hours (intervention) versus 161 hours (control). However, positive attitude and beliefs around PAP use was significantly higher in the intervention group compared with the control group. These positive responses around PAP may positively influence adherence.

Twenty couples were randomized to a couple-oriented education, patient-only education, or usual care.[108] Although this study was designed as an RCT, the target sample size was not reached and comparisons between the interventions were not made. However, within the couple-oriented intervention, PAP use improved by 1.6 hours between 1 week and 1 month but returned to baseline levels at 3 months, again highlighting how few studies maintain initial adherence.

A total of 118 PAP patients were randomized to either a targeted intervention exploring social cognitive perceptions (TI) around OSA and PAP usage or usual care (UC).[109] TIs are theory based

Table 1
An update on behavioral interventions for improving adherence with positive airway pressure in adults

Author	Study Design 1. Type 2. Intervention Group (IG) 3. Control Group (CG) 4. Assessment Time Point(s)	Subjects	Intervention Strategy and Description	Impact on CPAP Adherence
Bakker et al. 2016[101]	1. Psychosocial intervention 2. Standard care plus motivational enhancement therapy (MET) 3. Standard care 4. 6- & 12-mo follow-up	83 patients with moderate to severe OSA and established cardiovascular disease (CVD) or at risk of CVD (IG: n = 41; CG: n = 42)	Patients in the IG received 1-h face-to-face MET sessions at baseline and week 1 by a trained psychologist. Sessions included an educational video component. Patients also received a 10–30-minute telephone call from the same psychologist at weeks 3, 4, 8, 12, 20, and 32. Key components for intervention: assessing readiness and confidence to change; discussing current knowledge of OSA and CPAP on health and patient perception, as well as setting goals and identifying rewards for adherence.	6 mo: IG's average daily CPAP use was 99 min/night higher compared with CG (4.4 ± 2.9 vs 3.3 ± 2.7 h/night, respectively, $P = .003$). 12 mo: in a subset of 52 patients (IG: n = 26, CG: n = 26) who went on to use CPAP for 12 mo, adherence was higher in the IG by 97 min/night compared with CG (4.3 ± 2.9 vs 3.2 ± 2.8 h/night, respectively, $P = .006$).

Study		Sample	Intervention	Results

Fernandes et al. 2019[113]	1. Technological intervention
	2. Two intervention arms:
	  a. IG1: Phone-call support
	  b. IG2: Telemonitoring
	3. Usual care
	4. 4-wk follow-up
		51 patients with moderate to severe OSA (IG1: n = 18; IG2: n = 12; CG: n = 21)	IG1: Patients received regular phone calls by study staff over a 4-week period in which staff assessed patients' self-reported adherence and addressed issues relating to patients' clinical status/treatment. Each call lasted approximately 7 min. The number of calls made to each patient ranged from 4 to 7 (M = 4.4) over the 4-week period with the frequency determined by the study staff's perceptions of patient needs.
			IG2: Patient CPAP devices were fitted with a telemonitoring unit, which enabled CPAP data to be collected on a daily cycle and transmitted wirelessly to a secured Web portal accessible by study staff. If low daily compliance was detected, a management CPAP protocol was activated by a respiratory therapist. This protocol was based on an algorithm to detect and correct adverse effects and reinforce CPAP compliance in a timely manner. If necessary, a provider technician performed home visits and resolved issues (eg, changing interfaces, placement of humidifier).
				4-wk: No significant differences found in mean daily CPAP use between IG1, IG2, and CG (3.9 ± 2.6 vs 5.0 ± 1.8 vs 5.1 ± 2.5 h/d, respectively, $P = .296$)

Guralnick et al. 2017[104]	1. Educational intervention 2. Brief educational video 3. Usual care 4. 30-d follow-up	212 newly diagnosed patients with OSA (IG: n = 99; CG: n = 113)	Patients watched a 4-min educational video on consequences of untreated OSA and the importance/benefits of CPAP before undertaking a polysomnogram (PSG) for OSA diagnosis and receiving CPAP within 2 wk of the PSG.	30-d: No significant differences found between IG and CG on mean daily CPAP use (3.3 ± 2.5 vs3.5 ± 2.2 h/night, $P = .44$); number of days used (18.7 ± 10.6 vs21.5 ± 9.2, $P = .045$); percentage of days used ≥4 h (44.5% ± 35.4% vs 47.1% ± 34.6%, $P = .58$) and Medicare CPAP adherence rates (32.3% vs 31.9%, $P = 1$).

(continued on next page)

Table 1
(continued)

Author	Study Design 1. Type 2. Intervention Group (IG) 3. Control Group (CG) 4. Assessment Time Point(s)	Subjects	Intervention Strategy and Description	Impact on CPAP Adherence
Hoet et al. (2017)[102]	1. Technological intervention 2. Telemonitoring 3. Usual care 4. 3-mo follow-up	46 newly diagnosed patients with OSA (IG: n = 23; CG: n = 23)	Patient CPAP devices were linked to a telemonitoring unit that transmitted patient CPAP data (eg, daily report of usage, mask leaks, CPAP pressure, and residual apnea hypopnea index) to practitioners via a Web portal. Sleep laboratory technical staff connected to this Web portal and analyzed patient data twice per week. If problems were identified (eg, air leaks >50 L/min, residual AHI >10/h, or CPAP use <3 h on 3 consecutive days) patients were called to arrange a visit with staff to resolve.	3 mo: Average CPAP compliance was significantly better for the IG compared with CG (5.7 ± 1.6 vs 4.2 ± 1.9 h/night, respectively, $P = .018$) In all, 64% of CG and 82% of IG patients were considered to be adherent (ie, using CPAP for ≥4 h/night) at 3 mo ($P = .35$). In adherent patients, longer nightly use of CPAP was observed in the IG at 3 mo compared with CG (6.2 [4–8.1] vs 5.2 [4–7.5] h/night, respectively, $P = .027$).

| Hwang et al. 2018[103] | 1. Technological intervention
2. Three intervention arms:
a. IG1: Web-based educational program
b. IG2: CPAP telemonitoring with automated patient feedback
c. IG3: included both IG1 and IG2 intervention arms
3. Usual care
4. 90-d follow-up | 556 newly diagnosed patients with OSA (IG1: n = 164; IG2: n = 125; IG3: n = 138; CG: n = 129) | IG1: E-mailed link to the OSA educational program and received an appointment reminder call 2 wk before their Home Sleep Apnea Testing (HSAT) class. The OSA program included educational videos about the pathophysiology of OSA, health-related risks of OSA, an introduction to CPAP therapy, and assessment process details. Patients diagnosed with OSA were e-mailed a link to the CPAP educational program during their 1-wk trial of CPAP. It outlined information on how to properly use CPAP, potential benefits of treatment on health and daytime vigilance, methods of acclimating, and equipment care instructions. Both educational programs were self-paced, interactive and typically lasted 15 min.
IG2: Patient CPAP devices were linked to a Web-based application (U-Sleep; ResMed Corp), which receives and interprets device data and provides automated feedback through messages via the patients preferred method (ie, text messaging, e-mail, phone call, or a combination). For example, if CPAP usage thresholds were met, a message was automatically sent to the patient providing encouragement to improve use or positively reinforcing successful adherence.
IG3: included both IG1 and IG2 components | 90 d: Average daily CPAP use was significantly higher in the IG2 and IG3 groups compared with CG (4.4 ± 2.2, and 4.8 ± 2.3 vs 3.8 ± 2.5 h/d, respectively; P = .0002 for both), but not for IG1 (4.0 ± 2.4 vs 3.8 ± 2.5 h/d, P = .10). The IG2 and IG3 groups also showed a significant increase, compared with CG, in the proportion of days that CPAP was used (76.6% and 78.3% vs 64.8%; P = .0001 and P = .0004, respectively) and in Medicare adherence rates (65.6% and 73.2% vs 53.5%; P = .003 and P = .001, respectively). No significant differences found between IG1 and CG in proportion of days that CPAP was used (68.6 vs 64.8%, P = .28) and in Medicare adherence rates (61.0 vs 53.5%, P = .07). |

(continued on next page)

Table 1
(continued)

Author	Study Design 1. Type 2. Intervention Group (IG) 3. Control Group (CG) 4. Assessment Time Point(s)	Subjects	Intervention Strategy and Description	Impact on CPAP Adherence

Luyster et al. 2019[108] [a]	1. Pilot; Psychosocial intervention
	2. Two intervention arms:
	  a. IG1: Couples-oriented education and support
	  b. IG2: Patient-only education and support
	3. Usual care
	4. 1 and 3 mo
		30 newly diagnosed patients with OSA and their partners (IG1: n = 8; IG2: n = 10; CG: n = 12)	IG1: both patient and their partner attended two 1-h face-to-face sessions and then each person independently received a 20-min follow-up telephone call 1 wk after the completion of session 2. Both sessions and telephone calls were conducted by a trained respiratory therapist.
			Session 1: delivered before PAP setup and included educational videos about OSA and PAP, a demonstration of PAP, structured conversations about common and individual PAP concerns and goal setting with support of the partner in mind. Session 2: delivered 1-wk after PAP set up and included a review of patient data with a focus on identifying barriers of PAP use and further goal setting.
			Telephone call focused on reviewing goals, overcoming barriers, and tailoring support from their partner.
			IG2: same as IG1 but partners did not participate.
				IG1: a medium increase in hours of PAP use of 1.4 h from 1 wk to 1 mo was observed (95% CI; d = 0.52), but a medium to large decrease of 1.6 h occurred from 1 mo to 3 mo (95% CI; d = −0.63). A similar pattern was observed in IG1 for percentage of days with ≥4 h with a 16% increase of PAP use from 1 wk to 1 mo (95% CI; d = 0.38), and a 10.2% decrease from 1 mo to 3 mo (95% CI; d = −0.63).
				IG2: a medium increase in hours of PAP use of 0.5 h from 1 wk to 1 mo was observed (95% CI; d = 0.50) and a medium to large decrease of 0.5 h occurred from 1 mo to 3 mo (95% CI; d = −0.63). A similar pattern was observed in IG2 for percentage of days with ≥4 h with a 15.2% increase of PAP use from 1 wk to 1 mo (95% CI; d = 0.25), and a 8.9% decrease from 1 mo to 3 mo (95% CI; d = −0.63).
				CG: a large decrease in hours of PAP use of 0.7 h was observed from 1 wk to 1 mo (95% CI; d = 0.92) and a small decrease of 0.3 h was observed 1 mo to 3 mo (95% CI; d = 0.26). A similar pattern was observed in CG for percentage of days with ≥4 h with a 10.4% decrease of PAP use

Study	Intervention	Sample	Description	Findings
Munafo et al. 2016[105]	1. Technological intervention 2. Web-based automated telehealth messaging program 3. Standard care 4. 90-d follow-up	122 newly diagnosed patients with OSA (IG: n = 58; CG: n = 64)	Patients received CPAP device plus a pamphlet about U-sleep, a Web-based application that receives CPAP data and messages patients and providers via text and e-mail on customizable set rules (ie, no CPAP data from patient received for 2 consecutive days, CPAP usage <4 h for 3 consecutive nights, median mask leak >24 L/min for 2 consecutive days, AHI >15/h for 5 consecutive days, CPAP usage met Medicare criteria for adherence). When usage falls, messages are sent to encourage patients to use CPAP more regularly and alerts are triggered to providers to further assist patients in CPAP management.	from 1 wk to 1 mo (95% CI; d = 1.38), and a 5.2% decrease from 1 mo to 3 mo (95% CI; d = −0.30). 90 d: No statistically significant differences found between IG and CG on average daily CPAP use (5.1 ± 1.9 vs 4.7 ± 2.1 h/d, respectively, $P = .24$) or percentage of days used CPAP ≥4 h (70.2 ± 26.7 vs 63.3 ± 28.5%, respectively, $P = .17$).

(continued on next page)

Table 1
(continued)

Author	Study Design 1. Type 2. Intervention Group (IG) 3. Control Group (CG) 4. Assessment Time Point(s)	Subjects	Intervention Strategy and Description	Impact on CPAP Adherence
Nilius et al. 2019[106]	1. Technological intervention 2. Telemonitoring plus support 3. Standard care 4. 6-mo follow-up	80 patients with moderate to severe OSA and who had suffered an ischemic stroke within the past 3 mo (IG: n = 40; CG: n = 40)	Patients PAP devices transmitted PAP data (eg, adherence, leakage, pressure, AHI) to an online Web portal and was evaluated by researchers weekly. If mean PAP usage time had dropped below 4 h/night over a week, the patient was contacted via telephone to resolve problems and increase motivation through negatively framed educational messages and reinforcement of their knowledge about their OSA treatment by conducting a standardized semi-structured clinical interview questionnaire. Conversations were limited to 5 min and a personal visit by the service provider was offered, if problems could not be solved online or on the telephone.	6 mo: Average CPAP daily usage was significantly better for the IG compared with CG:(4.4 ± 2.5 vs 2.1 ± 2.2 h, respectively; P = .000063). Percentage of days of CPAP used for ≥4 h was significantly better in IG compared with CG (57.3% ± 34.5% vs 27.5% ± 32.5%, respectively, P = .00025).
Pengo et al. 2018[107]	1. Educational intervention 2. IG1: received positively framed messages about CPAP IG2: received negatively framed messages about CPAP 3. Standard care 4. 6-wk follow-up	112 newly diagnosed patients with OSA (IG1: n = 36; IG2: n = 37; CG: n = 39)	Patients were read out either positively (IG1) or negatively (IG2) framed messages during their CPAP collection appointment and during 6 weekly, 2–3-min, noninteractive phone calls by a researcher. During phone calls, patients listened to the researchers' messages and any questions were directed to the clinical team. Laminated labels with the printed framed messages were also attached to their CPAP machines.	6 wk: No significant differences found between IG1, IG2, or CG for average daily CPAP use (3.5 ± 2.7 h/night vs 2.6 ± 2.2 h/night vs 3.1 ± 2.7 h/night; respectively P = .679).

| Pepin et al. 2019[114] | 1. Technological intervention
2. Multimodal telemonitoring Web-based platform
3. Usual care
4. 6-mo follow-up | 306 patients with moderate to severe OSA and at least 1 cardiovascular disease (CVD) or at elevated risk of CVD
(IG: n = 157;
CG: n = 149) | Received remote home telemonitoring equipment that recorded systolic and diastolic home self-measured blood pressure, physical activity as well as CPAP adherence, leaks, and residual events. The data were transmitted to medical staff members via secured Web sites and provided an integrated care management system. The system allocated predefined interventions to home care providers when, for example, side effects, leaks, residual sleepiness, or persistent residual events were noted by either the patient via online questionnaires or the monitoring equipment and action would be taken to resolve these issues. Physicians were in charge of the appropriate management of residual events or CPAP lack of efficacy. Additional home or sleep clinic visits were organized when required. | 6 mo: Average daily CPAP use was significantly higher in IG compared with CG (5.28 ± 2.23 vs 4.75 ± 2.50 h/d, respectively; $P = .05$). |

(continued on next page)

Table 1
(continued)

Author	Study Design 1. Type 2. Intervention Group (IG) 3. Control Group (CG) 4. Assessment Time Point(s)	Subjects	Intervention Strategy and Description	Impact on CPAP Adherence
Sawyer et al. 2019[109]	1. Pilot psychosocial intervention 2. Tailored intervention targeting social cognitive perceptions of OSA/PAP treatment 3. Usual care 4. 1-wk and 1- and 3-month follow-up	118 newly diagnosed OSA adults (IG: n = 61; CG: n = 57)	Delivered in 4 phases: (1) prediagnosis, (2) postdiagnosis using PSG, (3) immediately post-PAP titration PSG, and (4) 1-wk post home PAP use; was 30–60 minutes in duration, was guided by a protocol and scripted templates and delivered by a trained registered nurse in either face-to-face sessions or by telephone. The content addressed cognitive perceptions of the diagnosis and treatment, outcome expectancies with PAP treatment and PAP treatment self-efficacy, all domains of Social Cognitive Theory. Participant scores from the Self-efficacy Measure in Sleep Apnea (SEMSA), Epworth Sleepiness Scale, and Functional Outcomes of Sleep Questionnaire were assessed at each of the 4 phases and used to tailor the intervention for each individual. For example, if a participant scored >3.0 on a SEMSA subdomain domain (eg, risk perception), the intervention activity addressing that domain was not addressed in the intervention phase.	No significant differences found in average PAP use between IG and CG at 1 wk (6.4 ± 2.01 vs 5.8 ± 1.35 h/night, respectively, $P = .20$), 1 mo (5.1 ± 2.05 vs 5.1 ± 1.66 h/night, respectively, $P = .90$), and at 3 mo (4.8 ± 2.27 vs 4.7 ± 1.85 h/night, respectively, $P = .89$).

Shapiro 2019[110]	1. Psychosocial intervention 2. CPAP-SAVER based on Theory of Planned Behavior plus Standard Care 3. Standard Care 4. 1-wk and 1-mo follow-up	66 newly diagnosed patients with OSA (IG: n = 33; CG: n = 33)	All intervention components (unless specified) were delivered during the first week of CPAP use and were scripted. It included (1) 2 support phone calls by a registered nurse during week 1 and 2 of CPAP use focusing on social pressure and building a subjective norm to adhere to CPAP; (2) a Web-based video and educational sheet delivered and reviewed by a trained research assistant (RA) with 21+y as a respiratory therapist. This focused on OSA risks and CPAP benefits; and (3) a report card updated and reviewed with participants by the RA at week 1 and 4 containing personal data on AHI, CPAP setting use, and self-CPAP adherence grades to improve self-efficacy.	1 wk: No significant differences found between IG and CG on weekly average CPAP use (37.9 vs 34.7 h, respectively, t = −0.834, P = .408) and adherence rates (78.8 vs 72.7%, respectively, $\chi^2(1, N = 66) = 0.083$, P = .774), which adherence was defined as ≥4 h per night for 70% of the nights. 1 mo: No significant differences found between IG and CG on weekly average CPAP use (154.1 vs 161.1 h, respectively, t = 0.426, P = .672) and adherence rates (69.7 vs 75.8%, respectively, χ^2 (1, N = 66) = .08, P = .782).

(continued on next page)

Table 1
(continued)

Author	Study Design 1. Type 2. Intervention Group (IG) 3. Control Group (CG) 4. Assessment Time Point(s)	Subjects	Intervention Strategy and Description	Impact on CPAP Adherence
Sweetman et al. 2019[111]	1. Cognitive behavioral intervention 2. Cognitive behavioral therapy for insomnia (CBT-I) plus CPAP usual care 3. Usual Care 4. 6-mo follow-up	145 participants with moderate to severe OSA and comorbid insomnia (IG: n = 72; CG: n = 73)	4 consecutive weekly 45-min individual or small-group sessions of CBT-I were delivered by a psychologist before starting CPAP. CBT-I components included bed restriction therapy, sleep psychoeducation and hygiene information, cognitive therapy, and relapse prevention. Participants were provided booklets to review concepts of therapy. Standard CPAP care was delivered after completion of CBT-I, which included a laboratory CPAP titration appointment with a sleep technician and CPAP set up appointments with qualified sleep nurses/technicians, who reviewed progress at 1 wk, and 3 and 6 mo using CPAP data.	6 mo: Average nightly CPAP use was 60.7 min higher (CI = 9–113) in IG (M = 265.2 min/night, CI = 226.2–304.2) compared with CG (M = 204.5 min/night, CI = 166.3–242.7; t(158.36) = 2.30, P = .023, d = 0.38).

Turino et al. 2017[112]	1. Technological intervention 2. Telemonitoring-based strategy 3. Standard care 4. 3-mo follow-up	100 newly diagnosed patients with OSA (IG: n = 52; CG: n = 48)	Received a CPAP device equipped with mobile 2G (GSM/GPRS) technology capable of sending information to a Web database relaying daily information on CPAP adherence, CPAP pressures, mask leak and residual respiratory events. Automatic alarms for the provider were generated and then followed-up by the pulmonary specialist medical officer of the CPAP provider who contacted the patient and provided individual problem solving. For example, providing suggestions on how to minimize unwanted symptoms such as dry mouth, providing specific interventions to improve compliance issues, such as mask changing or applying saline nasal sprays; and providing support for the patient with CPAP use.	3 mo: No significant differences between IG and CG on average nightly CPAP use (5.1 ± 2.1 vs 4.9 ± 2.2 h/night, respectively, $P = .627$)

Abbreviations: ±, standard deviation; AHI, apnea hypopnea index; CG, control group; CI, confidence interval; CPAP, continuous positive airway pressure; IG, intervention group; M, mean; MET, motivational enhancement therapy; OSA, obstructive sleep apnea; PAP, positive airway pressure; RCT, randomized control trial.
[a] This study was an RCT design, but it did not report between-group comparisons in analysis.

and customized toward the patients' specific characteristics. There were 4 x timed interventions from prediagnostic polysomnography (PSG), to 1 week of using PAP. A patient response of less than 3 on the SEMSA resulted in exploring that specific identified domain in the next session.[66] At 1 week, the TI group was using PAP for 35 minutes longer than the UC group, which was not maintained at 3 months. PAP usage was high at 1 week (6.1 hours) in both groups, which dropped to 4.8 hours at 3 months, highlighting support roles.

Motivational Enhancement

Motivational Enhancement previously used in PAP studies aims at empathetically and collaboratively directing ambivalence associated with change to enable a positive outcome, such as PAP adherence. An open-label parallel-arm of 83 patients with OSA and established or at-risk patients with CVD were randomized to PAP education or PAP education plus motivational enhancement.[101] Regular appointments were offered for both groups, whereas the motivational enhancement group had 2 psychologist-led appointments with 6 phone calls over 32 weeks. At 6 months, there was an 80-minute increase in adherence in the PAP plus motivational enhancement group, whereas at 12 months adherence was 97 minutes longer; however, there was considerable dropout at this time point. The motivational enhancement intervention was effective independently of baseline sleepiness, self-efficacy, depression, and insomnia symptoms and place of recruitment.

Cognitive Behavioral Therapy

Insomnia is a prevalent comorbid disorder in patients with OSA.[115] A CBT intervention for insomnia (CBT-I) involved 145 patients who had both diagnosed OSA and insomnia.[111] In this RCT, patients underwent 4 sessions of CBT-I or TAU. All patients received standard care for PAP. Follow-up was at 1 week, and 3 and 6 months, and data were downloaded and reviewed. The CBT-I group increased their adherence by 61 minutes, along with insomnia symptoms reducing to subclinical. Higher functional beliefs and sleep efficiency of 84% at 6 months were significant. Unequal face-to-face time for the TAU group was a limitation, with no significant differences in mood, sleepiness, or fatigue.

Educational Programs

A total of 212 at-risk patients for low adherence were randomized to attend either an educational video or UC before a split-night study for an OSA diagnosis and PAP titration.[104] The 4-minute video (SAVE-CPAP) contained information about untreated OSA, benefits of using PAP and what is a sleep study. At 30 days, there were no significant group differences in hours of PAP (3.3 vs 3.5 hours per night UC). CPAP adherence was greater if patients had attended college for ≥4 years and if they responded positively to a statement about using PAP every night. Targeting "at-risk" PAP nonusers early is important, but recruitment in this group is also difficult.

Telehealth Approaches

Seven studies have assessed the utility of telemonitoring to improve PAP adherence[102,103,105,106,112–114] with varying effects.

A multicenter RCT of 306 patients with moderate to severe OSA and high cardiovascular risk evaluated the effects of a multimodal telemonitoring program to reduce blood pressure (BP) after 6 months of auto-titrating PAP treatment.[114] The telemonitoring system included home-based measures of BP and physical activity/sleep duration (actimetry) for 3 days before PAP initiation and after 6 months of treatment; quality of life and symptom questionnaires at baseline and at 6 months; with PAP adherence and side-effects data. The telemonitoring did not reduce systolic BP compared with UC at 6 months; however, PAP usage was significantly higher (5.3 vs 4.8 hours per night). Other RCTs have shown that PAP treatment alone does not reduce cardiovascular morbidity or mortality,[9,10] which may in part be explained by poor adherence. Empowering patients to be engaged in and to monitor their own PAP management using telemonitoring appears to improve adherence, quality of life, and daytime sleepiness,[114] despite the lack of effect on cardiovascular risk.

In patients with post-ischemic stroke with comorbid moderate to severe OSA, a simpler telemonitoring intervention (Infomart Web, Fisher, and Paykel Healthcare) increased at-home auto-titrating PAP usage compared with UC at 6 months (4.4 vs 2.1 hours per night).[106] The intervention consisted of daily reports of PAP adherence, pressures, mask leak, and residual respiratory events, which were reviewed weekly by sleep laboratory staff. Patients were contacted via phone if the weekly mean usage time had dropped below 4 hours per night with 5-minute calls.[106] Telemonitoring reduced daytime sleepiness (Epworth Sleepiness Scale [ESS]) and systolic BP levels in patients post stroke, further supporting its use to address poor compliance in this vulnerable clinical population.

Telemonitoring (T4P Vision Web Portal) using similar daily reports delayed the time to the first technical intervention after PAP initiation, although the proportion of interventions was not different from UC.[102] In this study of 47 patients, the early monitoring of technical problems via the Web portal appeared to be an important factor in improving adherence at 3 months compared with UC (5.7 vs 4.2 hours per night).

In contrast, another telemonitoring system (MyOSA-OXigen Salud Web database) that also captured similar daily information (adherence, pressures, leak, and residual respiratory events) did not improve auto-titrating PAP usage (4.9 vs 5.1 hours per night), quality of life, or daytime sleepiness (ESS) compared with UC after 3 months.[112] The "alert" criteria for the sleep laboratory staff to intervene in this study did differ from Hoet and colleagues[102] (Turino, leak >30 L per minute for >30% of the night, or usage of <4 hours per night on 2 consecutive nights vs Hoet, leak >50 L per min, residual apnea hypopnea index [AHI] >10 per hour, or PAP use <3 hours on 3 consecutive nights), which may account for the inconsistent results, also patients in the latter study used auto-titrating PAP. Although telemonitoring did not improve adherence compared with UC in this trial, it was significantly less expensive and more cost-effective in terms of reducing the number of clinic visits. Patients did, however, report lower satisfaction with this intervention.[112]

The use of automated feedback messaging delivered alone, or in combination with telemedicine-delivered education improved PAP usage compared with UC or telemedicine education alone at 3 months.[103] In this 4-arm RCT of 556 patients, nightly average adherence was 4.4 versus 4.8 versus 3.8 versus 4.0 hours per night for telemonitoring alone (automated feedback messages based on device usage, U-Sleep), combined telemonitoring with telemedicine education (2 × 15 minutes Web-based OSA education sessions), UC, and telemedicine education alone, respectively. After the 3-month intervention had ceased, adherence gradually declined to similar levels as those observed in patients who had never received feedback when followed-up at 1 year, suggesting that sustained telemonitoring feedback was necessary to maintain higher adherence. Technology-based solutions that provide automated feedback directly from PAP devices may offer a cost-effective strategy to motivate patients to improve their adherence; however, their utility needs to be assessed over the longer term.

An earlier and smaller RCT[105] that tested the same telemonitoring system of text message feedback (U-Sleep, ResMed) over the same treatment period of 3 months, reported no difference in adherence compared with UC. However, the telehealth approach did positively affect health professionals' time, thus reducing pressure on health care services.[105] When adherence was assessed after a short follow-up period of 1 month using telemonitoring (Restraxx, ResMed), there was no significant difference in auto-titrating PAP usage, when compared with UC or weekly phone calls (5.0 vs 5.1 vs 3.9 hours per night); however, this 3-arm RCT did have a small sample size of 51 patients, which limits the interpretation of these results.[113]

SUMMARY

Innovative interventions to improve PAP adherence over the past 4 years have resulted in effective outcomes in the initial treatment (1 week to 1 month) or no significant effect over this period.[104,110] However, those studies that have assessed adherence over the longer term (3 months to 1 year) have produced minimal or negative adherence outcomes.[108,109] The exceptions were in 2 comorbid populations with interventions of motivational enhancement with follow-up at 12 months and CBT-I at 6 months.[111] Four[102,103,106,114] of the 7 telemonitoring RCTs increased adherence at 3 months[102,103] and 6 months,[106,114] whereas 3 studies showed no difference compared with UC at 1 month[113] or 3 months.[105,112]

CLINICS CARE POINTS

- Exploring baseline patient characteristics including self-efficacy, that is, SEMSA assessment, can be useful to identify those patients who are at risk of not taking up PAP or dropping out.
- Using targeted interventions based on a patient's cognitive perceptions to OSA and PAP treatment increases adherence.
- Being diagnosed with OSA is a time of considerable change, with associated stress. Motivational enhancement with a goal-oriented and very personal approach may be more useful for populations more at risk of nonadherence. Asking questions around "what is the patient prepared to do and how important is it for that person to learn to adapt to this chronic disorder?"
- Both CBT-I and motivational enhancement were effective in comorbid populations at 6

and 12 months of follow-up. Booster sessions (phone calls, telemedicine, face-to-face sessions) and ongoing contact with a known health professional appear to be crucial components of long-term adherence.
- The effectiveness of telehealth approaches was variable. Beneficial effects of telemonitoring may be dependent on several factors; for example, baseline patient characteristics, method and regularity of the feedback delivered, or alert criteria thresholds for triggering an "intervention." Reduced time commitment and costs for patients, that is, for clinic visits, and less burden on health services costs and professional input are factors requiring exploration in future telehealth interventions.

POINTS AROUND ENHANCING POSITIVE AIRWAY PRESSURE USAGE

- Health: stopping breathing has medical consequences.
- Relief of symptoms: waking with a headache, dry mouth, or bruised ribs!
- Partner disturbance: snoring and apneas; sleeping separately, explore the relationship?
- Weight loss: previously no energy to exercise and potentially explore diet to enhance weight loss, which may reduce PAP pressure.
- Education around normal sleep and aging: along with what happens when OSA is left untreated.
- Fear of the treatment and fear of the consequences of not treating the sleep disorder.
- Need for regular follow-ups.

DISCLOSURE

The authors have nothing to disclose.

ACKNOWLEDGMENT

This work was supported by an Australian National Health and Medical Research Council (NHMRC)/Australian Research Council (ARC) Fellowship to ALD (GNT1107716). Sincere thanks to Ms YuXin Kwan, CPAP Therapy Coordinator, Woolcock Clinic for sharing her experiences and providing input on the clinical care points.

REFERENCES

1. Heinzer R, Vat S, Marques-Vidal P, et al. Prevalence of sleep-disordered breathing in the general population: the HypnoLaus study. Lancet Respir Med 2015;3(4):310–8.
2. Benjafield AV, Ayas NT, Eastwood PR, et al. Estimation of the global prevalence and burden of obstructive sleep apnoea: a literature-based analysis. Lancet Respir Med 2019;7(8):687–98.
3. Ancoli-Israel S, Kripke DF, Klauber MR, et al. Sleep-disordered breathing in community-dwelling elderly. Sleep 1991;14(6):486–95.
4. Wickwire EM, Tom SE, Vadlamani A, et al. Older adult US Medicare beneficiaries with untreated obstructive sleep apnea are heavier users of health care than matched control patients. J Clin Sleep Med 2020;16(1):81–9.
5. Gaspar LS, Álvaro AR, Moita J, et al. Obstructive sleep apnea and hallmarks of aging. Trends Molecular Medicine 2017;23(8):675–92.
6. Ding Q, Kryger M. Greater health care utilization and cost associated with untreated sleep apnea. J Clin Sleep Med 2020;16(1):5–6.
7. Sullivan C, Issa F, al MB-Je. Reversal of obstructive sleep apnoea by continuous positive airway pressure applied through the nares. Lancet 1981;I:862–5.
8. McDaid C, Griffin S, Weatherly H, et al. Continuous positive airway pressure devices for the treatment of obstructive sleep apnoea-hypopnoea syndrome: a systematic review and economic analysis. Health Technol Assess 2009;13(4). iii-iv, xi-xiv, 1-119, 143-274.
9. Drager LF, McEvoy RD, Barbe F, et al. Sleep apnea and cardiovascular disease: lessons from recent trials and need for team science. Circulation 2017;136(19):1840–50.
10. McEvoy RD, Antic NA, Heeley E, et al. CPAP for prevention of cardiovascular events in obstructive sleep apnea. N Engl J Med 2016;375(10):919–31.
11. Javaheri S, Martinez-Garcia MA, Campos-Rodriguez F. CPAP treatment and cardiovascular prevention: we need to change the design and implementation of our trials. Chest 2019;156(3):431–7.
12. Weaver TE. Novel aspects of CPAP treatment and interventions to improve CPAP adherence. J Clin Med 2019;8(12):2220.
13. Antic NA, Catcheside P, Buchan C, et al. The effect of CPAP in normalizing daytime sleepiness, quality of life, and neurocognitive function in patients with moderate to severe OSA. Sleep 2011;34(1):111–9.
14. Peppard P, Szklo-Coxe M, Hla K, et al. Longitudinal association of sleep-related breathing disorder and depression. Arch Intern Med 2006;166:1709–15.
15. Weaver T, Maislin G, Dinges D, et al. Relationship between hours of CPAP use and achieving normal levels of sleepiness and daily functioning. Sleep 2007;30:711–9.
16. Chaiard J, Weaver TE. Update on research and practices in major sleep disorders: part I. Obstructive sleep apnea syndrome. J Nurs Scholarsh 2019;51(5):500–8.
17. Jackson ML, McEvoy RD, Banks S, et al. Neurobehavioral impairment and CPAP treatment response

in mild-moderate obstructive sleep apnea. J Clin Sleep Med 2018;14(01):47–56.

18. Stradling JR, Davies RJ. Is more NCPAP better? Sleep 2000;23(Suppl 4):S150–3.

19. Zhou J, Camacho M, Tang X, et al. A review of neurocognitive function and obstructive sleep apnea with or without daytime sleepiness. Sleep Med 2016;23:99–108.

20. Campos-Rodriguez F, Pena-Grinan N, Reyes-Nunez N, et al. Mortality in obstructive sleep apnea-hypopnea patients treated with positive airway pressure. Chest 2005;128(2):624–33.

21. Engleman H, Wild M. Improving CPAP use by patients with the sleep apnea/hypopnea syndrome (SAHS). Sleep Med Rev 2003;7:81–99.

22. Budhiraja R, Parthasarathy S, Drake CL, et al. Early CPAP use identifies subsequent adherence to CPAP therapy. Sleep 2007;30(3):320–4.

23. Kribbs NB, Pack AI, Kline LR, et al. Objective measurement of patterns of nasal CPAP use by patients with obstructive sleep apnea. Am Rev Respir Dis 1993;147(4):887–95.

24. Engleman HM, Martin SE, Douglas NJ. Compliance with CPAP therapy in patients with the sleep apnoea/hypopnoea syndrome. Thorax 1994;49(3): 263–6.

25. Reeves-Hoche MK, Meck R, Zwillich CW. Nasal CPAP: an objective evaluation of patient compliance. Am J Respir Crit Care Med 1994;149(1):149–54.

26. Mehrtash M, Bakker J, Ayas N. Predictors of continuous positive airway pressure adherence in patients with obstructive sleep apnea. Lung 2019; 197(2):115–21.

27. Inoue A, Chiba S, Matsuura K, et al. Nasal function and CPAP compliance. Auris Nasus Larynx 2019; 46(4):548–58.

28. Bailly S, Destors M, Grillet Y, et al. Obstructive sleep apnea: a cluster analysis at time of diagnosis. PLoS One 2016;11(6):e0157318.

29. Gagnadoux F, Le Vaillant M, Paris A, et al. Relationship between OSA clinical phenotypes and CPAP treatment outcomes. Chest 2016;149(1):288–90.

30. Pien GW, Ye L, Keenan BT, et al. Changing faces of obstructive sleep apnea: treatment effects by cluster designation in the Icelandic Sleep Apnea Cohort. Sleep 2018;41(3):zsx201.

31. Bachour A, Vitikainen P, Maasilta P. Rates of initial acceptance of PAP masks and outcomes of mask switching. Sleep Breathing 2015;20(2):733–8.

32. Krakow B, Melendrez D, Haynes P. Integrating psychosocial and biomedical CPAP adherence models. A commentary on: "Improving CPAP use by patients with the sleep apnea/hypopnea syndrome (SAHS)" (HM Engleman & MR Wild). Sleep Med Rev 2003;7(5):441–4.

33. Lebret M, Martinot JB, Arnol N, et al. Factors contributing to unintentional leak during CPAP treatment: a systematic review. Chest 2017; 151(3):707–19.

34. Lettieri CJ, Williams SG, Collen JF, et al. Treatment of obstructive sleep apnea: achieving adherence to positive airway pressure treatment and dealing with complications. Sleep Med Clin 2017;12(4): 551–64.

35. Chasens ER, Pack AI, Maislin G, et al. Claustrophobia and adherence to CPAP treatment. West J Nurs Res 2005;27(3):307–21.

36. Edmonds JC, Yang H, King TS, et al. Claustrophobic tendencies and continuous positive airway pressure therapy non-adherence in adults with obstructive sleep apnea. Heart Lung 2015;44(2): 100–6.

37. Anderson FE, Kingshott RN, Taylor DR, et al. A randomized crossover efficacy trial of oral CPAP (Oracle) compared with nasal CPAP in the management of obstructive sleep apnea. Sleep 2003;26(6):721–6.

38. Rowland S, Aiyappan V, Hennessy C, et al. Comparing the efficacy, mask leak, patient adherence, and patient preference of three different CPAP interfaces to treat moderate-severe obstructive sleep apnea. J Clin Sleep Med 2018;14(1): 101–8.

39. Chai CL, Pathinathan A, Smith B. Continuous positive airway pressure delivery interfaces for obstructive sleep apnoea. Cochrane Database Syst Rev 2006;(4):CD005308.

40. Boyer L, Philippe C, Covali-Noroc A, et al. OSA treatment with CPAP: randomized crossover study comparing tolerance and efficacy with and without humidification by ThermoSmart. Clin Respir J 2019; 13(6):384–90.

41. Massie CA, Hart RW, Peralez K, et al. Effects of humidification on nasal symptoms and compliance in sleep apnea patients using continuous positive airway pressure. Chest 1999;116(2):403–8.

42. Bakker JP, Marshall NS. Flexible pressure delivery modification of continuous positive airway pressure for obstructive sleep apnea does not improve compliance with therapy: systematic review and meta-analysis. Chest 2011;139(6):1322–30.

43. Kushida CA, Berry RB, Blau A, et al. Positive airway pressure initiation: a randomized controlled trial to assess the impact of therapy mode and titration process on efficacy, adherence, and outcomes. Sleep 2011;34(8):1083–92.

44. Kennedy B, Lasserson TJ, Wozniak DR, et al. Pressure modification or humidification for improving usage of continuous positive airway pressure machines in adults with obstructive sleep apnoea. Cochrane Database Syst Rev 2019;2019(12): CD003531.

45. Goh KJ, Soh RY, Leow LC, et al. Choosing the right mask for your Asian patient with sleep apnoea: a

randomized, crossover trial of CPAP interfaces. Respirology 2019;24(3):278–85.

46. Ma Z, Drinnan M, Hyde P, et al. Mask interface for continuous positive airway pressure therapy: selection and design considerations. Expert Rev Med Devices 2018;15(10):725–33.

47. Craig P, Dieppe P, Macintyre S, et al. Developing and evaluating complex interventions: the new Medical Research Council guidance. BMJ 2008; 337:a1655.

48. Smith CE, Mayer LS, Metsker C, et al. Continuous positive airway pressure: patients' and caregivers' learning needs and barriers to use. Heart Lung 1998;27(2):99–108.

49. Brostrom A, Johansson P, Albers J, et al. 6-month CPAP-treatment in a young male patient with severe obstructive sleep apnoea syndrome - a case study from the couple's perspective. Eur J Cardiovasc Nurs 2008;7(2):103–12.

50. Ayow TM, Paquet F, Dallaire J, et al. Factors influencing the use and nonuse of continuous positive airway pressure therapy: a comparative case study. Rehabil Nurs 2009;34(6):230–6.

51. Zarhin D, Oksenberg A. Ambivalent adherence and nonadherence to continuous positive airway pressure devices: a qualitative study. J Clin Sleep Med 2017;13(12):1375–84.

52. Brostrom A, Nilsen P, Johansson P, et al. Putative facilitators and barriers for adherence to CPAP treatment in patients with obstructive sleep apnea syndrome: a qualitative content analysis. Sleep Med 2010;11(2):126–30.

53. Dickerson SS, Akhu-Zaheya L. Life changes in individuals diagnosed with sleep apnea while accommodating to continuous positive airway pressure (CPAP) devices. Rehabil Nurs 2007;32(6):241–50.

54. Luyster FS, Dunbar-Jacob J, Aloia MS, et al. Patient and partner experiences with obstructive sleep apnea and CPAP treatment: a qualitative analysis. Behav Sleep Med 2016;14(1):67–84.

55. Aalaei S, Rezaeitalab F, Tabesh H, et al. Factors affecting patients' adherence to continuous positive airway pressure therapy for obstructive sleep apnea disorder: a multi-method approach. Iran J Med Sci 2019;45(3):170–8.

56. Baron KG, Gunn HE, Wolfe LF, et al. Relationships and CPAP adherence among women with obstructive sleep apnea. Sleep Sci Pract 2017;1(1):10.

57. Ward K, Gott M, Hoare K. Mastering Treatment for Sleep Apnoea: The Grounded Theory of Bargaining and Balancing Life With Continuous Positive Airway Pressure (CPAP), in the Context of Decisional Conflict and Change Theories. 2019. 2019; 20(3).

58. Sawyer AM, Deatrick JA, Kuna ST, et al. Differences in perceptions of the diagnosis and treatment of obstructive sleep apnea and continuous positive airway pressure therapy among adherers and nonadherers. Qual Health Res 2010;20(7): 873–92.

59. Crawford MR, Vallieres A. The dark side of adherence-a commentary on Palm et al. (2018) factors influencing adherence to continuous positive airway pressure treatment in obstructive sleep apnea and mortality associated with treatment failure - a national registry-based cohort study. Sleep Med 2018;51:85–91. Sleep Med. 2019;59:96.

60. Wozniak DR, Lasserson TJ, Smith I. Educational, supportive and behavioural interventions to improve usage of continuous positive airway pressure machines in adults with obstructive sleep apnoea. Cochrane Database Syst Rev 2014;1: Cd007736.

61. Bandura A. Social learning theory. Englewood Cliffs (NJ): Prentice Hall; 1977.

62. Bandura A. Human agency in social cognitive theory. Am Psychol 1989;44(9):1175–84.

63. Aloia M, Arendt J, Stepnowski C. Predicting treatment adherence in obstructive sleep apnea using principles of behaviour change. J Clin Sleep Med 2005;1:346–53.

64. Stepnowsky C, Marler M, Ancoli-Israel S. Determinants of nasal CPAP compliance. Sleep Med 2002;3:239–47.

65. Stepnowsky CJ Jr, Bardwell WA, Moore PJ, et al. Psychologic correlates of compliance with continuous positive airway pressure. Sleep 2002;25(7): 758–62.

66. Weaver T, Maislin G, Dinges D, et al. Self efficacy in sleep apnea: instrument development and patient perceptions of obstructive sleep apnea risk, treatment benefit and volition to use continuous positive airway pressure. Sleep 2003;26:727–32.

67. Sawyer AM, Canamucio A, Moriarty H, et al. Do cognitive perceptions influence CPAP use? Patient Educ Couns 2011;85(1):85–91.

68. Olsen S, Smith S, Oei T, et al. Health belief and model predicts adherence to CPAP before experience with CPAP. Eur Respir J 2008;32:710–7.

69. Richards D, Bartlett D, Wong K, et al. Increased adherence to CPAP with a group cognitive behavioural treatment intervention: a randomized trial. Sleep 2007;30:635–40.

70. Bartlett D, Wong K, Richards D, et al. Increasing adherence to obstructive sleep apnea treatment with a group social cognitive therapy treatment intervention: a randomized trial. Sleep 2013; 36(11):1647–54.

71. Saconi B, Yang H, Watach AJ, et al. Coping processes, self-efficacy, and CPAP use in adults with obstructive sleep apnea. Behav Sleep Med 2020; 18(1):68–80.

72. Baron KG, Berg CA, Czajkowski LA, et al. Self-efficacy contributes to individual differences in

subjective improvements using CPAP. Sleep Breath 2011;15(3):599–606.

73. Aloia MS, Di Dio L, Ilniczky N, et al. Improving compliance with nasal CPAP and vigilance in older adults with OAHS. Sleep Breath 2001;5(1):13–21.

74. Aloia M, Smith K, Arendt J, et al. Brief behavioral therapies reduce early positive airway pressure discontinuation rates in sleep apnea syndrom: preliminary findings. Behav Sleep Med 2007;5(2):89–104.

75. Olsen S, Smith S, Oei T, et al. Cues to starting CPAP in obstructive sleep apnea: development and validation of the cues to CPAP use questionnaire. J Clin Sleep Med 2010;6:229–37.

76. Olsen S, Smith SS, Oei TP, et al. Motivational interviewing (MINT) improves continuous positive airway pressure (CPAP) acceptance and adherence: a randomized controlled trial. J consulting Clin Psychol 2012;80(1):151–63.

77. Aloia MS, Arnedt JT, Strand M, et al. Motivational enhancement to improve adherence to positive airway pressure in patients with obstructive sleep apnea: a randomized controlled trial. Sleep 2013;36(11):1655–62.

78. Sawyer AM, King TS, Hanlon A, et al. Risk assessment for CPAP nonadherence in adults with newly diagnosed obstructive sleep apnea: preliminary testing of the Index for Nonadherence to PAP (I-NAP). Sleep Breathing 2014;18(4):875–83.

79. Lai AY, Fong DY, Lam JC, et al. The efficacy of a brief motivational enhancement education program on CPAP adherence in OSA: a randomized controlled trial. Chest 2014;146(3):600–10.

80. Deng T, Wang Y, Sun M, et al. Stage-matched intervention for adherence to CPAP in patients with obstructive sleep apnea: a randomized controlled trial. Sleep Breath 2013;17(2):791–801.

81. Cvengros JA, Rodríguez VM, Snyder S, et al. An adaptive treatment to improve positive airway pressure (PAP) adherence in patients with obstructive sleep apnea: a proof of concept trial. Behav Sleep Med 2017;15(5):345–60.

82. Epstein LJ, Kristo D, Strollo PJ Jr, et al. Clinical guideline for the evaluation, management and long-term care of obstructive sleep apnea in adults. J Clin Sleep Med 2009;5(3):263–76.

83. Sawyer AM, Gooneratne NS, Marcus CL, et al. A systematic review of CPAP adherence across age groups: clinical and empiric insights for developing CPAP adherence interventions. Sleep Med Rev 2011;15(6):343–56.

84. Hoy C, Vennelle R, Kingshott R, et al. Can intensive support improve continuous positive airway pressure use in patients with the sleep apnea/hypopnea syndrome? Am J Respir Crit Care Med 1999;159:1096–100.

85. Delanote I, Borzée P, Belge C, et al. Adherence to cpap therapy: comparing the effect of three educational approaches in patients with obstructive sleep apnoea. Clin Respir J 2018;12(1):91–6.

86. Stepnowsky C, Sarmiento KF, Amdur A. Weaving the internet of sleep: the future of patient-centric collaborative sleep health management using web-based platforms. Sleep 2015;38(8):1157–8.

87. Sedkaoui K, Leseux L, Pontier S, et al. Efficiency of a phone coaching program on adherence to continuous positive airway pressure in sleep apnea hypopnea syndrome: a randomized trial. BMC Pulm Med 2015;15:102.

88. Lo Bue A, Salvaggio A, Isidoro SI, et al. Usefulness of reinforcing interventions on continuous positive airway pressure compliance. BMC Pulm Med 2014;14:78.

89. Soares Pires F, Drummond M, Marinho A, et al. Effectiveness of a group education session on adherence with APAP in obstructive sleep apnea–a randomized controlled study. Sleep Breath 2013;17(3):993–1001.

90. Sin DD, Mayers I, Man GC, et al. Long-term compliance rates to continuous positive airway pressure in obstructive sleep apnea: a population-based study. Chest 2002;121(2):430–5.

91. Bouloukaki I, Giannadaki K, Mermigkis C, et al. Intensive versus standard follow-up to improve continuous positive airway pressure compliance. Eur Respir J 2014;44(5):1262–74.

92. Chen X, Chen W, Hu W, et al. Nurse-led intensive interventions improve adherence to continuous positive airway pressure therapy and quality of life in obstructive sleep apnea patients. Patient Prefer Adherence 2015;9:1707–13.

93. Parthasarathy S, Wendel C, Haynes PL, et al. A pilot study of CPAP adherence promotion by peer buddies with sleep apnea. J Clin Sleep Med 2013;9(6):543–50.

94. Lewis KE, Seale L, Bartle IE, et al. Early predictors of CPAP use for the treatment of obstructive sleep apnea. Sleep 2004;27(1):134–8.

95. Baron KG, Smith TW, Berg CA, et al. Spousal involvement in CPAP adherence among patients with obstructive sleep apnea. Sleep Breathing 2011;15(3):525–34.

96. McArdle N, Kingshott R, Engleman H, et al. Partners of patients with sleep apnoea/hypopnoea syndrome: effect of CPAP treatment on sleep quantity and quality of life. Thorax 2001;56:513–8.

97. Ye L, Malhotra A, Kayser K, et al. Spousal involvement and CPAP adherence: a dyadic perspective. Sleep Med Rev 2015;19:67–74.

98. Golay A, Girard A, Grandin S, et al. A new educational program for patients suffering from sleep apnea syndrome. Patient Educ Couns 2006;60(2):220–7.

99. Sawyer AM, King TS, Sawyer DA, et al. Is inconsistent pre-treatment bedtime related to CPAP non-adherence? Res Nurs Health 2014;37(6):504–11.

100. D'Rozario AL, Galgut Y, Bartlett DJ. An update on behavioural interventions for improving adherence with continuous positive airway pressure in adults. Curr Sleep Med Rep 2016;2(3):166–79.

101. Bakker JP, Wang R, Weng J, et al. Motivational enhancement for increasing adherence to CPAP: a randomized controlled trial. Chest 2016;150(2):337–45.

102. Hoet F, Libert W, Sanida C, et al. Telemonitoring in continuous positive airway pressure-treated patients improves delay to first intervention and early compliance: a randomized trial. Sleep Med 2017;39:77–83.

103. Hwang D, Chang JW, Benjafield AV, et al. Effect of telemedicine education and telemonitoring on continuous positive airway pressure adherence. The tele-OSA randomized trial. Am J Respir Crit Care Med 2018;197(1):117–26.

104. Guralnick AS, Balachandran JS, Szutenbach S, et al. Educational video to improve CPAP use in patients with obstructive sleep apnoea at risk for poor adherence: a randomised controlled trial. Thorax 2017;72(12):1132–9.

105. Munafo D, Hevener W, Crocker M, et al. A telehealth program for CPAP adherence reduces labor and yields similar adherence and efficacy when compared to standard of care. Sleep Breath 2016;20(2):777–85.

106. Nilius G, Schroeder M, Domanski U, et al. Telemedicine improves continuous positive airway pressure adherence in stroke patients with obstructive sleep apnea in a randomized trial. Respiration 2019;98(5):410–20.

107. Pengo MF, Czaban M, Berry MP, et al. The effect of positive and negative message framing on short term continuous positive airway pressure compliance in patients with obstructive sleep apnea. J Thorac Dis 2018;10:S160–9.

108. Luyster FS, Aloia MS, Buysse DJ, et al. A couples-oriented intervention for positive airway pressure therapy adherence: a pilot study of obstructive sleep apnea patients and their partners. Behav Sleep Med 2019;17(5):561–72.

109. Sawyer AM, King TS, Weaver TE, et al. A tailored intervention for PAP adherence: the SCIP-PA trial. Behav Sleep Med 2019;17(1):49–69.

110. Shapiro AL. Effect of the CPAP-SAVER intervention on adherence. Clin Nurs Res 2019. https://doi.org/10.1177/1054773819865875.

111. Sweetman A, Lack L, Catcheside PG, et al. Cognitive and behavioral therapy for insomnia increases the use of continuous positive airway pressure therapy in obstructive sleep apnea participants with comorbid insomnia: a randomized clinical trial. Sleep 2019;42(12):zsz178.

112. Turino C, De Batlle J, Woehrle H, et al. Management of continuous positive airway pressure treatment compliance using telemonitoring in obstructive sleep apnoea. Eur Respir J 2017;49(2):1601128.

113. Fernandes M, Antunes C, Martinho C, et al. Evaluation of telemonitoring of continuous positive airway pressure therapy in obstructive sleep apnoea syndrome: TELEPAP pilot study. J Telemed Telecare 2019. https://doi.org/10.1177/1357633X19875850.

114. Pépin J-L, Jullian-Desayes I, Sapène M, et al. Multimodal remote monitoring of high cardiovascular risk patients with OSA initiating CPAP: a randomized trial. Chest 2019;155(4):730–9.

115. Zhang Y, Ren R, Lei F, et al. Worldwide and regional prevalence rates of co-occurrence of insomnia and insomnia symptoms with obstructive sleep apnea: a systematic review and meta-analysis. Sleep Med Rev 2019;45:1–17.

Where to Next for Optimizing Adherence in Large-Scale Trials of Continuous Positive Airway Pressure?

Amy M. Sawyer, PhD, RN[a,b,c,]*, Douglas M. Wallace, MD[d,e],
Luis F. Buenaver, PhD[f], Alexa J. Watach, PhD, RN[c,g], Amy Blase, CCRA[h],
Bruno Saconi, MS, RN[i], Sanjay R. Patel, MD, MS[j], Samuel T. Kuna, MD[c,k],
Naresh M. Punjabi, MD, PhD[l]

KEYWORDS

- Obstructive sleep apnea • Continuous positive airway pressure • Patient compliance
- Health behavior • Telemedicine • Health education • Controlled clinical trial • Behavioral economics

KEY POINTS

- Large-scale, randomized trials to evaluate the efficacy of positive airway pressure (PAP) for improving patient-reported outcomes and clinical end points associated with obstructive sleep apnea (OSA), including cardiovascular and metabolic disease, have been largely negative.
- Several design-related criticisms have plagued the large-scale PAP trials, with a common focus on PAP nonadherence among trial participants.
- Advancing large-scale PAP trial methods to optimize PAP adherence is crucial if the field is to be successful in generating valid knowledge of the causal effect of OSA on comorbid outcomes.
- Best trial practices that focus on optimizing PAP adherence in large-scale trials are needed.
- Opportunities to enhance PAP adherence in large-scale trials include methodological and operational recommendations and reporting guidance that, in sum, are consistent with scientific requirements for rigor, reproducibility, and transparency.

[a] Department of Biobehavioral Health Science, University of Pennsylvania School of Nursing, 418 Curie Boulevard, Claire Fagin Hall, Room 349, Philadelphia, PA 19104, USA; [b] Corporal Michael J. Crescenz Veterans Affairs Medical Center, Philadelphia, PA, USA; [c] University of Pennsylvania Perelman School of Medicine, Center for Sleep and Circadian Neurobiology, Philadelphia, PA, USA; [d] Department of Neurology, Sleep Medicine Division, University of Miami Miller School of Medicine, 1201 Northwest 16th Street, Room A212, Miami, FL 33125, USA; [e] Miami Veterans Affairs HealthCare System, Miami, FL, USA; [f] Johns Hopkins Behavioral Sleep Medicine Program, Johns Hopkins University School of Medicine, 5510 Nathan Shock Drive, Suite 100, Baltimore, MD 21224-6823, USA; [g] University of Pennsylvania School of Nursing, 418 Curie Boulevard, Claire Fagin Hall, Room 349, Philadelphia, PA 19104, USA; [h] ResMed Corporation, 9001 Spectrum Center Boulevard, San Diego, CA 92123, USA; [i] University of Pennsylvania School of Nursing, 418 Curie Boulevard, Claire Fagin Hall, Philadelphia, PA 19104, USA; [j] Center for Sleep and Cardiovascular Outcomes Research, University of Pittsburgh, 3609 Forbes Avenue, 2nd Floor, Room 108, Pittsburgh, PA 15213, USA; [k] Sleep Medicine, Sleep Medicine Section (111P), Corporal Michael J. Crescenz Veterans Affairs Medical Center, 3900 Woodland Avenue, Philadelphia, PA 19104, USA; [l] Division of Pulmonary, Critical Care, and Sleep Medicine, University of Miami, Miller School of Medicine, 1951 NW 7th Avenue, Miami, FL 33136, USA
* Corresponding author. Department of Biobehavioral Health Science, University of Pennsylvania School of Nursing, 418 Curie Boulevard, Claire Fagin Hall, Room 349, Philadelphia, PA 19104.
E-mail address: asawyer@nursing.upenn.edu

Sleep Med Clin 16 (2021) 125–144
https://doi.org/10.1016/j.jsmc.2020.10.007
1556-407X/21/Published by Elsevier Inc.

INTRODUCTION

Clinical trials are defined as experiments in humans designed to evaluate the effects of specific treatments, or exposure condition that by design reduce random error and bias.[1] Effects or outcomes evaluated in clinical trials commonly include safety, dosing, efficacy, and effectiveness. Phase III trials that evaluate efficacy and/or effectiveness of a treatment compared with a standard, alternative, or placebo are often designed as large-scale trials to ensure adequate statistical power and potentiate the ability to generalize to the defined target population.[1] For the purpose of this article, large-scale trial characteristics include the following: (1) multisite; (2) total sample size greater than 300 participants; and (3) a primary outcome evaluation period greater than or equal to 3 months.

In sleep medicine, large-scale trials that meet these criteria and examined the effects of positive airway pressure (PAP) are recent to the literature. Driven in part by prior large epidemiologic or observational studies of obstructive sleep apnea (OSA) and associated comorbidities,[2–6] these large-scale trials[7–12] examined the effects of PAP on comorbid outcomes, OSA outcomes, and/or preventive effects for associated comorbidities such as cardiovascular, metabolic, and neurologic outcomes. Although such trials would expectedly provide confirmatory evidence and advance the cycle of research for translation to practice, there have instead been questions raised about the validity of the results because of design and methodological concerns. PAP adherence has consistently been an area of concern for many of these trials, expressed clearly in noteworthy editorials that have accompanied, or followed, the publication of the large-scale trials of PAP.[13–18] This article uses the recent large-scale trial experience to (1) identify opportunities for increasing rigor, reproducibility, and transparency of forthcoming and future large-scale, prospective trials of PAP effects; and (2) set forth best trial practices that directly address PAP adherence while also considering key methodologies and opportunities relative to implementing health behavior strategies embedded within a larger trial design.

LARGE-SCALE CLINICAL TRIALS OF POSITIVE AIRWAY PRESSURE

In a systematic database search of PubMed Plus, Scopus, and ClinicalTrials.gov that used a keyword search strategy (OSA, continuous positive airway pressure [CPAP], randomized controlled trial [RCT], or trial) with delimiters for adult and publication date from 2000 to current (February 1, 2020), 6 trials were identified that additionally met criteria for (1) the large-scale definition used herein, (2) an objective measurement of PAP use/adherence, and (3) reported PAP use in the primary results publication (**Table 1**). Most excluded trials did not meet the review-specific large-scale definition for sample size or outcome interval duration or failed to fully report PAP use with the primary results. Across the included trials, PAP use ranged from 2.3 to 5.0 h/night (mean or median). In trials reporting a PAP adherence criterion, approximately half of the samples met the commonly reported PAP adherence criterion of greater than or equal to 4 h/night. The trial samples were characteristically similar, with the exception of 2 trials that had target populations without excessive daytime sleepiness[11] (ie, by Epworth Sleepiness Score criterion) and/or minimally symptomatic individuals with OSA[8] (ie, absence of other patient-reported OSA symptoms). Studied samples were predominantly male, middle-aged, obese adults with moderate to severe OSA. All trials set forth a primary objective to evaluate PAP effects, absent explicit use of the term "efficacy." PAP was compared with at least 1 other exposure condition, to evaluate the primary outcome assessed at or after 3 months of exposure. Primary outcome results were largely negative, or supportive of the null hypothesis, across the trials.

Evaluation of efficacy, or the true biological effect of a treatment,[1] necessitates exposure to the test and comparator conditions to permit the exploration of patient-reported outcomes and/or clinical end points that are the efficacy outcomes. Efficacy is evaluated in the trial setting wherein internal validity is prioritized, notably to the detriment of external validity, or the ability to generalize to practice.[19] Evaluation of effectiveness, or outcomes of the test and comparator relative to usual, real-world conditions, may similarly examine biomedical end points but, by design, prioritize external validity for addressing practice and policy priorities.[19] Effectiveness is the "effect of a treatment when widely used in practice."[1]

The identified large-scale trials of PAP all report a primary objective to evaluate the effect of PAP on a primary end point and report designs and analytical methods (eg, intention to treat) consistent with efficacy evaluation. However, when the published protocols and primary results with supporting documents (ie, supplement, appendix) are carefully scrutinized, the methodologies and procedures specific to the PAP exposure condition are likened to protocol methods consistent with effectiveness evaluation. Such methods are reflective of standard practice, or usual care. For

Table 1
Published large-scale trials (n = 6)

Trial (Project Years)	Location (Sites)	Primary End Point	Follow-up	Study Sample	Intervention (N)	Comparator (N)	PAP Use Criterion	Adherence h/night	Adherence % ≥ 4 h	Primary Outcome (+ or −)
APPLES[7] 2003–2008	United States (5)	Neurocognitive function	6 mo	Patients with OSA	CPAP (n = 556)	Sham PAP (n = 542)	≥4	4.2	56.2	−
Spanish Cohort[11] 2004–2009	Spain (14)	Incident HTN and CV events	3 y	Patients with OSA (nonsleepy)	CPAP (n = 358)	No treatment (n = 367)	≥4	5.0	64.4	−
MOSAIC[8] 2006–2010	United Kingdom/ Canada (10)	CV risk score	6 mo	Patients with OSA (nonsleepy)	CPAP (n = 195)	Usual care (n = 196)	≥4	2.4	NR	−
HeartBEAT[12] 2010–2012	United States (4)	24-h blood pressure	3-mo	Cardiology patients with OSA	CPAP (n = 106) Oxygen (n = 106)	Lifestyle education (n = 106)	NR	3.5	NR	+
SAVE[9] 2008–2015	Australia, China, New Zealand, India, Spain, United States, Brazil (89)	MACE	4 y	Patients with CVD with OSA	CPAP (n = 1359)	Usual care (n = 1358)	≥4	3.3	42	−
ISAACC[10] 2011–2018	Spain (15)	MACE	≥1 y	Patients with ACS with OSA	CPAP (n = 633)	Usual care (n = 631)	≥4	2.8	37.5	−

Abbreviations: ACS, acute coronary syndrome; CV, cardiovascular; CVD, cardiovascular disease; HTN, hypertension; MACE, major adverse cardiovascular event; NR, not reported.

example, a trial that reports providing participants with contact information for device troubleshooting after providing standard OSA and PAP patient education, including device setup and mask fitting for longer large-scale trials, assumes participants will acknowledge and recognize specific barriers to PAP use and then initiate contact. This example is more consistent with standard practice and is thereby better aligned with effectiveness evaluation wherein the effect of treatment in practice is the trial objective. Although effectiveness trials are imperative to the field, efficacy evaluations cannot and should not be forgone, because knowledge of PAP efficacy is central to defining treatment standards of OSA by varied outcomes, including comorbid outcomes of physiologic and clinical importance. Furthermore, efficacy evaluations from randomized trials are viewed as among the strongest evidence toward answering questions of causality (ie, does OSA cause comorbid outcomes of clinical importance?).

RIGOR AND REPRODUCIBILITY OF POSITIVE AIRWAY PRESSURE ADHERENCE PROTOCOLS IN LARGE-SCALE TRIALS OF POSITIVE AIRWAY PRESSURE

Critical insights from the large-scale PAP trials published to date provide the field with an opportunity to consider how efficacy trials will need to explicitly address PAP adherence within the larger trial protocol to better meet the requirements for rigor and reproducibility as defined by the National Institutes of Health (NIH)[20] and similarly emphasized by other federal agencies.[21,22] Trials included herein were designed by teams of interdisciplinary scientific investigators with relevant expertise (**Table 2**) and supported by at least 1 federal or regional agency. Resources for trial conduct and oversight (internal and external) were clearly explicated in half of the trial reports,[7,9,12] suggesting careful attention to trial

operations that is consistent with the safe, ethical, and rigorous conduct of efficacy trials.

There are noteworthy gaps, specific to PAP exposure and PAP adherence protocols, across the included trials that can be leveraged for optimizing PAP adherence in the next generation of large-scale trials of PAP efficacy. For example, an absence of evidence-based behavioral approaches to support PAP use was observed. Some of these gaps are likely attributed to the state of PAP adherence science at the time of planning and conducting the trials. Other gaps may be relative to a myriad of contributors, including the absence of clear guidance and/or expectancies for reporting efficacy trial PAP adherence protocols at the time of grant submission and subsequent publications related to the trial.

Methods specific to PAP adherence were abstracted from all available published sources for each trial, including primary results publications, design and methodology publications, publicly accessible protocols, trial registry data, grant databases (eg, RePORTER for NIH-funded studies), and secondary results publications if available (**Table 3**; **Table S1** for detailed methods). Corresponding authors identified on the primary results publication were also contacted when published or publicly available sources lacked information or data specific to PAP adherence methods reported in **Table 3**. Sorting the reported PAP adherence methods by study period revealed important similarities and differences between these trials for PAP adherence protocols (**Boxes 1** and **2**).

Positive Airway Pressure Adherence Criterion

All trials but 1[12] identified a PAP adherence criterion, most often defined in the analysis or results section of the respective published articles. This criterion was consistently reported as greater than or equal to 4 h/night of average PAP use without explicit rationale. There were no

---

Table 2
Scientific trial team members by discipline or specialty[a]

Discipline Involved	APPLES	Spanish Cohort	MOSAIC	HeartBEAT	SAVE	ISAACC
Sleep medicine	+	+	+	+	+	+
Respiratory medicine	+	+	+	+	+	+
Clinical trialist and/or statistics	+	−	+	+	+	+
Study- specific discipline relative to biomedical focus	+	−	−	+	+	+
Behavioral science	−	−	+	−	−	−

[a] Identified by author affiliations in methodology and/or result publication.

Table 3
Concentration of methods specific to positive airway pressure adherence by large-scale trial study period (n = 6)

Trial Name	Screening Criteria[a] Or Other Prerandomization Methods	Random Assignment[b]	PAP Initiation	Week 1	Month 1 PAP Exposure	> Month 1
APPLES	+	+	+	++	+	++
Spanish Cohort Trial	–	–	++	–	–	–
MOSAIC	+	–	++	–	+	+
HeartBEAT	+	–	+++	–	–	–
SAVE	+++	+	+++	++	+++	++
ISAACC	+	–	+++	++	++	+

–, zero reported method; +, 1 reported method; ++, 2 reported methods; +++, 3+ reported methods. See Supplemental table for detailed reported methods.
[a] Inclusion and exclusion criteria that are specified for PAP adherence in methodology and/or result publication and/or supplemental/appendix materials and/or publicly availably protocol materials.
[b] Reported protocol activities specific to PAP use/initiation/adherence conducted concurrently with randomization.

methodological details provided for the specified protocol periods during which the criterion was to have been met, and, if the criterion was not met in any specific interval, there were no reports of specific PAP adherence protocols that were used other than that study contact was initiated. All trials reported designated visits at which time PAP adherence was electronically retrieved or downloaded. Two trials[7,9] reported using a PAP adherence criterion to guide study contact with participants; these interactions were either by phone and/or at an additional research visit to address low PAP adherence. No protocol-based, prespecified actions were reported for the low PAP adherence interactions.

Trial Positive Airway Pressure Exposure Less than or Equal to 4 Months and Adherence Protocols

All trials reported that mask fitting, equipment review, and education were provided by trained or experienced study personnel. Only 1 trial reported the educational approach used with participants, using 3 education modalities to deliver the information.[12] No trials reported specific educational content that was provided to the trial participants. Mask and/or humidification choice was prioritized relative to adherence in 1 trial,[8] whereas others specified that humidification and best-fit mask were provided.[9,12] In some trials,[7-10] troubleshooting, support for adapting to PAP, and advice were reported as protocol activities in the first several weeks to 4 months.

Trial Positive Airway Pressure Exposure Greater than 4 Months and Adherence Protocols

All included trials except 1[12] assessed a primary end point with PAP exposure greater than 4 months. The Sleep Apnea Cardiovascular Endpoints Study (SAVE)[9] was the only trial that

reported using a specific PAP adherence protocol extending beyond 4 months. This trial, with a large number of sites extending around the globe, was also unique in that a centralized study structure, sleep laboratory core, was charged with monitoring PAP use across sites and provided

---

> **Box 2**
> **Exceptional[a] positive airway pressure adherence methods in large-scale positive airway pressure efficacy trials**
>
> - Exclusion criteria
>   - Other household member with PAP use[7-9]
> - Other criteria at screening or enrollment
>   - One-week run-in with greater than or equal to 3 h/night average use[9]
> - Random assignment
>   - Twenty-minute acclimatize-to-PAP session[7]
> - PAP initiation
>   - Education about OSA and PAP provided by verbal, audiovisual, and written methods[12]
>   - Behavioral sleep medicine specialist provided pretreatment information about PAP[10,b]
>   - Mask and humidification choice[8]
> - Exposure intervals
>   - PAP use criterion during auto-PAP titration period[9]
>   - PAP frequently asked questions for study staff to reduce risk of unblinding participants (sham vs CPAP)[7]
>   - Core sleep laboratory remote review of PAP use, leak data at regular defined intervals[9]
>   - Core sleep laboratory provides corrective advice to sites, study team as needed[9]
>   - Sleep hygiene advice specified by investigators as relevant to PAP adherence (alcohol and tobacco use, short sleep duration)[10]
>   - Week 1 phone follow-up[7,9]
>   - Week 2 phone follow-up[10]
>   - Phone follow-up based on PAP usage criterion[7,9]
>   - Motivational and cognitive strategies used to increase PAP use[10,b]
>
> [a]Exceptional defined as reported in less than or equal to 50% of included trials. [b]Not reported in published methodology or results; provided by corresponding author in response to electronic mail query requesting any additional protocol activities specific to PAP adherence.

> **Box 1**
> **Consistent positive airway pressure adherence methods in large-scale positive airway pressure efficacy trials (n = 6)**
>
> - Exclusion criteria
>   - Prior PAP use
> - PAP initiation
>   - By trained (or experienced) study personnel
> - PAP use measurement
>   - Objective at varied study intervals

centralized expert advice to sites when PAP adherence was less than the study-defined criterion. The SAVE trial also used PAP use, leak, and residual apnea-hypopnea index (AHI) criteria from PAP initiation to study end with PAP remote monitoring.[9]

When the trials are considered collectively, PAP adherence protocols are generally under-reported, which limits reproducibility and affects evaluation of the rigor for the reported work. This weakness limits the potential for other investigators to address the challenge of optimizing PAP adherence in subsequent large-scale PAP trials. The included trials report methods that are seemingly consistent with earlier published clinical practice guidelines[23] and with what the field considered standard practice at the time of these trials. The PAP adherence achieved in the included trials is therefore expected given (1) the modest trial PAP adherence protocols; and (2) the observation that, across PAP clinical trials and clinical trial follow-up observational studies, the weighted average of PAP use was 4.46 h/night and the average nonadherence rate was 36.3%.[24] These observed metrics of PAP adherence are consistent with other reviews that have addressed summary PAP adherence across studies.[25,26] The obvious concern is that this level of PAP adherence is suboptimal for a rigorous assessment of efficacy.

The overwhelmingly negative results across the large-scale trials coupled with the minimalist approaches to PAP adherence within the conduct of the efficacy trials provide the evidence and the necessary motivation for future large-scale trials to carefully design and report PAP adherence protocols in great detail. These protocols will need to use the current PAP adherence evidence to potentiate higher PAP adherence across study participants. Such adherence protocols should be embedded within the larger trial protocol to ensure reproducibility and strengthen rigor relative to PAP adherence. This approach will best position large-scale efficacy trials to test PAP by providing results that are unbiased relative to adherence.

STATE OF THE SCIENCE: POSITIVE AIRWAY PRESSURE ADHERENCE

Since the earliest large-scale trial[7] was conducted, PAP adherence intervention studies have been increasingly represented in the literature. The body of evidence has recently been systematically examined, resulting in a meta-analysis[27] that supports the current American Academy of Sleep Medicine's clinical practice guideline for the PAP treatment of adults with OSA.[28] The meta-analyses addressed PICO (Population, Intervention, Comparison, Outcome) questions of which 8 of the 11 questions included PAP adherence as an outcome (**Box 3**). The cumulative set of reviewed evidence (n = 1512) was reduced to a final set of 184 studies that addressed 1 or more of the PICO questions[27]; for each PICO question, a subset of studies were eligible for meta-analysis. With a prespecified clinical threshold of significance for the PAP adherence outcome set at 0.5 h/night or 10% patient use greater than 4 h/night, the results of the meta-analysis support the accompanying practice guidelines.[28] Explicit PAP adherence interventions addressed by the meta-analyses and subsequent practice guidelines include educational, behavioral, and telemonitoring recommendations; on average, these interventions, individually, result in an estimated PAP use effect of 1.0 h/night (**Fig. 1**). The available cumulative evidence provides guidance for designing evidence-based PAP adherence protocols for future large-scale efficacy trials.

Box 3
Summary of population, intervention, comparison, outcome questions and evidence density and quality for meta-analyses of positive airway pressure adherence outcome in Patil and colleagues 2019[27]

Question 4: in-laboratory versus ambulatory PAP titration based on 10 RCTs of high quality

Question 5: autotitrating versus continuous PAP based on 23 RCTs of moderate to high quality

Question 6: bilevel PAP or autobilevel PAP versus CPAP based on 4 RCTs of low quality

Question 7: modified pressure profile versus no modified pressure profile based on 6 RCTs of low quality

Question 8: oral versus nasal PAP mask based on 2 crossover RCTs and 1 RCT of low quality

Question 9: PAP with humidity versus no humidity based on 9 RCTs of low to moderate quality

Question 10: educational intervention based on 7 RCTs of moderate quality, or

Behavioral intervention based on 6 RCTs of moderate to high quality versus no intervention (interventions delivered before or during PAP)

- Troubleshooting plus education intervention based on 9 RCTs of moderate quality was separately meta-analyzed

Question 11: telemonitor guided intervention versus no telemonitoring based on 5 RCTs of high quality

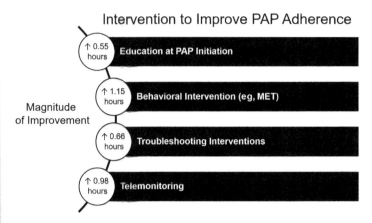

Fig. 1. Evidence-based PAP adherence interventions and their estimated improvement for PAP adherence. Estimated effects for PAP adherence (ie, use) are meta-analyses results reported in Patil and colleagues, 2019.[27] MET, Motivational Enhancement Therapy. (*Adapted from* Patil SP, Ayappa IA, Caples SM, Kimoff RJ, Patel SR, Harrod CG. Treatment of Adult Obstructive Sleep Apnea With Positive Airway Pressure: An American Academy of Sleep Medicine Systematic Review, Meta-Analysis, and GRADE Assessment. *J Clin Sleep Med* 2019;15(2):301-334; with permission.)

ADVANCING POSITIVE AIRWAY PRESSURE ADHERENCE PROTOCOLS IN LARGE-SCALE POSITIVE AIRWAY PRESSURE TRIALS

Recommendations for using evidence-based PAP adherence protocols in large-scale trials include (1) telemonitoring, (2) behavioral approaches, and (3) education. In addition, other methodologies can be leveraged to improve PAP adherence, including (1) using a PAP run-in period, and (2) considering sampling criteria specific to PAP adherence. Because of the well-recognized heterogeneity in PAP adherence behavior and factors that are associated with this behavior,[25,26] a multicomponent PAP adherence protocol is best suited for large-scale trials. Investigative teams will need to carefully balance the complexity and required expertise for these protocols with feasibility and resource considerations. This requirement is particularly poignant because the large-scale PAP trials to date have been severely underfunded (**Box 4**).

Telemonitoring

With the advancement of PAP technology by industry, the field is well positioned to objectively measure PAP adherence and capitalize on near-real-time treatment usage and effectiveness data. Future large-scale trials will leverage this technology in PAP adherence protocols to guide PAP interventions. Study-defined criteria for PAP adherence by study intervals (eg, first week, first month) and by near-real-time intervals (eg, within

---

Box 4
Publicly reported funding of large-scale positive airway pressure efficacy trials (n = 6)

Trial Name	Funding Sources[a]	Publicly Available Total Costs[b] ($)
APPLES	NIH/NHLBI	14,094,332
Spanish Cohort Trial	Sociedad Española de Neumología y Cirugía Torácica	Not available
MOSAIC	British Heart Foundation Oxford Radcliffe Hospitals NHS Trust (United Kingdom)	Not available
HeartBEAT	NIH/NHLBI	3,679,973
SAVE	National Health and Medical Research Council Philips Respironics (industry) Respironics Foundation	8,904,248
ISAACC	ResMed (industry) Fondo de Investigacion Sanitaria (Fondo Europeo de Desarrollo Regional)	Not available

Abbreviation: NHLBI, National Heart, Lung, and Blood Institute.[a]Funding source identified in methodology and/or result publication and/or in trial registry.[b]Data retrieved from funding agency database, when publicly available.

consecutive days) can be established. This approach, if combined with a response-to-PAP-use plan (eg, telecoaching), supports early intervention for PAP nonadherence[29] and conservation of resources within the trial. This approach is important because evidence from observational studies has consistently identified that early PAP use is a predictor of long-term PAP use[30,31]; similarly, analyses of PAP trial data have shown the same.[32,33] The recommendation for using a telemonitoring and response-to-PAP-use protocol within large-scale trials also potentiates engagement, which is a relevant consideration for improving or changing health behaviors.[34–37] Using both participant-facing and trial-facing applications and/or Web-based portals that may be industry supported or study specific are strategies that support PAP use during the active engagement period[37–42]; importantly, PAP use may attenuate after engagement concludes.[38] When using industry-supported applications and telemonitoring platforms, industry partners bring knowledge on how these digital solutions work as well as experience from other trials to support streamlined data acquisition and integration.

When designing the PAP adherence telemonitoring protocol, the following factors should be carefully considered: (1) predefined usage thresholds in industry-supported telemonitoring solutions and the alignment of these thresholds with trial-defined usage criteria; (2) centralized and/or site-level telemonitoring and response-to-PAP-use responsibilities and protocols; (3) resources necessary to maintain telemonitoring protocols; (4) participant burden, including ethical considerations for informed consent language addressing the schedule of interactions (ie, intensity); and (5) innovative approaches that can be used to automate telemonitoring response actions by the trial team, whether at a centralized or site level, with specific intention to deliver response actions by communication methods that are defined by participant preference (eg, video visits, text messaging, online chat access as opposed to telephone calls and face-to-face visits).

Behavioral Approaches

Several behavioral approaches for PAP adherence can be considered for large-scale trials. Behavioral sleep medicine has significantly grown over the past 10 years, as has the interdisciplinary field of experts in behavioral sciences who can provide required expertise for planning and delivering behavioral approaches for PAP adherence in large-scale trials. Determining which behavioral approaches to embed in a large-scale PAP trial

is guided by the evidence at the time of planning the trial, expertise of the trial team, schedule of research visits and/or interactions, and the target population/sample of the trial.

Behavioral interventions tested with positive effects for PAP adherence to date have been delivered at the outset of PAP treatment (eg, at PAP initiation) to PAP-naive adults with OSA.[43–47] Included in this review, 1 large-scale trial indicated by corresponding author communication that motivational or cognitive strategies were used to encourage PAP adherence without further details; this protocol activity was not reported in the study publications.[10,48] Based on the publications and corresponding author communications, it is unknown whether other trials included in this review also used behavioral approaches for PAP adherence. It is recommended that these behavioral protocol activities be fully reported by future large-scale trials. Reporting guidance that can be used include the SPIRIT guidelines[49] (Standard Protocol Items: Recommendations for Interventional Trials) and TIDier[50] (Template Intervention Description and Replication) checklist and guide; both available at https://www.equator-network.org/. Other important considerations for embedding behavioral approaches include (1) timing and format of delivery; (2) centralized and/or site-level oversight, training, and management of behavioral approaches; (3) resources required to maintain delivery of behavioral approaches during trial execution, including fidelity assessments; (4) participant burden, including informed consent language addressing the schedule of interactions (ie, intensity); and (5) including a behavioral scientist as a team member with expertise specific to the phenomenon of PAP adherence, or health behavior.

Education

Disease and treatment education is a practice norm at diagnosis and treatment initiation in OSA, consistently set forth by consensus[23] or strong recommendation.[28] Although the effect of education on PAP adherence is notably modest,[27] it is an essential component of behavior change.[51] Education about OSA and PAP was a consistent protocol activity in the trial setting based on our review of large-scale PAP trials. Considering the diverse (eg, geographic, literacy, culture) nature of participants in PAP randomized trials, and to minimize the risk of excluding subgroups with different or special needs (eg, language, visual impairment, low health and general literacy), the content and delivery modes of education materials should be designed with attention to these needs.

Recent evidence suggests commonly used sleep education materials that are widely available from the American Thoracic Society and American Academy of Sleep Medicine have high health literacy demands, requiring high school level or higher education.[52] Understandability and clear communication indices of the materials were also scored low.[52] The Centers for Disease Control and Prevention and Agency for Healthcare Research and Quality provide explicit guides and information for designing and delivering health information to varied audiences[53,54]; trial teams are urged to use such resources when designing educational materials (see also: http://centerforhealthguidance.org/health-literacy-principles-checklist.pdf). If selecting publicly or commercially available materials for trial use, evaluation of the materials with more than readability procedures is important (eg, Flesch-Kincaid tests). Other recommendations include (1) consulting with or having a team member with education expertise specific to the delivery of health information; (2) pilot testing trial education materials with a representative group of patients and revising materials as indicated; and (3) exploring multimodal delivery of educational materials to trial participants at varied study intervals so as to off-load demands at the outset of PAP initiation.

Incentives

The behavioral economics framework assumes that people make decisions with error and nudges are needed to increase the likelihood of good decisions, or decisions that are in a person's best self-interest.[55,56] Nudges can take many forms, including, but not limited to, incentives and rewards, which may be financial. Using incentives and rewards as an intervention approach for health behavior is an emerging area of study across the literature; however, a small body of evidence exists for PAP adherence in patients, and no studies, to our knowledge, report on incentives directed to research sites/teams for PAP behavioral intervention delivery. Use of incentives in large-scale PAP trials for participants and/or sites and staff must be considered with caution because the effects, ethics, and methodologies are not well understood. As has been recently acknowledged,[57] financial incentives do not always work. There are a myriad of details that must be understood before embedding such incentives in a study; "the devil is in the detail, because the magnitude of effects differs substantially based on the nature of the behavior, the size of the incentive, the population involved, the social context and the design [of the incentive]."[58]

However, if incentives and rewards are conceptualized as nonfinancial, the ethical concern for coercive effects and distributive inequity are lessened.[58] For example, such incentives and rewards might include deidentified performance metrics with comparative ratings and messages (eg, kudos reports), goal tracking worksheets/visualizations to explicate incremental progress with digital badges, and personal rewards to self that are based on self-appraisal metrics. These examples are but a few derived from both behavioral economics theory and the existing PAP adherence evidence that address goal-directed behavior change, engagement, and motivation. Although the state of the science for financial incentives for PAP adherence is still underdeveloped, incentives are likely to be a consideration for future large-scale trials with scientific advancement in behavioral economics for sleep and PAP adherence.[59]

Run-in Methods

Randomized trials may use a run-in, or a prerandomization exposure period to the active or placebo conditions, in order to exclude nonadherers, placebo responders, active condition nonresponders, or active condition intolerance.[60] Run-in methods are common in industry and/or pharmacologic trials, but are less common in PAP trials,[46] including large-scale trials.[9] Using run-in periods is controversial, because external validity is compromised when a run-in period is used[61] because the representativeness of the trial sample necessarily differs from the clinical target population. However, when efficacy is the primary aim of the trial, internal validity is prioritized, unlike in effectiveness trials. Another concern to be carefully considered in implementing a run-in period is the impact that a positive PAP experience, and positive treatment effects, may have on crossover rates, wherein subjects having done well with PAP and then randomized to the comparator condition may decide to obtain PAP therapy outside the trial. Similarly, in trials where active PAP is compared with placebo, or sham PAP, and sham PAP or a modified PAP profile (eg, mask/headgear only) is used during the run-in, subsequent use of PAP, or adherence, may be affected by the run-in experience. For example, cognitive perceptions of PAP are different (eg, lower outcome expectancies) with sham vs active PAP.[62] In addition, when a placebo is the trial comparator, such as with sham PAP, the risk of unblinding must be carefully navigated when using run-in methods.

There are important considerations when planning a run-in period for a large-scale PAP trial, which include (1) monitoring run-in data to support fully reporting the number of run-in exposures conducted, failed run-in rate, and run-in participants' (failed and completed) characteristics compared with the trial sample; (2) determining and reporting run-in PAP adherence criteria, which should be consistent with the postrandomization PAP adherence criteria if the run-in is designed to reduce the overall risk of bias introduced by nonadherence; and (3) determining whether a failed run-in will be repeated based on prespecified criteria. Most trials that have reported run-in periods have not adequately described the run-in protocol or run-in results to address concerns about sample representativeness.[63] As of the writing of this article, there are no published guidelines for run-in period reporting; until such are available, large-scale trials that use a run-in period need to carefully consider the implications of the run-in methods on the overall trial results. Statistical expertise and trial methodologists are recommended to best guide these considerations.

Sampling Criteria Methods

A robust evidence set exists that addresses influential factors on PAP adherence.[25,26,64] The evidence suggests that these factors may be measurable at baseline in the efficacy trial setting and used as sampling criteria to potentiate PAP adherence. When considering this approach, it is important to reflect on how the selected factors may affect enrollment rates and trial sample characteristics. The measurement, or screening, for such factors must also be feasible using validated instruments. Consideration must be given to the burden of measurement, ethical decision-making for sampling criteria, and timing of measuring such factors. If predictive factors of PAP adherence are used as sampling criteria to potentiate PAP use in the efficacy trial setting, this will necessarily have implications on the ability to generalize. For this reason, investigators might examine site-level target population characteristics and determine the effect of imposing the sampling criteria specific to PAP adherence on sample accrual and characteristics at the trial design phase. This approach may best reduce sampling feasibility concerns and also provide data-based insights for statements of the ability to generalize.

Future large-scale trial teams will need to remain abreast of emerging evidence for PAP adherence interventions and use innovative and tested approaches to best optimize PAP adherence in the setting of an efficacy trial. No single approach to PAP adherence interventions within any trial is recommended; instead, evidence-based interventions should be embedded that are aligned with:

- Trial team expertise (discussed next)
- The a priori threshold for PAP adherence for the end point
- The estimated PAP use in the target population based on prior published observational studies or pilot trials
- Trial resources

Both investigators and funding agencies will necessarily embrace increasingly complex trial designs that necessitate thoughtful trial planning periods and nuanced trial management plans/processes and structures for successfully conducting these trials.

WHAT DOES THE FUTURE OF LARGE-SCALE TRIALS OF POSITIVE AIRWAY PRESSURE LOOK LIKE?

Designing and conducting the next generation of large-scale PAP trials is a critical consideration for the field based on recent trial experiences. Explicit opportunities that are germane to addressing the rigor and reproducibility aspects of large-scale prospective PAP trials and thereby reducing concerns for internal validity specific to PAP adherence include (1) trial team composition, (2) operational structure, (3) protocol-within-protocol design, (4) protocol execution, and (5) trial reporting. By setting forth these recommendations for large-scale PAP trials, the stage is set for substantive dialogue among investigators, funding agencies, and trial partners (eg, industry, technology/innovation) in order that best trial practices for large-scale PAP adherence efficacy trials become commonplace.

Trial Team Composition

Adherence to a new health behavior, such as in the trial setting with assignment to PAP among treatment-naive adults with OSA, is challenging for both participants and the trial team. Trial investigators and site staff may have substantial clinical and/or practical experience with introducing PAP and managing PAP adherence but this is not necessarily transferrable to a trial setting. For example, unlike research participants, who should have equipoise about receiving PAP therapy, patients presenting for clinical care, by virtue of seeking care, are motivated to initiate treatment. Also, unlike the clinical setting, time to adherence is of high importance in large-scale PAP trials because of predefined outcome assessments and study resource constraints. Active adherence interventions that consist of more than device/equipment troubleshooting and advice may not be well-developed skills among staff and investigators with primarily practice-based experience who manage a wide range of sleep disorders and treatments.

Behavioral science is a distinct field. Although investigators of these large-scale trials may have practical health behavior experience, this does not necessarily equate to depth and breadth of knowledge and application of behavioral health interventions that are scientifically derived; nor does such practical experience equate to measurable performance outcomes as are necessary in these trials. Trial team composition must therefore be carefully considered at the earliest planning stages of the trial. At the investigator level, a behavioral scientist with expertise in PAP adherence will ideally be included and lead the protocol for PAP adherence. This approach potentiates a scientifically sound protocol specific to PAP adherence and an investigator with committed time and focus for this methodological and implementation work.

Another key consideration for team composition is successfully recruiting and retaining site-level staff members that may, or may not, have relevant experience but who are amenable to learning and consistently applying behavioral protocol activities as prescribed. Retention of staff ensures consistency of contact between the trial site and participants. This point is similarly applicable if a centralized structure, or core, is designated for PAP adherence in the trial. Staff with strong communication skills, including skills for developing rapport and active listening, are imperative to the success of delivering health behavior interventions such as those with positive effects for PAP adherence (see **Fig. 1**). These team composition recommendations are directly supportive of behavioral and implementation science approaches that address partnership, engagement, and collaboration as the cornerstone of health behavior change,[34,65,66] including recent work in the PAP adherence field addressing technology-driven patient engagement,[37] a vision for patient-centered approaches to OSA and PAP management,[67] and emphasis on team approaches for PAP adherence.[68]

The introduction of stakeholder advisory boards, which may include patients, community leaders, and/or clinical providers, has emerged as a research priority in many countries, including the United States, United Kingdom, Canada, and Europe.[69] Designing PAP adherence protocols for use within an efficacy trial with patient stakeholders has yet to be reported to our knowledge; patient engagement across published RCTs has been limited to date.[69] However this approach may be an innovative opportunity for large-scale PAP trials. Patient preferences for protocol activities, such as communication frequency and mechanism, can be accounted for from the outset of the trial with input from patient stakeholders or advisors. This approach may potentiate participant acceptability of the PAP adherence methods and protocols[70] and, thereby, trial enrollment and retention. Resources for researchers considering engagement approaches at any study phase, but as suggested here at the trial design level, can be found at the Patient-Centered Outcomes Research Institute Web site (https://www.pcori.org/engagement/engagement-resources/Engagement-Tool-Resource-Repository).

Operational Structure

From the outset of trial planning, the investigative team should consider the development of a PAP adherence core, a centralized operating structure specific to PAP adherence. Consistent with the more commonly reported trial structure of a sleep reading core or sleep laboratory core, the PAP adherence core investigators who have scientific and implementation expertise in health behavior change and PAP adherence will design protocols specific to PAP adherence that are embedded within the larger trial protocol. Oversight for adherence protocols is a central responsibility of the core, including training, protocol fidelity, and quality of protocol implementation. By centralizing these functions among a dedicated core, the necessary knowledge and skill to support site-based staff and investigators for PAP adherence can be efficiently managed. Increasingly focused intervention approaches to PAP adherence that are evidence based can be designed with an expert core; these approaches can be carefully aligned with the larger trial protocol (ie, protocol within protocol, or a nested protocol). In order for this approach to be successful, the PAP adherence core investigators must be engaged with the trial investigators/team from the earliest point possible in the design of the trial and function as active trial team members. This approach will ensure that all trial activities that bear influence on participants' use of the test condition will be addressed from a behavioral perspective from design through results reporting.

Trial Execution

A dedicated PAP adherence core will necessarily design and deliver training specific to PAP adherence protocols. Because most large-scale trials include a training or education committee, the core will work collaboratively with the larger committee to ensure all trial-specific standards and expectations are met with delivery of PAP adherence training. In the setting of large-scale trials that have numerous geographically dispersed sites, training approaches need to be increasingly innovative but effective in the delivery to conserve trial resources (**Box 5**). Areas of training consideration by the core will include training content, delivery modes and styles of training content, performance standards relative to training sessions and ongoing monitoring performance standards, and certification and recertification of staff for all procedures. Contingency training plans for newly hired staff and for those previously certified staff who show a need for booster training identified during the protocol fidelity monitoring procedure are also recommended.

Fidelity monitoring procedures should be designed by the PAP adherence core and monitoring intervals and procedures established in collaboration with relevant trial entities, most likely to include the Data Coordinating Center (DCC). By establishing partnerships between the core and the DCC, which is a cornerstone of efficient data monitoring in large-scale trials, fidelity monitoring of PAP adherence intervention protocols and performance metrics for quality protocol delivery will be meticulously tracked and communicated to the core and study investigators. Thresholds for fidelity and protocol delivery, established by the core and trial investigators, will subsequently guide remediation, or booster, training decisions, adjustment of monitoring intervals, and trial site evaluation and feedback. Although these thresholds are directly aligned with suboptimal performance, the core will also ideally recognize and reward consistent performance above the threshold and exceptional performance.

Trial Reporting

Reporting of PAP adherence protocols in large-scale trials should be included with the methodology publication and/or with the primary results publication. Although page limitations may be prohibitive of a complete reporting of PAP adherence protocols, supplemental or appendix materials can be used to fully report the protocol. To support both rigor and reproducibility guidelines, a minimum description of PAP adherence protocols should include:

- All intervention approaches used by protocol period/interval
- Complete description of all intervention methods
- PAP adherence criterion and rationale

- Measurement methods of PAP adherence used and measurement intervals
- Description of training for delivery of interventions
- Fidelity monitoring plan, including performance thresholds at study and site levels

---

Box 5
Training approaches for site staff in large-scale positive airway pressure trials: leveraging innovation in delivery, format, and style

- Baseline protocol training
  - Face-to-face delivery
    - Didactic for general protocol information
    - Written materials to reinforce didactically delivered content
    - Diagrammatic materials for protocol scheme, decision making
    - Teach–teach back for protocol delivery to participants
    - Role play for protocol delivery to participants with peer-to-peer evaluation
    - Case-based learning with participant scenarios
  - Review of manual of operations for PAP adherence protocol
- Protocol training refreshers
  - Pocket card deck for PAP adherence protocols and procedures
  - Web-based portal with baseline training materials and access to refresher training materials
  - PAP adherence protocol and procedure checklists
- Periodic booster training (PBT) and new staff training after baseline training (NST)
  - Web-based synchronous videoconferences: challenging scenarios, case-based learning approach (PBT)
  - Web-based asynchronous case-based learning (PBT)
  - Web-based or nudge-based push notifications to Web-based link: brief training modules ($\leq$5 minutes) (PBT)
  - Web-based synchronous and asynchronous training sessions (NST)
  - Peer-to-peer training within sites with expert staff (NST)
  - Simulation training by remote access portal/teleeducation (NST)

When reporting trial results, PAP adherence should be reported as a summary continuous research variable (mean hours per night) at trial end point and by study interval for trial-relevant periods (eg, scheduled recurrent research visits). Because PAP adherence is usually not normally distributed, reporting PAP use by only mean and standard deviation can be misleading. Therefore, the PAP adherence criterion for the trial should also be reported as a frequency at trial end point and by study interval at trial-relevant periods. Any prespecified per-protocol analyses based on PAP adherence should also be reported with trial results. Protocol-based results that are of importance to report include summary fidelity results at the study level and training completion rates, including booster/remediation training conducted throughout the trial period.

SUMMARY

Prospective efficacy trials are requisite to setting forth treatment standards and guidelines and generating causal effects knowledge. Although innovative comparative methodologies that use big data and precision health scientific methods are likely to also contribute treatment standards and guidelines, prospective efficacy trials of a large-scale nature will continue to be necessary. Recent efficacy trials of PAP therapy have been challenged by concerns for validity relative to low PAP use, or nonadherence. Careful scrutiny of these precedents shed light on opportunities to address PAP adherence in forthcoming and subsequent trials. In order that PAP adherence is optimized, evidence-based protocols focused on PAP use should be embedded within the larger trial protocol. In doing so, investigators will need to carefully balance numerous factors relative to feasibility, ethical trial conduct, and overall study rigor. Important considerations are highlighted in this article to facilitate dialogue for best trial practices that are specific to PAP adherence, including reporting guidance at the time of funding application, methodology, and results/protocol publications. It is with attention to these opportunities that there will be reduced concern for the validity of large-scale PAP trial results and these trials will meet expectancies for rigor and reproducibility.

ACKNOWLEDGMENTS

This work was supported in part by NIH/NIDDK (DK120051, principal investigator N.M. Punjabi). The views expressed in this article are those of the authors and do not necessarily reflect the position or policy of the Department of Veterans Affairs or the US government.

DISCLOSURE

Dr A.M. Sawyer has received grant support from NIH, American Nurses Foundation, American Lung Association, and VA HSR&D. Dr D.M. Wallace has no disclosures. Dr L.F. Buenaver discloses grant support from NIH and American Sleep Medicine Foundation. Ms A. Blase is an employee of ResMed Corp. Dr A.J. Watach discloses research training support from NIH (HL07953). Mr B. Saconi has no disclosures. Dr S.R. Patel discloses grant support from NIH (DK120051) and has received grant support from NIH, Bayer Pharmaceuticals, Philips Respironics, and Respicardia. Dr S.T. Kuna discloses grant support from NIH (DK120051). Dr N.M. Punjabi discloses grant support from NIH (NL117167, HL146709, DK120051) and from ResMed and Philips Respironics to Johns Hopkins University.

CLINICS CARE POINTS

- When designing PAP efficacy trials, PAP adherence protocol-in-protocol should be included early in the trial planning process.
- Behavioral specialist with scientific expertise relevant to PAP adherence, or health behavior, will be a trial team member and lead the PAP adherence protocol and, if indicated, centralized adherence core.
- PAP adherence protocol must be feasible and sustainable for large-scale efficacy trials that span multiple sites, include diverse sample members, and that have long-term endpoints.
- Determine and report PAP use (ie, adherence) criterion relative to the primary outcome.

REFERENCES

1. Piantadosi S. Clinical trials: a methodologic perspective. 2nd edition. Hoboken (NJ): John Wiley & Sons, Inc.; 2005.
2. Gottlieb DJ, Yenokyan G, Newman AB, et al. Prospective study of obstructive sleep apnea and incident coronary heart disease and heart failure. Circulation 2010;122(4):352–60.
3. Nieto FJ, Young TB, Lind BK, et al. Association of sleep-disordered breathing, sleep apnea, and hypertension in a large community-based study. JAMA 2000;283:1829–36.
4. Yaggi HK, Concato J, Kernan WN, et al. Obstructive sleep apnea as a risk factor for stroke and death. N Engl J Med 2005;353(19):2034–41.
5. Drager LF, Togeiro SM, Polotsky VY, et al. Obstructive sleep apnea: a cardiometabolic risk in obesity

and the metabolic syndrome. J Am Coll Cardiol 2013;62(7):569–76.

6. Marshall NS, Wong KK, Cullen SR, et al. Sleep apnea and 20-year follow-up for all-cause mortality, stroke, and cancer incidence and mortality in the Busselton Health Study cohort. J Clin Sleep Med 2014;10(4):355–62.

7. Kushida CA, Nichols DA, Holmes TH, et al. Effects of continuous positive airway pressure on neurocognitive function in obstructive sleep apnea patients: the Apnea Positive Pressure Long-term Efficacy Study (APPLES). Sleep 2012;35(12):1593–602.

8. Craig SE, Kohler M, Nicoll D, et al. Continuous positive airway pressure improves sleepiness but not calculated vascular risk in patients with minimally symptomatic obstructive sleep apnoea: the MOSAIC randomised controlled trial. Thorax 2012; 67(12):1090–6.

9. McEvoy RD, Antic NA, Heeley E, et al. CPAP for prevention of cardiovascular events in obstructive sleep apnea. N Engl J Med 2016;375(10):919–31.

10. Sanchez-de-la-Torre M, Sanchez-de-la-Torre A, Bertran S, et al. Effect of obstructive sleep apnoea and its treatment with continuous positive airway pressure on the prevalence of cardiovascular events in patients with acute coronary syndrome (ISAACC study): a randomised controlled trial. Lancet Resp Med 2019. https://doi.org/10.1016/52213-2600(19)30271-1.

11. Barbe F, Duran-Cantolla J, Capote F, et al. Long-term effect of continuous positive airway pressure in hypertensive patients with sleep apnea. Am J Resp Crit Care Med 2010;181(7):718–26.

12. Gottlieb D, Punjabi NM, Mehra R, et al. CPAP versus oxygen in obstructive sleep apnea. N Engl J Med 2014;370(24):2276–85.

13. Collop N, Stierer TL, Shafazand S. SAVE Me from CPAP. J Clin Sleep Med 2016;12(12):1701–4.

14. Furlow B. SAVE trial: no cardiovascular benefits for CPAP in OSA. Lancet Resp Med 2016;4(11):860.

15. Gildeh N, Rosenzweig I, Kent BD. Lessons from randomised controlled trials of continuous positive airways pressure therapy in the prevention of cardiovascular morbidity and mortality. J Thorac Dis 2017; 9(2):244–6.

16. Mokhlesi B, Ayas NT. Cardiovascular events in obstructive sleep apnea — can CPAP therapy SAVE Lives? N Engl J Med 2016;375(10):994–6.

17. Schwartz SW, Cimino CR, Anderson WM. CPAP or placebo-effect? Sleep 2012;35(12):1585–6.

18. Berlowitz DJ, Shafazand S. CPAP and cognition in OSA (APPLES). J Clin Sleep Med 2013;9(5):515–6.

19. Helms RW. Precise definitions of some terminology for longitudinal clinical trials: subjects, patient populations, analysis sets, intention to treat, and related terms. Pharm Stat 2016;15(6):471–85.

20. National Institutes of Health. Guidance: rigor and reproducibility 2019. Available at: https://grants.nih. gov/policy/reproducibility/index.htm. Accessed February 1, 2020.

21. Australian Government National Health and Medical Research Council. NHMRC's research quality strategy 2019. Available at: https://www.nhmrc.gov.au/ research-policy/research-quality. Accessed February 1, 2020.

22. Medical Research Council. Policies and guidance for researchers: research integrity, rigour and reproducibility 2020. Available at: https://mrc.ukri. org/research/policies-and-guidance-for-researchers/. Accessed February 1, 2020.

23. Epstein LJ, Kristo D, Strollo PJ Jr, et al. Clinical guideline for the evaluation, management and long-term care of obstructive sleep apnea in adults. J Clin Sleep Med 2009;5(3):263–76.

24. Rotenberg BW, Murariu D, Pang KP. Trends in CPAP adherence over twenty years of data collection: a flattened curve. J Otolaryngol Head Neck Surg 2016;45:1–9.

25. Crawford MR, Espie CA, Bartlett DJ, et al. Integrating psychology and medicine in CPAP adherence–new concepts? Sleep Med Rev 2014;18(2): 123–39.

26. Sawyer AM, Gooneratne NS, Marcus CL, et al. A systematic review of CPAP adherence across age groups: clinical and empiric insights for developing CPAP adherence interventions. Sleep Med Rev 2011;15:343–56.

27. Patil SP, Ayappa IA, Caples SM, et al. Treatment of adult obstructive sleep apnea with positive airway pressure: an American Academy of sleep medicine systematic review, meta-analysis, and GRADE assessment. J Clin Sleep Med 2019; 15(2):301–34.

28. Patil SP, Ayappa IA, Caples SM, et al. Treatment of adult obstructive sleep apnea with positive airway pressure: an American Academy of sleep medicine clinical practice guideline. J Clin Sleep Med 2019; 15(2):335–43.

29. Aardoom JJ, Loheide-Niesmann L, Ossebaard HC, et al. Effectiveness of eHealth interventions in improving treatment adherence for adults with obstructive sleep apnea: meta-Analytic review. J Med Internet Res 2020;22(2):e16972.

30. Chai-Coetzer CL, Luo YM, Antic NA, et al. Predictors of long-term adherence to continuous positive airway pressure therapy in patients with obstructive sleep apnea and cardiovascular disease in the SAVE study. Sleep 2013;36(12):1929–37.

31. Budhiraja R, Parthasarathy S, Drake CL, et al. Early CPAP use identifies subsequent adherence to CPAP therapy. Sleep 2007;30:320–4.

32. May AM, Gharibeh T, Wang L, et al. CPAP adherence predictors in a randomized trial of moderate-to-severe OSA enriched with women and minorities. Chest 2018;154(3):567–78.

33. Budhiraja R, Kushida CA, Nichols DA, et al. Impact of randomization, clinic visits, and medical and psychiatric cormorbidities on continuous positive airway pressure adherence in obstructive sleep apnea. J Clin Sleep Med 2016;12(3):333–41.

34. Graffigna G, Barello S. Spotlight on the Patient Health Engagement model (PHE model): a psychosocial theory to understand people's meaningful engagement in their own health care. Patient Prefer Adherence 2018;12:1261–71.

35. Greene J, Hibbard JH, Sacks R, et al. When patient activation levels change, health outcomes and costs change, too. Health Aff (Millwood) 2015;34(3):431–7.

36. Gruman J, Rovner MH, French ME, et al. From patient education to patient engagement: implications for the field of patient education. Patient Educ Couns 2010;78(3):350–6.

37. Woehrle H, Arzt M, Graml A, et al. Effect of a patient engagement tool on positive airway pressure adherence: analysis of a German healthcare provider database. Sleep Med 2018;41:20–6.

38. Kuna ST, Shuttleworth D, Chi L, et al. Web-based access to positive airway pressure usage with or without an initial financial incentive improves treatment use in patients with obstructive sleep apnea. Sleep 2015;38(8):1229–36.

39. Malhotra A, Crocker ME, Willes L, et al. Patient engagement using new technology to improve adherence to positive airway pressure therapy: a retrospective analysis. Chest 2018;153(4):843–50.

40. Stepnowsky CJ, Palau JJ, Marler MR, et al. Pilot randomized trial of the effect of wireless telemonitoring on compliance and treatment efficacy of obstructive sleep apnea. J Med Internet Res 2007;9(2):e14.

41. Hwang D, Chang JW, Benjafield AV, et al. Effect of telemedicine education and telemonitoring on continuous positive airway pressure adherence. the tele-osa randomized trial. Am J Resp Crit Care Med 2018;197(1):117–26.

42. Pepin JL, Jullian-Desayes I, Sapene M, et al. Multimodal remote monitoring of high cardiovascular risk patients with OSA Initiating CPAP: a randomized trial. Chest 2019;155(4):730–9.

43. Richards D, Bartlett DJ, Wong K, et al. Increased adherence to CPAP with a group cognitive behavioral treatment intervention: a randomized trial. Sleep 2007;30(5):635–40.

44. Aloia MS, Arnedt JT, Millman RP, et al. Brief behavioral therapies reduce early positive airway pressure discontinuation rates in sleep apnea syndrome: preliminary findings. Behav Sleep Med 2007;5:89–104.

45. Aloia MS, Arnedt JT, Strand M, et al. Motivational enhancement to improve adherence to positive airway pressure in patients with obstructive sleep apnea: a randomized controlled trial. Sleep 2013;36(11):1655–62.

46. Bakker JP, Wang R, Weng J, et al. Motivational enhancement for increasing adherence to CPAP: a randomized controlled trial. Chest 2016;150(2):337–45.

47. Lai AYK, Fong DYT, Lam JCM, et al. The efficacy of a brief motivational enhancement education program on CPAP adherence in OSA: a randomized controlled trial. Chest 2014;146(3):600–10.

48. Esquinas C, Sanchez-de-la Torre M, Aldoma A, et al. Rationale and methodology of the impact of continuous positive airway pressure on patients with ACS and nonsleepy OSA: the ISAACC Trial. Clin Cardiol 2013;36(9):495–501.

49. Chan AW, Tetzlaff JM, Gotzsche PC, et al. SPIRIT 2013 explanation and elaboration: guidance for protocols of clinical trials. BMJ 2013;346:e7586.

50. Hoffmann TC, Glasziou PP, Boutron I, et al. Better reporting of interventions: template for intervention description and replication (TIDieR) checklist and guide. BMJ 2014;348:g1687.

51. Lauver DR, West R, Johnson JE. Nursing science and psychological phenomena. In: Suls JM, Davidson KW, Kaplan RM, editors. Handbook of health Psychology and behavioral medicine. New York: The Guilford Press; 2010. p. 260–76.

52. Dudley KA, Rovnak A, Bertisch SM, et al. High Health Literacy Demands of Patient Education Materials for Obstructive Sleep Apnea. Paper presented at: American Thoracic Society (ATS) International Conference. Washington, DC, May 23, 2017.

53. Centers for Disease Control and Prevention. Health literacy. 2019. Available at: https://www.cdc.gov/healthliteracy/index.html. Accessed February 1, 2020.

54. Agency for Healthcare Research and Quality. AHRQ health literacy universal precautions toolkit 2019. Available at: https://www.ahrq.gov/health-literacy/quality-resources/tools/literacy-toolkit/index.html. Accessed February 1, 2020.

55. Thaler RH. Nudge: improving decisions about health, wealth, and happiness. New Haven: Yale University Press; 2008.

56. Volpp KG, Asch DA. Make the healthy choice the easy choice: using behavioral economics to advance a culture of health. QJM 2017;110(5):271–5.

57. Thirumurthy H, Asch DA, Volpp KG. The uncertain effect of financial incentives to improve health behaviors. JAMA 2019;321(15):1451–2.

58. Vlaev I, King D, Darzi A, et al. Changing health behaviors using financial incentives: a review from behavioral economics. BMC Public Health 2019;19(1):1059.

59. Stevens J. Behavioral economics strategies for promoting adherence to sleep interventions. Sleep Med Rev 2015;23:20–7.

60. Fralick M, Avorn J, Franklin JM, et al. Application and impact of run-in studies. J Gen Intern Med 2018;33(5):759–63.

61. Pablos-Mendez A, Barr RG, Shea S. Run-in periods in randomized trials: implications for the application of results in clinical practice. JAMA 1998;279(3): 222–5.

62. Reid ML, Gleason KJ, Bakker JP, et al. The role of sham continuous positive airway pressure as a placebo in controlled trials: best Apnea Interventions for Research Trial. Sleep 2019;42(8):zsz099.

63. Laursen DRT, Paludan-Muller AS, Hrobjartsson A. Randomized clinical trials with run-in periods: frequency, characteristics and reporting. Clin Epidemiol 2019;11:169–84.

64. Weaver TE, Sawyer A. Adherence to continuous positive airway pressure treatment for obstructive sleep apnoea: implications for future interventions. Indian J Med Res 2010;131:245–58.

65. Huang K-Y, Kwon SC, Cheng S, et al. Unpacking partnership, engagement, and collaboration research to inform implementation strategies development: theoretical frameworks and emerging methodologies. Front Public Health 2018;6:190.

66. Higgins T, Larson E, Schnall R. Unraveling the meaning of patient engagement: a concept analysis. Patient Educ Couns 2017;100(1):30–6.

67. Hilbert J, Yaggi HK. Patient-centered care in obstructive sleep apnea: a vision for the future. Sleep Med Rev 2018;37:138–47.

68. Weaver TE. Novel aspects of CPAP treatment and interventions to improve CPAP adherence. J Clin Med 2019;8(12):2220.

69. Fergusson D, Monfaredi Z, Pussegoda K, et al. The prevalence of patient engagement in published trials: a systematic review. Res Involv Engagem 2018;4:17.

70. Redline S, Baker-Goodwin S, Bakker JP, et al. Patient partnerships transforming sleep medicine research and clinical care: perspectives from the sleep apnea patient-centered outcomes network. J Clin Sleep Med 2016;12(7):1053–8.

TABLE S1: LARGE-SCALE TRIALS: METHODS SPECIFIC TO POSITIVE AIRWAY PRESSURE ADHERENCE BY STUDY PERIOD

Trial Name	Screening Criteria[a] Or Other Prerandomization Methods	Random Assignment[b]	PAP[c] Initiation	Exposure Week 1	Month 1	>Month 1
APPLES[7]	Exclusion: Prior PAP use Other house member with PAP use (current or past)	20-min PAP habituation exercise before titration PSG	CPAP dispense by study personnel after titration PSG	1 wk: phone by RS times 2 • Ensure use •Manage problems •Protocol guide for PAP FAQs (reduce risk of unblinding)[d] Contact with <4 h/night use	Regular contact with <4 h/night use	Regular contact with <4 h/night use 4 mo: FTFV with study physician • Discuss PAP use
Spanish Cohort Trial[11]	NR	NR	CPAP dispensed at home after PSG or unattended HST at sleep center • 5 h sleep • Leak criteria	NR	NR	NR
MOSAIC[8]	Exclusion: prior PAP use	NR	PAP dispensed by study staff after randomization • APAP • Trained staff • Humidity optional • Mask choice	NR	3-wk FTFV •PAP f/u	2-mo phone •Advice •Supplies 4-mo phone •Advice •Supplies PAP use data download minimum once between initiation and end •Residual AHI •Air leaks

HeartBEAT[12]	Exclusion: prior PAP use	NR	APAP dispense by site coordinator with random assign • Autotitrate for 7 d • Then set pressure Instruction by coordinator for use of assigned treatment • Humidity • Mask fit by expert technician Healthy lifestyle and sleep education to both groups by slide presentation, hard copy of slides, publicly available education materials (AHA): • Regular sleep schedule • Avoid ETOH at bedtime • Sleep duration 7–8 h/night	NR	NR	NR
SAVE[9]	Exclusion: Neurologic deficit prevents PAP mask use Prior PAP use Other house member on PAP Other: 1-wk sham run-in to exclude unlikely/unwilling to adhere to PAP; patients informed of run-in purpose; sham device used; phone call run-in day 2–3; run-in criterion ≥3 h/night average	Written information about PAP View DVD: trial importance and adherence to PAP	APAP dispense by study staff at FTFV • Best mask fit • Humidity • Autotitrate for 7 d • Set pressure • Autotitrate criteria: ≥3 h/night average use, average leak <60 L/min • If autotitration criterion not met: Address issues and repeat titration for 7 d	1 wk: phone RS contact • Manage problems Additional phone contact if problems	1 mo: remote review of PAP data by core sleep laboratory • PAP use < 3 h/night • Air leak > 60 L/min • AHI>15/h 1 mo: FTFV as needed for PAP problems Core sleep laboratory monitors PAP use, provides corrective advice to sites, study team	3 mo and 6 mo: Remote review of PAP data by core sleep laboratory • PAP use <3 h/night • Air leak >60 L/min • AHI>15/h Every 6 mo: phone

(continued on next page)

(continued)

Trial Name	Screening Criteria[a] Or Other Prerandomization Methods	Random Assignment[b]	PAP[c] Initiation	Exposure			
				Week 1	Month 1	> Month 1

Trial Name	Screening Criteria[a] Or Other Prerandomization Methods	Random Assignment[b]	PAP[c] Initiation	Week 1	Month 1	> Month 1
ISAACC[10]	Exclusion: prior PAP use	NR	In-hospital (enrolled inpatients) APAP by trained nurse followed by fixed-pressure PAP Behavioral sleep medicine specialist provided pretreatment information; motivational and cognitive strategies to increase PAP use[d]	15 d: phone • Resolve problems • Phone number provided to access study staff any time for PAP problems • FTFV schedule PRN	1 mo: FTFV • Adapt to PAP support • Support PAP adherence using cognitive and motivational strategies[d] • Sleep hygiene advice by sleep unit staff at all scheduled visits; health behavior advice includes avoid evening ETOH, reducing tobacco use, avoiding short sleeps	3 mo: FTFV • Adapt to PAP support • Support PAP adherence

Trial names are in chronologic order by publication date.

Abbreviations: AHA, American Heart Association; AHI, apnea-hypopnea index; APAP, autoadjusting positive airway pressure; APPLES, Apnea Positive Pressure Long-term Efficacy Study; DVD, digital versatile disk; ETOH, alcohol; FAQs, Frequently Asked Questions; FTFV, face-to-face visits; f/u, follow-up; HeartBEAT, Heart Biomarker Evaluation in Apnea Treatment; ISAACC, Impact of Sleep Apnea Syndrome in the Evolution of Acute Coronary syndrome; MOSAIC, Multicenter Obstructive Sleep Apnea Interventional Cardiovascular Trial; NR, none reported; PRN, as needed; PSG, polysomnogram; RS, research staff; SAVE, Sleep Apnea Cardiovascular Endpoints Study.

[a] Inclusion and exclusion criteria that are specified for PAP adherence in methodology and/or supplemental/appendix materials and/or publicly availably protocol materials.

[b] Reported protocol activities specific to PAP use/initiation/adherence conducted concurrent with randomization;

[c] PAP terminology used generically to represent all forms of PAP treatment. Where trials specified type of PAP treatment, the specified type/mode is reported;

[d] Additional information provided by corresponding authors.

What Do We Know About Adherence to Oral Appliances?

Kate Sutherland, PhD[a,b],*, Oyku Dalci, DDS, PhD[c,d], Peter A. Cistulli, MD, PhD[a,b]

KEYWORDS

- Obstructive sleep apnea • Mandibular advancement device • Oral appliance
- Treatment adherence • Compliance monitoring

KEY POINTS

- Oral appliance (OA) therapy for obstructive sleep apnea (OSA) appears to have equivalent short-term health effects to positive airway pressure (PAP) therapy, despite overall lower efficacy.
- OSA patients often report preference of OA over PAP therapy and greater hours of nightly usage; however, until recently, objective adherence data have not been reported.
- Temperature microsensors embedded in appliances have allowed objective assessment of OA usage.
- To date, a small number of studies and participants suggest nightly usage over 6 hours and greater than 80% adherence after 1 year of OA therapy.
- Objective adherence monitors provide opportunity for further research into factors relating to adherence patterns in individual OSA patients and relationship to treatment effectiveness.

INTRODUCTION

Oral appliances (OA) of the mandibular advancement splint variety are recommended for treatment of obstructive sleep apnea (OSA) in patients who are intolerant of positive airway pressure (PAP) therapy or prefer an alternate therapy.[1] PAP has long been the mainstay of OSA therapy because of its high efficacy in preventing obstructive breathing events when worn. OA are generally reserved for second-line therapy, as it is well recognized that OA are variably efficacious in reducing AHI between individuals.[2] In some it works as well as PAP, but in others there may be minimal benefit, which would seem unlikely to translate into health benefit. There are multiple reasons for this variability in the effect of OA on reducing OSA, including individual differences in factors such as obesity, craniofacial structure, and OSA pathophysiology.[3]

When PAP- and OA-treated groups are compared, the mean Apnea-Hypopnea Index (AHI) reduces to less than 5 events per hour on PAP (amelioration of OSA), but tends to remain in the mild range on OA treatment (residual OSA still present).[4] Despite this discrepancy in average efficacy, there are several studies suggesting that health benefits, such as blood pressure reduction,

a Sleep Research Group, Charles Perkins Centre, University of Sydney, Camperdown, Sydney, New South Wales, Australia; b Department of Respiratory & Sleep Medicine, Royal North Shore Hospital, 8A, Acute Services Building, Reserve Road, St Leonards, Sydney, New South Wales 2065, Australia; c Department of Orthodontics and Paediatric Dentistry, University of Sydney, Surry Hills, New South Wales, Australia; d Department of Orthodontics, Sydney Dental Hospital, 2 Chalmers Street, Surry Hills, New South Wales 2010, Australia
* Corresponding author. Department of Respiratory & Sleep Medicine, Royal North Shore Hospital, 8A, Acute Services Building, Reserve Road, St Leonards, Sydney, New South Wales 2065, Australia.
E-mail address: kate.sutherland@sydney.edu.au

Sleep Med Clin 16 (2021) 145–154
https://doi.org/10.1016/j.jsmc.2020.10.004
1556-407X/21/© 2020 Elsevier Inc. All rights reserved.

are similar, at least following short-term therapy.[5,6] It has long been recognized that there can be issues with PAP adherence, with many OSA patients using it at suboptimal nightly usage hours, below the level needed to evoke health outcomes.[7,8] In cross-over trials where participants have experienced both PAP and OA therapies and are asked which therapy they prefer at the end of the trial, in most cases most participants select OA as their preferred therapy over PAP. This finding raises the possibility that the equivalent health effects seen with PAP and OA could be explained by preference for and hence better usage of OA. An OSA patient may have residual OSA with the OA but wear it all night for most nights, which may be more effective than using the highly efficacious PAP occasionally, or for only a few hours of total sleep time. However, solid evidence to support this premise as the explanation for equivalent health outcomes is still needed.

Most of the information on OA usage has been collected from self-report (eg, diaries, questionnaires). It is known that self-report PAP usage is discrepant with objective data from machine download.[9] However, we have only recently entered an era whereby OA adherence can be widely objectively measured, and there is still much to understand about how this treatment is used, particularly over the long term, and how this affects health outcomes. This review summarizes what is known about adherence to OA, particularly what is emerging from objective adherence studies.

ORAL APPLIANCE THERAPY FOR OBSTRUCTIVE SLEEP APNEA BY SELF-REPORT
Long-Term Adherence

Adherence to medical therapy is of utmost importance in the management of chronic conditions, whether in the form of medication or a medical device. It is important to understand long-term OA therapy use. However, systematic information on long-term usage is limited. **Fig. 1** shows discontinuation rates in follow-up of participants in prospective clinical studies. Most studies have followed participants out to 2 years, with an average discontinuation rate of around 40%. There is limited information beyond 2 years of follow-up. Most other information on long-term adherence comes from review and survey of clinical populations by questionnaire.

In a large-scale follow-up, 619 of 630 patients (98%) who received treatment for OSA and snoring with a mono-bloc OA in a single center in Sweden (between years 1989 and 2000) were followed up after 1 year, and some were reevaluated after 10 years.[10] After 1 year, 148 of the 619 patients (24%) had discontinued treatment. A phone survey of OSA patients treated with OA therapy 4 years previously was conducted from a center in Turkey.[11] Sixty-nine of 77 were contactable, and of these, 32% reported regular OA use. Most nonadherent patients stopped within the first year (55%), with an additional 10% in the second year, and 15% in the fourth year of treatment. de Almeida and colleagues[12] in Canada followed up OA-treated patients for an average of 5.7 ± 3.5 years. Of those that returned the mailed questionnaire, 161 (64.1%) were still wearing their OA (users) and 90 patients (35.9%) had stopped treatment (nonusers). Among the users, 82.3% of patients reported wearing their OA every night, and 10.3% of patients used it 4 to 6 nights per week. From the nonusers, 18% stopped wearing their appliance during the first month, 32% in the following 6 months, and another 22% before the end of the first year. The remaining 27% of nonusers stopped using their OA after 1 to 4 years of use. These examples illustrate varying long-term adherence rates, which likely relate to many factors.

Factors Related to Adherence

Patient adherence to different types of OA, including orthodontic appliances, relates to multiple parameters, such as social life, activities, personal preferences, and possible dissatisfactions regarding treatment, and psychological status.[13] Self-reported factors related to poor adherence and discontinuation of OA treatment have included "bothersome to use" and "little or no effect," "tooth discomfort or pain," and "difficulty sleeping" with the appliance and "stifling feeling."[14] Appliance design factors can contribute to comfort, and by extension, adherence. Appliances with less vertical opening and that are titratable were found to be more comfortable for patients.[15] However, there are no randomized clinical trials that investigate adherence to different types of OA with different designs in the long term. Another factor is the amount of mandibular advancement provided by the appliance. There is a relationship with the amount of advancement and the success of OA for therapeutic effect.[16] However, increased mandibular advancement may then increase the risk of having temporomandibular discomfort in some patients in the initial stages of treatment, affecting adherence.

Patients followed for 9 to 24 months after using a bi-bloc appliance most frequently reported side effects of hypersalivation (44%), mucosal dryness (42.3%), and tooth pain (40.6%).[17] However, reported side effects, including subjective occlusal

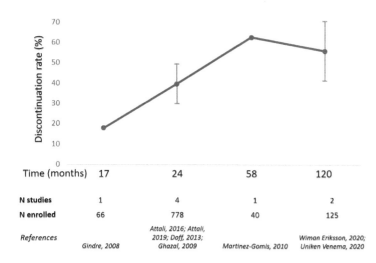

Fig. 1. Discontinuation rates of OA therapy over long-term use. Reported discontinuation rates of OA therapy by follow-up time. Error bars are standard deviation of the mean discontinuation rates of studies (unweighted) reporting that time point. Studies included prospectively enrolled participants in research study (clinical audits not included). (*Date from* Refs.[17,19,43–48])

Time (months)	17	24	58	120
N studies	1	4	1	2
N enrolled	66	778	40	125
References	Gindre, 2008	Attali, 2016; Attali, 2019; Doff, 2013; Ghazal, 2009	Martinez-Gomis, 2010	Wiman Eriksson, 2020; Uniken Venema, 2020

changes, were found to be of mild intensity and did not constitute an obstacle to long-term regular use of OA in this patient cohort. Discomfort, poor effect on snoring, and odontologic problems were the main reasons for discontinuation in the study of greater than 600 OA-treated patients.[10] Tolerability of OA therapy was unrelated to severity of disease, supine-dependent OSA, age, gender, obesity, or pretreatment symptoms. Personal preferences, side effects from the treatment, or the relief of symptoms were suggested as the main reasons for poor or good tolerance.[10]

Over longer follow-up (~5 years), other common reasons for discontinuing treatment included uncomfortable (44.9%), had little or no effect (36.0%), switched to nasal PAP (23.6%), or had experienced a dry mouth (20.2%).[12] Similarly, factors of sex, age, body mass index (BMI), posttitration respiratory disturbance index, and increase in temporomandibular joint (TMJ) symptoms did not show statistically significant difference between OA users and nonusers. When looking at those who discontinued OA therapy early (<6 months), the most common complaints were the OA being uncomfortable and inconvenient,[12] whereas in those who stopped therapy after longer use, changes in occlusion was the most commonly reported reason. The effectiveness of the OA may also decline with the dental changes that take place,[18] and less stability of the appliance has been associated with discontinuation of OA therapy at 2 years.[19] This finding also feeds back to the issue of amount of advancement, which could also increase in dental side effects, causing the appliances to be less effective.[20]

Other factors studied in relation to OA adherence include personality. A type D "distressed" personality (negative affectivity and social inhibition) has been shown to negatively impact

adherence to OA therapy.[21] Personality type may be related to these patients perceiving a higher frequency and magnitude of side effects, decreasing their self-efficacy (confidence to engage in treatment) and objective adherence, and hence their perceived benefit. In this study, 45% of type D patients discontinued OA therapy compared with 15% of non-type D patients.[21] The reasons reported included discomfort and a self-estimated insufficient treatment effect on clinical symptoms like daytime sleepiness and snoring. In regards to OSA treatment, PAP adherence is known to be influenced by the bed partner.[22,23] A bed partner could also influence OA usage, but this has not been investigated.

Adherence to Oral Appliance Therapy Versus Positive Airway Pressure

Treatment effects of OA and PAP appear equivalent on health outcomes, such as quality of life and blood pressure.[4,6] Metaanalysis of treatment usage in 6 trials comparing OA and PAP therapies shows that OA usage is greater than PAP in these short-term studies (1–3 months), with 4 individual trials indicating higher OA usage.[4] The summation of these trials indicates that PAP is used 1.1 hours per night less than OA over the trial period. Greater OA usage could contribute to the equivalent health effects observed despite the presence of higher residual OSA. However, the caveat is that PAP usage was obtained by machine download and OA therapy by self-report.

TEMPERATURE MICROSENSORS FOR OBJECTIVE ADHERENCE DATA

Objective usage monitoring for OA therapy uses temperature data to impute wear of the appliance. Temperature microsensors are embedded or attached to the appliance to collect continual temperature data. When the temperature is within a certain range (generally 31.5–33°C to 38.5–39.2°C), it is assumed that the appliance is in the mouth and hence being used. Outside of this temperature range, the appliance is designated to be in the external environment and not being used. Safety investigations of these microsensors have shown no cytotoxicity[24] or adverse events (oral burn injuries, lesions to the oral mucosa, microsensor detachment) for wear.[25]

There are several temperature microsensor chips available for monitoring OA therapy adherence.[26] All are light in weight (~0.4 g), with sampling intervals from 5 to 15 minutes and storage capacity of a minimum of 100 days of data. Data presentation in software varies by brand. In addition to summary data (h/d), more granular time-stamped data to view daily usage patterns are possible, and 1 brand of microsensor also records head position and how much of usage time was in the supine versus nonsupine position. A base station is required to place on the OA to read the data from the chip. Battery life is reported at around 18 to 24 months, and some sensors have additional capabilities to record head position to designate supine and nonsupine sleep time.[26] Kirshenblatt and colleagues[26] conducted a validation study of 3 different brands of temperature microsensors used by using in vitro short and long wear-time protocols in a water bath set to temperatures to indicate OA wear. All 3 microsensors were deemed to be highly accurate with the differences to water bath time generally less than 5 minutes.

At this time, these adherence monitors are not widely used in clinical practice, and there is a cost associated with adding them to standard therapy and in infrastructure (reading stations, software) for the clinician. Without requirements for adherence monitoring for OA therapy reimbursement, they remain primarily in the realm of a research tool in dental sleep medicine.

OBJECTIVE ADHERENCE MONITORING OF ORAL APPLIANCES

Orthodontic appliances have used objective adherences monitors and provide information of OA adherence, outside the setting of OSA. Orthodontic appliances also potentially need to be worn over many years. Reported adherence to different orthodontic appliances includes extra-oral headgear, intra-OA, such as retainers, that are typically only worn at night, or removable appliances, including functional appliances, which are similar to mandibular advancement

devices used for OSA patients. Timers placed on orthodontic appliances to check adherence date back to 1979.[27] Temperature microsensors, described above, are now commonly used in functional appliances with and without headgear.[28–30] A significant discrepancy between objective and subjective reports in orthodontic appliance use has been shown in systematic review of these indwelling devices with a mean discrepancy of 5 hours a day between self-reported and objectively assessed appliance wear, ranging from nearly 6 hours a day for extra-oral headgears to just more than 3 hours for upper removable appliances that attach on a single jaw.[31] Factors that influence patient adherence to nighttime orthodontic retainers looked into the effects of age, sex, type of retention device (single-jaw Hawley retainer or functional appliance retainer), place of treatment (university hospital or private orthodontic practice), and health insurance status (statutory health insurance or private health insurance).[13] Women, younger patients, and patients from private practices were more adherent, and these parameters influenced the participants' adherence to a greater or lesser extent, but none was statistically significant. For orthodontic appliances the relationship between the clinician and patient plays a key role in patient adherence to the appliance.[32]

OBJECTIVE DATA ON ORAL APPLIANCE THERAPY ADHERENCE FOR OBSTRUCTIVE SLEEP APNEA
Initial Treatment Phase

An early study using a protype temperature sensor showed an average 6.8 hours per night (range 5.6–7.5 hours) in 6 subjects with OSA over a 2-week period.[33] The currently available information on average objective treatment usage time for OA therapy for OSA is summarized in **Table 1**. Most published objective adherence data for OA therapy capture the initial treatment period (up to 3 months). On average, these studies suggest daily adherence greater than 6 hours a night in this early phase of treatment.

Adequate OSA treatment usage is commonly defined as a minimum of 4 hours of daily usage on more than 70% of days.[9] A covert monitoring study (participants not aware of monitoring capabilities of the appliance) from Belgium found 84% of participants, termed "regular users," meet this usage criteria across a 3-month period. This study also collected self-reported sleep time via a daily diary found that treatment usage time as a percent of total sleep time over the 3 months was greater

Table 1
Published objective adherence data for oral appliance therapy

	Study (First Author, Year)	Inclusion Criteria	Microsensor	Covert Monitoring	Time-frame (mo)	N with Data	% Data Loss from Technical issues[a]	Average Daily Usage (Mean ± SD)	Adherence, %
Initial treatment phase (≥3 mo)	Gagnadoux et al,[35] 2017	Age <70 y, PAP intolerant, AHI >30 (exclude BMI >32, ESS >16)	TheraMon	Unclear	2	52	15	6.6 ± 1.4	(1) 96.1
	Vanderveken,[25] 2012	No OA contraindications	TheraMon	Yes	3	43	15.7	6.6 ± 1.3	(2) 84
	de Vries et al,[34] 2019	AHI (15–30), no OA contraindications, no previous OSA treatment	TheraMon	No	3	15	26.7	7.4 (5.2–8.2)[b]	(1) 91.9
	Mullane & Loke,[37] 2019	PAP intolerant	Dual sensor with idle/active modes[49]	Yes	1	21	9.5	5.49 ± 2.93	(2) 33
	Inoko et al,[24] 2009	AHI >5	Thermochron iButton	Yes	1	6	0	6.5 ± 0.71	NR
							TOTAL	6.5 ± 0.7	
Long-term follow-up (1 y)	Dieltjens,[38] 2013	No OA contraindications	TheraMon	Yes	12	37	16	6.4 ± 1.7	(1) 85 (2) 82
	de Vries et al,[34] 2019	AHI (15–30), no OA contraindications, no previous OSA treatment	TheraMon	No	12	14	7.1	6.9 (3.5–7.9)[b]	(1) 88.7
							TOTAL	6.7 ± 0.4	

Data presented are mean ± standard deviation (SD), unless otherwise indicated.

Abbreviation: NR, not reported; apnea.

[a] Data loss of objective usage occurred for various reasons in these studies, including failure to retrieve data from chip, exceeding data storage and recording over previous data, and chip activation failure or delay.

[b] Median (interquartile range). The total reflects the mean of average usage data reported in these studies. Adherence was reported by various definitions: (1) percentage of participants that used therapy for ≥4 h per day across the treatment period, (2) percentage of participants using therapy for ≥4 h per day on 70% of days across the treatment period. Whether the purpose of the microsensor in recording adherence was concealed from the participants (covert monitoring) is indicated.

than 90%. In a parallel group randomized trial, 15 participants on OA therapy showed that 91.9% were meeting a daily usage target of 4 hours after 3 months of therapy.[34] Objective usage was reported for both active and sham (upper plate only) appliances in a 2-month parallel group study.[35] Active therapy average usage was greater than the sham device (6.6 vs 5.6 hours), and active therapy was associated with high rates of users achieving greater than 4 hours per night (96.1% vs 73.6%). However, in a series of PAP-intolerant men over 1 month of OA therapy, only 33% could be classified as "regular users." There are likely to be different subtypes of users in clinical samples. The authors used objective OA data from the initial 60 days of OA therapy.[36] Cluster analysis was used to identify subgroups with similar usage patterns. Of the 58 OA-treated OSA patients, 48.3% could be termed "consistent" users, 32.8% "patchy" users, and 19% "nonusers."[36] Further investigation of treatment user subtypes may have important clinical implications for early intervention in nonusers.

Treatment Usage Trajectories

Treatment usage could follow different trajectories, for example, a user may increase usage of OA therapy as they become accustomed to the device and initial side effects subside. In examination of trajectories in the initial treatment period, a month-by-month analysis of the first 3 months showed stability in daily usage hours for each month.[25] The proportion of regular users ($\geq$4 hours per night on $\geq$70% of nights) decreased slightly from 90% after the first month to 84% in month 3. However, 84% of participants remained regular users at each month, suggesting most users are good adherers from the start and remain so. In contrast, a small Texan study of the first 4 weeks of OA therapy in PAP failures overall showed a much lower rate of regular users across the study (33%).[37] This study did appear to show an early usage trajectory with regular usage rates in the first week at 26%, which increased to 50% in the fourth week of treatment.

To date, 2 studies have followed participants with OA with embedded microsensors out to 12 months after implementation.[34,38] The data suggest relatively stable hours of usage in those still on therapy, with no statistical difference between months 3 and 12 (see **Table 1**). The discontinuation rate for OA therapy was reported at 9.8% at 1 year of those eligible for 1-year follow-up.[38] Therefore, daily usage in treatment adherers remains relatively constant long term, at least out

to 1 year after initiation in the relatively small number of participants assessed.

Self-Report Usage Versus Objective Data

A daily usage and sleep time diary was completed by participants during 3 months of covert collection of objective usage data.[25] There was no significant difference between self-report usage and microsensor data for average daily hours of usage at each monthly interval. At the 12-month follow-up, participants provided estimates of subjective hours of OA usage in hours per night and days per week[38]; again no significant difference between objective and self-reported OA usage was found.

In the sham-controlled trial,[35] participants completed a diary for the 2-month trial period indicating hours used each day for their active or sham therapy. There was a slight overestimation compared with objective data with the active therapy (7.3 subjective hours per night vs 6.6 objective hours per night). Over-reporting of usage was more pronounced in the sham therapy (6.8 subjective hours per night vs 5.6 objective hours per night). When comparing objective to subjective nightly hours, there was a moderate correlation between the two for active therapy, with no relationship between subjective and objective usage hours for the sham arm. Other studies have reported strong correlation between objective and subjective measures over 4 weeks[37] and no difference in average usage time at 12 months.[34] Available data suggest that subjective estimates of OA therapy usage are relatively concordant.

Oral Appliances Versus Positive Airway Pressure

Commercially available compliance monitors will make objective comparisons of OA and PAP therapies possible for future studies. To date, objective adherence data for both therapies are available from 1 parallel group study.[34] In this study of adherence data from 21 PAP-treated participants and 14 OA-treated participants, there was no difference in objective daily usage hours or adherence rates between the 2 treatments at 3 months (median usage hours OA 7.4 vs PAP 6.8), 6 months (OA 6.8 vs PAP 6.9 hours per night), or 12 months (OA 6.9 vs PAP 6.8 hours per night). Although there was a suggestion of more hours of usage with OA on days when worn compared with PAP during the initial period (although did not reach statistical significance),[34] participants in this study were aware their treatment adherence was being recorded and were fed back information about their usage at study visits. The impact of this will need to be investigated in future comparative studies.

Predictors of Oral Appliance Adherence

One use of objective adherence data is to understand adherence patterns to OA therapy and what factors may contribute to poor adherence in order to intervene. Dieltjens and colleagues[39] explored association of 3 months of objective usage data with anthropometric and polysomnographic data, as well as OA-associated side effects and OSA symptoms and snoring. No associations with anthropometric or polysomnographic data were found. Treatment usage was not associated with baseline or posttreatment changes in AHI or subjective daytime sleepiness (Epworth Sleepiness Scale [ESS]) but showed a moderate correlation with improvement in snoring on a visual analogue scale. The frequency of side effects was assessed for hypersalivation, xerostomia, tooth pain or discomfort, TMJ pain, generally or in the morning. Dry mouth was the only side effect to show a modest correlation with reduced usage hours. Mullane and Loke[37] asked participants to grade the severity of their side effects (none, mild, moderate, severe). There was an association with nonmild severity side effects to have greater usage (>5.5 hours), with severe reporting of side effects mean usage time less than 4 hours per night. The side effects significantly related to noncompliance were "noises in jaw joint," "jaw discomfort," and "gum discomfort." This study also did not find association with treatment usage and baseline AHI or ESS.

FUTURE DIRECTIONS

Temperature microsensors embedded in OA for objective adherence data have the potential to open avenues to understand OA treatment effects, and subsequent tailoring of therapy. Collection of digital health data also opens up "big data" opportunities for OA research.

Evidence of equivalent health outcomes between OA and PAP, at least in the short term, suggests that real-world treatment effectiveness is not necessarily captured by AHI on treatment. However, currently, this remains the metric on which clinical decisions are primarily made. The different treatment profiles of PAP (high efficacy/low adherence) and OA (moderate efficacy/high adherence) may conceptually result in similar profiles of treatment effectiveness.[40] Treatment effectiveness is a composite of efficacy (degree to which the treatment reduces the AHI) and adherence (hours of sleep used). Hence, the advent of objective monitoring capabilities for OA therapy enables the ability to assess this component of effectiveness. A measurement of "Mean Disease Alleviation" has been proposed,[25] in which efficacy and time on treatment for the sleep period are combined to give an estimate of effectiveness (**Fig. 2**). Such effectiveness calculations could be a more suitable means to compare OSA treatments with different efficacy and adherence profiles and between individuals. To date, these metrics of measuring disease alleviation have not been measured and compared with health outcomes. A step further on assessing treatment effectiveness is to incorporate components of real-time efficacy for sleep time on and off treatment. Digital innovations that integrate objective information about efficacy, compliance, and sleep duration will enhance the ability to assess treatment effectiveness and its links to health outcomes. Future comparative effectiveness research of PAP and OA treatment could allow patients more freedom to choose their preferred treatment over all aspects of treatment effectiveness and health outcomes.

In addition, objective monitors for OA therapy could create "big data" and patient engagement opportunities, similar to those that have emerged for PAP therapy. The latest generation of PAP devices has an on-board mobile communication that connects to a secure cloud infrastructure automatically, thereby enabling continuously wireless connectivity on a daily basis to capture compliance and therapy data. Wirelessly collected data can also be shared with the patient, either through a Web portal or through the use of mobile phone applications ("Apps") that aim to enhance patient engagement with therapy. Such digital capabilities have been used to draw large-scale "real-world" insights about PAP compliance[41] and the positive influence of patient engagement tools.[42] The OA field is lagging behind in such capabilities, but there are positive signs on the horizon. Efforts are underway to develop additional intraoral and/or wearable sensors that will augment the compliance data that are currently available. Nightly objective information about treatment efficacy and sleep duration is feasible and will generate big data opportunities for the field.

SUMMARY

The emergence of objective adherence monitors for OA therapy has provided initial data on average usage time, now out to 1 year of treatment. However, to date, these studies remain small, and more information is needed to understand OA adherence patterns in different populations and

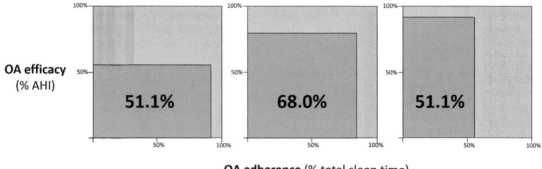

OA adherence (% total sleep time)

☐ Mean Disease Alleviation

Fig. 2. Mean disease alleviation (MDA) measurement. Treatment effectiveness depends on how well a therapy works (*efficacy*) but also how it is used (*adherence*). Traditionally, OSA therapy has only been assessed by the AHI, an efficacy metric. Treatment effectiveness measures aim to incorporate both efficacy and adherence into a single metric. The MDA percentage expresses both usage over the sleep period and efficacy while on treatment. The MDA is given by the area of the rectangle bounded by the efficacy and adherence values (*green*). Adherence is adjusted to a proportion of total sleep time. The MDA percentage for various combinations of adherence and efficacy. An equivalent MDA can be seen with different efficacy and adherence profiles. Temperature microsensors for OA therapy could provide objective usage information for treatment effectiveness metrics. Further work is needed to compare these metrics to health outcomes to determine if they are a more useful way of understanding OSA therapy outcomes. (*Adapted from* Vanderveken OM, Dieltjens M, Wouters K, De Backer WA, Van de Heyning PH, Braem MJ. Objective measurement of compliance during oral appliance therapy for sleep-disordered breathing. *Thorax.* 2013;68(1):91-96; with permission.)

across individuals. An outstanding question is an objective comparison to PAP adherence; an initial small study has not identified a difference in average nightly usage rates at 1 year, in contrast to studies using self-report data. However, larger samples are needed. Technology, such as adherence microsensors, in combination with other sensors, provides a means to more completely measure treatment effectiveness. Objective monitoring will facilitate comparative effectiveness studies between these 2 OSA therapies. As more objective adherence data for OA are collected, an opportunity to identify individual patterns and relate these to clinical outcomes will ultimately facilitate participatory care and patient-centered outcomes as part of a future of precision sleep medicine.

CLINICS CARE POINTS

- Data on objective usage hours of oral appliances for OSA is limited but suggests nightly adherence remains high (>6 hours) out to one year of follow-up.
- Patient report of daily usage hours of oral appliance therapy appears to be relatively consistent with objective data.
- Initial frequency and severity of side effects related to device wear are likely to reduce usage hours.

- Usage data beyond a year is not currently available but increasing discontinuation rates over time warrants yearly clinical follow-up of patients undergoing oral appliance therapy.

DISCLOSURE

K. Sutherland has received in kind support from SomnoMed Australia in the form of donation of oral appliances for investigator-initiated research. P.A. Cistulli holds an endowed academic Chair at the University of Sydney, established through funding from ResMed. P.A. Cistulli has received research support from ResMed, SomnoMed, Zephyr Sleep Technologies, and Bayer. He is a consultant/adviser to Zephyr Sleep Technologies, ResMed, and SomnoMed. He has a pecuniary interest in SomnoMed related to a previous role in R&D (2004). He has received speaker fees from Nox Medical and ResMed. O. Dalci has no conflicts to disclose.

REFERENCES

1. Ramar K, Dort LC, Katz SG, et al. Clinical practice guideline for the treatment of obstructive sleep apnea and snoring with oral appliance therapy: an update for 2015. J Clin Sleep Med 2015;11(7): 773–827.
2. Sutherland K, Takaya H, Qian J, et al. Oral appliance treatment response and polysomnographic

phenotypes of obstructive sleep apnea. J Clin Sleep Med 2015;11(8):861–8.

3. Chen H, Eckert DJ, van der Stelt PF, et al. Phenotypes of responders to mandibular advancement device therapy in obstructive sleep apnea patients: a systematic review and meta-analysis. Sleep Med Rev 2020;49:101229.

4. Schwartz M, Acosta L, Hung YL, et al. Effects of CPAP and mandibular advancement device treatment in obstructive sleep apnea patients: a systematic review and meta-analysis. Sleep Breath 2018; 22(3):555–68.

5. Phillips CL, Grunstein RR, Darendeliler MA, et al. Health outcomes of continuous positive airway pressure versus oral appliance treatment for obstructive sleep apnea: a randomized controlled trial. Am J Respir Crit Care Med 2013;187(8): 879–87.

6. Bratton DJ, Gaisl T, Wons AM, et al. CPAP vs mandibular advancement devices and blood pressure in patients with obstructive sleep apnea: a systematic review and meta-analysis. JAMA 2015; 314(21):2280–93.

7. Weaver TE, Maislin G, Dinges DF, et al. Relationship between hours of CPAP use and achieving normal levels of sleepiness and daily functioning. Sleep 2007;30(6):711–9.

8. Antic NA, Catcheside P, Buchan C, et al. The effect of CPAP in normalizing daytime sleepiness, quality of life, and neurocognitive function in patients with moderate to severe OSA. Sleep 2011; 34(1):111–9.

9. Kribbs NB, Pack AI, Kline LR, et al. Objective measurement of patterns of nasal CPAP use by patients with obstructive sleep apnea. Am Rev Respir Dis 1993;147(4):887–95.

10. Marklund M, Stenlund H, Franklin KA. Mandibular advancement devices in 630 men and women with obstructive sleep apnea and snoring: tolerability and predictors of treatment success. Chest 2004; 125(4):1270–8.

11. Saglam-Aydinatay B, Taner T. Oral appliance therapy in obstructive sleep apnea: long-term adherence and patients experiences. Med Oral Patol Oral Cir Bucal 2018;23(1):e72–7.

12. de Almeida FR, Lowe AA, Tsuiki S, et al. Long-term compliance and side effects of oral appliances used for the treatment of snoring and obstructive sleep apnea syndrome. J Clin Sleep Med 2005; 1(2):143–52.

13. Schott TC, Schlipf C, Glasl B, et al. Quantification of patient compliance with Hawley retainers and removable functional appliances during the retention phase. Am J Orthod Dentofacial Orthop 2013; 144(4):533–40.

14. Nishigawa K, Hayama R, Matsuka Y. Complications causing patients to discontinue using oral appliances for treatment of obstructive sleep apnea. J Prosthodont Res 2017;61(2):133–8.

15. Pitsis AJ, Darendeliler MA, Gotsopoulos H, et al. Effect of vertical dimension on efficacy of oral appliance therapy in obstructive sleep apnea. Am J Respir Crit Care Med 2002;166(6):860–4.

16. Bamagoos AA, Cistulli PA, Sutherland K, et al. Dose-dependent effects of mandibular advancement on upper airway collapsibility and muscle function in obstructive sleep apnea. Sleep 2019; 42(6):zsz049.

17. Gindre L, Gagnadoux F, Meslier N, et al. Mandibular advancement for obstructive sleep apnea: dose effect on apnea, long-term use and tolerance. Respiration 2008;76(4):386–92.

18. Marklund M. Update on oral appliance therapy for OSA. Curr Sleep Med Rep 2017;3(3):143–51.

19. Doff MH, Hoekema A, Wijkstra PJ, et al. Oral appliance versus continuous positive airway pressure in obstructive sleep apnea syndrome: a 2-year follow-up. Sleep 2013;36(9):1289–96.

20. Doff MH, Veldhuis SK, Hoekema A, et al. Long-term oral appliance therapy in obstructive sleep apnea syndrome: a controlled study on temporomandibular side effects. Clin Oral Investig 2012;16(3): 689–97.

21. Dieltjens M, Vanderveken OM, Van den Bosch D, et al. Impact of type D personality on adherence to oral appliance therapy for sleep-disordered breathing. Sleep Breath 2013;17(3):985–91.

22. Gagnadoux F, Le Vaillant M, Goupil F, et al. Influence of marital status and employment status on long-term adherence with continuous positive airway pressure in sleep apnea patients. PLoS One 2011; 6(8):e22503.

23. Baron KG, Smith TW, Berg CA, et al. Spousal involvement in CPAP adherence among patients with obstructive sleep apnea. Sleep Breath 2011; 15(3):525–34.

24. Inoko Y, Yoshimura K, Kato C, et al. Efficacy and safety of temperature data loggers in measuring compliance with the use of oral appliances. Sleep Biol Rhythms 2009;7(3):188–92.

25. Vanderveken OM, Dieltjens M, Wouters K, et al. Objective measurement of compliance during oral appliance therapy for sleep-disordered breathing. Thorax 2013;68(1):91–6.

26. Kirshenblatt S, Chen H, Dieltjens M, et al. Accuracy of thermosensitive microsensors intended to monitor patient use of removable oral appliances. J Can Dent Assoc 2018;84:i2.

27. Clemmer EJ, Hayes EW. Patient cooperation in wearing orthodontic headgear. Am J Orthod 1979;75(5): 517–24.

28. Pauls A, Nienkemper M, Panayotidis A, et al. Effects of wear time recording on the patient's compliance. Angle Orthod 2013;83(6):1002–8.

29. Schott TC, Meyer-Gutknecht H, Mayer N, et al. A comparison between indirect and objective wear-time assessment of removable orthodontic appliances. Eur J Orthod 2017;39(2):170–5.

30. Arponen H, Hirvensalo R, Lindgren V, et al. Treatment compliance of adolescent orthodontic patients with headgear activator and twin-block appliance assessed prospectively using microelectronic wear-time documentation. Eur J Orthod 2020;42(2):180–6.

31. Al-Moghrabi D, Salazar FC, Pandis N, et al. Compliance with removable orthodontic appliances and adjuncts: a systematic review and meta-analysis. Am J Orthod Dentofacial Orthop 2017;152(1):17–32.

32. Schafer K, Ludwig B, Meyer-Gutknecht H, et al. Quantifying patient adherence during active orthodontic treatment with removable appliances using microelectronic wear-time documentation. Eur J Orthod 2015;37(1):73–80.

33. Lowe AA, Sjoholm TT, Ryan CF, et al. Treatment, airway and compliance effects of a titratable oral appliance. Sleep 2000;23(Suppl 4):S172–8.

34. de Vries GE, Hoekema A, Claessen J, et al. Long-term objective adherence to mandibular advancement device therapy versus continuous positive airway pressure in patients with moderate obstructive sleep apnea. J Clin Sleep Med 2019;15(11):1655–63.

35. Gagnadoux F, Pepin JL, Vielle B, et al. Impact of mandibular advancement therapy on endothelial function in severe obstructive sleep apnea. Am J Respir Crit Care Med 2017;195(9):1244–52.

36. Sutherland K, Almeida FR, Kim T, et al. Treatment usage patterns across the first 60 days of oral appliance therapy: a cluster analysis. Paper presented at: Sleep Down Under 2019. Sydney, October 19, 2019.

37. Mullane S, Loke W. Influence of short-term side effects on oral sleep appliance compliance among CPAP-intolerant patients: an objective monitoring of compliance. J Oral Rehabil 2019;46(8):715–22.

38. Dieltjens M, Braem MJ, Vroegop A, et al. Objectively measured vs self-reported compliance during oral appliance therapy for sleep-disordered breathing. Chest 2013;144(5):1495–502.

39. Dieltjens M, Verbruggen AE, Braem MJ, et al. Determinants of objective compliance during oral appliance therapy in patients with sleep-disordered breathing: a prospective clinical trial. JAMA Otolaryngol Head Neck Surg 2015;141(10):894–900.

40. Sutherland K, Phillips CL, Cistulli PA. Efficacy versus effectiveness in the treatment of obstructive sleep apnea: CPAP and oral appliances. J Dent Sleep Med 2015;2(4):175–81.

41. Cistulli PA, Armitstead J, Pepin JL, et al. Short-term CPAP adherence in obstructive sleep apnea: a big data analysis using real world data. Sleep Med 2019;59:114–6.

42. Malhotra A, Crocker ME, Willes L, et al. Patient engagement using new technology to improve adherence to positive airway pressure therapy: a retrospective analysis. Chest 2018;153(4):843–50.

43. Attali V, Chaumereuil C, Arnulf I, et al. Predictors of long-term effectiveness to mandibular repositioning device treatment in obstructive sleep apnea patients after 1000 days. Sleep Med 2016;27-28:107–14.

44. Attali V, Vecchierini MF, Collet JM, et al. Efficacy and tolerability of a custom-made Narval mandibular repositioning device for the treatment of obstructive sleep apnea: ORCADES study 2-year follow-up data. Sleep Med 2019;63:64–74.

45. Ghazal A, Sorichter S, Jonas I, et al. A randomized prospective long-term study of two oral appliances for sleep apnoea treatment. J Sleep Res 2009;18(3):321–8.

46. Martinez-Gomis J, Willaert E, Nogues L, et al. Five years of sleep apnea treatment with a mandibular advancement device. Side effects and technical complications. Angle Orthod 2010;80(1):30–6.

47. Uniken Venema JAM, Doff MHJ, Joffe-Sokolova D, et al. Long-term obstructive sleep apnea therapy; a 10-year follow-up of mandibular advancement device and continuous positive airway pressure. J Clin Sleep Med 2020;16(3):353–9.

48. Wiman Eriksson E, Leissner L, Isacsson G, et al. A prospective 10-year follow-up polygraphic study of patients treated with a mandibular protruding device. Sleep Breath 2015;19(1):393–401.

49. Smith YK, Verrett RG. Evaluation of a novel device for measuring patient compliance with oral appliances in the treatment of obstructive sleep apnea. J Prosthodont 2014;23(1):31–8.

Adherence to Cognitive Behavior Therapy for Insomnia
An Updated Systematic Review

Sommer Agnew, MSc[a], Annie Vallières, PhD[b], Ailie Hamilton, MSc[a],
Stephanie McCrory, MSc[a], Marek Nikolic, MSc[a], Simon D. Kyle, PhD[c],
Leanne Fleming, PhD[a], Megan R. Crawford, PhD[a],*

KEYWORDS

• Adherence • Compliance • Insomnia • Cognitive behavior therapy

KEY POINTS

• Adherence to cognitive behavior therapy for insomnia (CBT-I) is complex and requires clear definitions.
• The literature on adherence to CBT-I is heterogeneous and researchers/clinicians need to work towards a consensus on how to measure and operationalize adherence.
• Studies need to examinie the relationship between adherence and treatment outcome.

INTRODUCTION

Chronic insomnia is a major public health concern, being the most prevalent sleep problem, and estimated to affect 6% to 10% of adults.[1] The current treatment of choice for chronic insomnia is cognitive behavior therapy for insomnia (CBT-I), a multicomponent intervention typically involving strategies such as cognitive restructuring, sleep restriction, stimulus control, sleep hygiene education, and relaxation therapy (**Table 1**).[2,3] CBT-I is effective in reducing insomnia symptoms, improving self-reported sleep onset latency (SOL), and reducing wakefulness after sleep onset (WASO), with improvements still present at postintervention follow-ups.[4,5] Although CBT-I has considerable empirical support, it often requires behavioral and lifestyle changes that are intrusive and may be difficult to implement. For example, sleep restriction involves reducing time spent in bed to a therapist-prescribed sleep window, in order to increase sleep efficiency (the proportion of time in bed [TIB] spent sleeping).[6] Patients reportedly struggle to implement sleep restriction therapy (SRT) because of the initial reduction in sleep opportunity leading to temporary sleep deprivation, increased daytime sleepiness, and impaired daytime functioning.[6,7] Adherence may be particularly difficult when insomnia treatment involves lifestyle changes that require modification of habit, which in the case of insomnia can often be long standing.

Patient adherence is important for establishing which aspects of therapy are particularly effective. The term adherence (vs the outdated term compliance) acknowledges the patient's ability to decide whether to follow recommendations, and thus typically encapsulates the patient's behavior as well as beliefs, attitudes and motivations.[8] Conceptualizing something like adherence to

[a] School of Psychological Sciences and Health, Graham Hills Building, 40 George Street, Glasgow, G1 1QE, UK;
[b] École de psychologie, Pavillon Félix-Antoine-Savard, Université Laval, 2325 rue des bibliothèques, Félix-Antoine-Savard Local 1044, Québec, QC G1V 0A6, Canada; [c] Sleep and Circadian Neuroscience Institute, Nuffield Department of Clinical Neurosciences, University of Oxford, Oxford OX3 9DU, UK
* Corresponding author.
E-mail address: megan.crawford@strath.ac.uk
Twitter: @MeganRDC (M.R.C.)

Sleep Med Clin 16 (2021) 155–202
https://doi.org/10.1016/j.jsmc.2020.11.002
1556-407X/21/© 2020 Elsevier Inc. All rights reserved.

Table 1
Description of cognitive behavior therapy for insomnia components

CBT-I Components	Definition
Cognitive restructuring	Identifying and challenging negative/maladaptive thoughts about sleep
Sleep restriction	Reducing overall time spent in bed to increase homeostatic drive for sleep
Stimulus control	Ensuring bed/bedroom is a strong cue for sleep by reducing time spent in bed for nonsleep behaviors; getting out of bed at night if unable to sleep after 15 min, no daytime naps
Sleep hygiene education	Learning about behaviors conducive to good sleep, such as reducing caffeine consumption; relaxing for a set amount of time before bed (creating a buffer zone); and ensuring the bedroom is a quiet, dark space at a comfortable temperature
Relaxation therapy	May include progressive muscle relaxation, breathing exercises, and guided imagery

medication is simple; the question is whether the patient has taken the medication or not. Adherence to CBT-I is more complex, because it is a multicomponent intervention; the "dose" of therapy is ill defined, so optimal levels of adherence cannot be determined; and there are variations in the way that treatment is delivered (eg, different combinations of components). Consequently, it is not clear which elements of the intervention are the mechanistic drivers of improvement, and which factors predict nonadherence. A 2013 systematic review of adherence to CBT-I[9] identified considerable heterogeneity in the way adherence to CBT-I was operationalized and measured. The current literature review therefore discusses whether clinical trials involving CBT for patients with insomnia published since Matthews and colleagues'[9] review in 2013 have (1) measured adherence and whether this has been more homogeneous, (2) reported any relationship between adherence and CBT-I outcomes, and (3) identified any consistent factors influencing adherence to CBT-I.

METHODS
Searches

The protocol for this review was registered at OSF (https://osf.io/tf7hp/). A systematic literature search was performed with the assistance of a trained social sciences librarian. Searches were performed in November 2019, in the databases PsychInfo, MEDLINE, and Scopus. PubMed was not used as a search engine, based on advice by the librarian, because it is similar to MEDLINE and might have generated several duplicates. In PsychInfo and Scopus, full texts were searched for combinations of: ("cognitive behavio* therap*" or "sleep restriction" or "sleep hygiene" or "stimulus control" or "sleep education" or relaxation or

"cognitive therap*"), ("sleep disorder*" or insomnia), and (adherence or compliance or nonadherence or noncompliance or attrition). Searches were filtered to include only journal articles including human samples, written in English or German. The search in the MEDLINE database included the same search terms as keywords and relevant subject headings. Searches were limited to articles published from May 2012 onward, because the most recent systematic review in this area[9] was conducted until this point. The search terms and criteria used in the Matthews and colleagues[9] review were used for this review. References of articles were reviewed to determine any articles that were missed in the literature searches. Articles that were published since the end of our literature search were reviewed and included where appropriate.

Inclusion/Exclusion Criteria

Studies that met the following criteria were included within the review: (1) peer-reviewed articles; (2) written in English or German; (3) measured adherence, meaning implementing behavior change (not simply attrition or session attendance/engagement with the digital intervention); (4) assessed a CBT-I intervention; (5) adult participants with insomnia (either characterized as sleep difficulties or measured via clinical assessment). The following exclusion criteria were used: (1) pediatric or adolescent samples; (2) or having only measured participant attendance or attrition/engagement in the digital intervention; and (3) qualitative articles, editorials, single case studies, and literature reviews. When choosing a reason for exclusion, we used the hierarchy of (1) no insomnia, (2) no CBT-I, (3) pediatric/adolescent sample, (4) ongoing study, (5) measured attrition (not adherence), thus almost following PICO (patient, intervention, comparison, outcome) order.

Screening Procedures

Search results were uploaded to the screening platform Covidence (https://www.covidence.org/), which is an online platform provided by the Cochrane Community, to facilitate systematic reviews. Titles and abstracts were screened by 2 reviewers (M.C. or S.A. and either M.K., A.H., or S.M. who were blind to each other's decisions), and conflicts were resolved by a third reviewer. The full texts of the articles included at this stage were then screened by 2 independent reviewers (M.C. and then either S.A., M.K., A.H., or S.M.), with conflicts resolved by a third author to determine which articles should be included in the final review.

Quality Assessment

Studies were assessed for quality of adherence data by considering the description of measures and whether the data were direct (self-reported), indirect, or clinician/spouse reported. Self-report questionnaires (validated or not) were included in the direct category. Any measure of adherence that was not directly assessed (eg, whether patients adhere to their bedtimes), but was derived from reports of behavior on the sleep diary (ie, what time patients go to bed) was classified as indirect. Such an assessment of adherence would be less likely to be influenced by social desirability. If the spouse or therapist rated the patient's level of treatment implementation, this was classed as clinician reported or spouse reported, because it did not derive from the patients themselves. The description of adherence measure was rated as high or low based on the clarity of the method of measurement and calculation of magnitude. Self-reported data were given a quality rating of low, whereas indirect or spouse/clinician-reported data were rated as high. The reason for this is that the authors believe that the patients' reporting whether they were adherent may be influenced by social desirability (wanting to report that they followed the recommendations of their therapists). However, we do acknowledge that spouse/clinician-reported measures (such as the therapist-ratings considered here) are also amenable to certain biases. Furthermore, even measures such as actigraphy, which some might consider gold standard for measuring adherence, often rely on the participant pressing an event marker or accurately completing a sleep diary, and therefore might also not be an error-free measure of behavior. Quality ratings were made by 2 reviewers (M.C. and then either S.A.,

M.K., A.H., or S.M.) and conflicts were discussed between the 2 reviewers.

Data Extraction

The following data were extracted from the included studies: definition of insomnia, comorbidities, the type of intervention implemented (including CBT-I components, whether this was delivered face to face or online, individual or group format, whether the treatment was combined with another CBT-I intervention, length of sessions, and duration of CBT-I). Data were also collected about study setting, participant demographics, measurement and magnitude of adherence, relationship between adherence and outcome (eg, a correlation coefficient), and potential predictors or nonpredictors of adherence. Data extraction was performed by 2 independent reviewers (M.C. and then either S.A., M.N., A.H., or S.M.) and conflicts were resolved by M.C.

RESULTS
Search Results

Database searches identified 1901 articles, 2 of which were included in the Matthews and colleagues[9] review. One-hundred and sixty-seven duplicates were removed; a further 1579 were deemed irrelevant at the title and abstract screening stage. The most frequent reasons for exclusion at this stage were a noninsomnia sample, no CBT-I intervention, and nonprimary research. Full-text screening excluded 155 articles. Reasons for exclusions are outlined in **Fig. 1**. Twelve articles from Matthews and colleagues'[9] review that were published before 2013 were added at the full text review/extraction stage. Three studies that were included in Matthews and colleagues'[9] review were not added to ours. Two articles did not include a sample of individuals with insomnia, and 1 study examined use of CBT-I components long term (as opposed to adherence). One study was added after reviewing reference lists of included studies, and thus, 53 studies were included for data extraction.

Sample Characteristics

Table 2 summarizes the 53 studies included in the final review.

Sample sizes in the included studies showed a wide variety, with a range from 6 to 696 participants. Most studies were from adult samples, with ages ranging from 18 to 95 years. Female-only samples were recruited by 4 studies,[10–13] and these were studies on female patients with cancer or survivors. Three studies recruited male

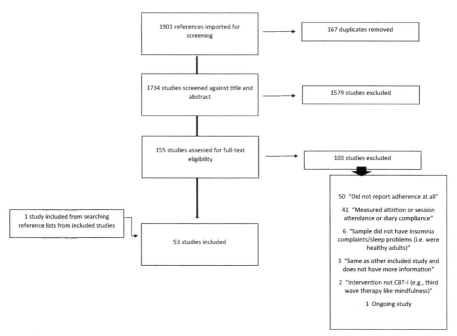

Fig. 1. Study exclusion/inclusion process.

samples,[14–16] 2 samples of veterans and 1 prison sample. Of 45 studies that included mixed male/female samples, the percentage of female participants ranged from 5% to 94%. Overall, most studies recruited mainly female participants, which is reflective of the higher prevalence of insomnia in women.[17] In 16 studies, individuals with insomnia and a comorbid condition were recruited; in 8, the comorbid condition was cancer.[10–13,18–21] Other comorbidities included depression,[22] bipolar disorder,[23] alcohol dependency,[14] cardiac rehabilitation,[24] war veterans with blast exposure/head injury,[25] human immunodeficiency virus (HIV),[26] chronic migraine,[27] and chronic obstructive pulmonary disease.[28] Most studies defined presence of insomnia by using diagnostic criteria (eg, Diagnostic and Statistical Manual of Mental Disorders [DSM]-IV,[29] International Classification of Sleep Disorders [ICSD],[30] or research diagnostic criteria[31]). Screening questionnaires included the Insomnia Severity Index[12,32–34] and the Pittsburgh Sleep Quality Index.[10,18,28] Several studies set a minimum SOL and WASO score[13,20,35–37] in addition to daytime dysfunction/impairment.[23,25,26,38–45] Some studies required only a subjective complaint of insomnia or sleep problems.[46,47]

Intervention Characteristics

There was a variety of combinations of treatment components. Two studies focused on progressive muscle relaxation,[28,47] or focused on breathing and visualisation.[18] Several studies evaluated cognitive and behavioral CBT-I components separately and as a combined intervention.[44,48] Three studies focused on sleep restriction as a standalone treatment.[36,45,49] One study evaluated stimulus control and sleep restriction separately and as a combined intervention.[39] In several studies, only behavioral components were delivered.[26,27,32,37,41,50] Additional interventions that were implemented alongside CBT-I were mindfulness meditation,[50] armodafinil,[20,21] modafinil,[51] cardiac-relevant information,[24] 1 session of mindfulness,[52] reminders to improve adherence,[47] and CBT-I coach mobile app.[53]

Most studies focused on individual, face-to-face interventions; 9 studies evaluated group CBT-I, and 10 evaluated digital CBT-I interventions. One study implemented a combination of group and individual sessions.[54] Several studies included both face-to-face and digital treatment arms[12,53]; 1 study included separate telehealth and digital interventions[52]; and 1 comprised an individual, group, and telephone treatment arm.[35] Of the 10 studies using digital interventions, only 4 included therapist support such as feedback and ability to message the therapist[12,22,38,55]; 5[33,38,47,55,56] were adapted to individual patients based on their progress and/or feedback throughout. Some studies used a combination of face-to-face and telephone sessions,[11,20,21,26,49] and some

Table 2
Study characteristics of reviewed studies

Author, Year	Sample	Intervention	Setting	Insomnia Inclusion Criteria
Absolon et al,[18] 2016	N = 28 Age = mean 54.14 y (SD = 11.3) 85.7% female Comorbidity: cancer	Breathing and visualizations	Ambulatory radiation center	PSQI>5, self-identified as having insomnia over the last 4 wk
Arem et al,[10] 2019	N = 11 Age = 52.8 y (7.1) 100% female Comorbidity: cancer (survivor)	CBT-I, 90-min sessions over 8 wk	Community and cancer centers	PSQI ≥, self-identified as having problems sleeping since cancer diagnosis
Bernatchez et al,[19] 2019	N = 6 Age range = 57–88 y 33% female Comorbidity: cancer	CBT-E, 60-min sessions over 3 wk	Community	DSM-IV diagnosis of insomnia or hypersomnolence
Birling et al,[54] 2018	N = 72 Age = 46.9 y (12.77) 79% female	CBT-I, 8 × 50–90-min sessions (some in group, some individual)	Community and sleep center	DSM-V diagnostic criteria for insomnia
Blom,[22] 2016	N = 18 Age = 46.1 y (13.6) 51% female Comorbidity: depression	Digital CBT-I, 9 wk	Community	Research diagnostic criteria and ISI>10
Bouchard et al,[35] 2003	N = 39 Age = 41.44 y 59% female	CBT-I, 8 wk (50 min, individual; 90 min, group; 30 min, telephone)	Community	Complaint of insomnia, SOL/WASO >30 min per night, ≥3 nights a week during a 2-wk baseline assessment; insomnia duration of ≥6 mo; daytime dysfunction
Boullin et al,[57] 2017	N = 25 Age: 39.62 y (13.64 group arm); 42.00 y (17.83, individual arm) 76% female	CBT-I, 1 session	Community	DSM-V criteria for acute insomnia (between 2 wk and 3 mo)

(continued on next page)

Table 2
(continued)

Author, Year	Sample	Intervention	Setting	Insomnia Inclusion Criteria
Buchanan et al. (2018)[26]	N = 22 Age = 46 y (range 30–59 y) 23% female Comorbidity: HIV	Brief behavioral therapy, 4 sessions (2 face to face, 2 telephone)	Community	SOL or WASO or EMA reports ≥3 nights per week, ≥1 mo, and associated with daytime dysfunction
Chakravorty et al,[14] 2019	N = 11 Age = 52 y (7) 0% female Comorbidity: alcohol dependence	CBT-I, 8 sessions	Community and local health clinics	ISI ≥ 8
Chambers & Alexander,[46] 1992	N = 103 Age = 39.9 y (range 19–75 y) 67% female	CBT-I, 1–4 sessions (most first sessions 2–3 h)	Sleep clinic	Subjective complaint of insomnia
Cui & Fiske,[64] 2019	N = 108 Age = 50.5 y (14.6) 72% female	CBT-I, 6 × 60-min sessions	Sleep clinic	DSM-IV-TR criteria
Cvengros et al,[50] 2015	N = 30 Age = 36.4 y (14.1) 60% female	Behavioral treatment and mindfulness meditation 6 weekly sessions (90–120 min)	Community	ICSD-2 diagnosis of psychophysiologic insomnia and SOL/WASO >30 min ≥3 nights per week for at least 1 mo

Study	Sample	Intervention	Recruitment	Diagnostic Criteria
Dolsen et al,[44] 2017	N = 188 Age = 47.4 y (12.6) 62% female	Cognitive therapy, behavioral therapy, or CBT-I, 8 weekly sessions (behavioral and cognitive therapy 45–60 min, CBT-I 75 min)	Community and referral	SOL, WASO ≥30 min, TST ≤6.5 h per night established with 2-wk sleep diary, insomnia ≥3 nights per week, >6 mo significant daytime impairment
Dong et al,[48] 2018	N = 188 Age = 48.5 y (13.6, behavioral therapy), 46.7 y (12.8, cognitive therapy), 46.9 y (11.3, CBT) 63.4% female for BT, 70% female for CT, 53% female for CBT	Cognitive therapy, behavioral therapy, or CBT-I, 8 weekly sessions (behavioral and cognitive therapy 45–60 min, CBT-I 75 min)	Community and referral	DSM-IV-TR criteria
Ebert et al,[33] 2015	N = 64 Age = 48.4 y (9.9) 70.3% female	Digital CBT-I, 6 sessions (45–60 min)	Schools	ISI ≥ 15
Edinger et al,[61] 2009	N = 41 Age = 56.9 y (16.3, primary insomnia), 52.0 y (11.1, comorbid insomnia) 15% female	CBT-I, 4 biweekly sessions, 30–60 min	Community and referral (health centers and VA outpatient mailing lists)	Research Diagnostic Criteria and SOL + WASO time of >60 min per night
Ellis et al,[58] 2015	N = 20 Age = 32.9 y (14.02) 55% female	CBT-I and self-help leaflet, 1 session, 60–70 min	Community	DSM-V diagnostic criteria for acute insomnia

(continued on next page)

Table 2
(continued)

Author, Year	Sample	Intervention	Setting	Insomnia Inclusion Criteria
Epstein et al,[39] 2012	N: SCT = 44, SRT = 44, MCI = 41 Age = 70.95 y (8.33 for stimulus control), 68.00 y (8.25 for sleep restriction), 67.22 y (6.55 for multicomponent therapy) SCT: 71% female, SRT: 57% female, MCI: 66% female	Stimulus control, sleep restriction, or both, 6 wk (4 groups face to face, 2 telephone)	Community	SOL or WASO ≥45 min for at least 3 nights per week as determined by 14-d sleep diary, ≥6 mo and daytime dysfunction
Epstein et al,[25] 2013	N = 41 Age = 30.32 y (7.73) range = 20–58 y 5% female Comorbidity: war veteran with blast exposure and/or other injury with loss of consciousness	CBT-I, 4 wk (1 face to face, 3 telephone), initial group session (M = 69.51 min), telephone sessions (M = 15.73 min)	Trauma clinic	SOL or WASO >1 mo and ISI ≥10 and impairment in daytime functioning
Garland et al,[20] 2016	N = 43 Age = 57.5 (average of CBT-I groups) 90% female (just CBT-I groups) Comorbidity: cancer (survivor)	CBT-I and armodafinil, 7 weekly individual sessions (face to face and telephone)	Community and cancer centers	Insomnia >3 mo, SOL/WASO >30 min on ≥3 d/wk for at least 1 mo; started or became worse with diagnosis/cancer treatment
Hebert et al,[59] 2010	N = 94 62% female	Digital CBT-I	Community and referral	Problems with SOL/WASO or EMA >30 min on 4 d/wk for at least 6 mo
Heenan et al,[24] 2019	N = 47 Age = 62.11 y (12.12), range 22–88 y 47% female Comorbidity: cardiac rehabilitation	CBT-I, including some cardiac-relevant information, 6 × 90-min group sessions	Cardiac rehabilitation center	DSM-V diagnostic criteria

Study	Sample	Intervention	Setting	Diagnostic criteria
Ho et al,[38] 2014	N = 207, Age = 36.9 y (13.0 self-help with support), 38.6 y (11.8 self-help without support), 69% female	Digital CBT-I self-help (without vs with support), 6 wk (4 face to face, 2 by phone)	Community	SOL or WASO, EMA, or nonrestorative sleep with daytime impairment on ≥3 nights for ≥3 mo
Holmqvist et al,[52] 2014	N: Web based = 39, Telehealth based = 34, 71.8% female (Web) 79.4% female(telehealth)	Telehealth and digital CBT-I, 6 sessions, 1 mindfulness session	Community and referral	Research diagnostic criteria
Horsch et al,[47] 2017	N = 45, Age = 35 y (14), 67% female	Digital behavioral treatment (progressive muscle relaxation exercises), with reminders to improve adherence	Community	Individuals with insomnia
Horsch et al,[56] 2017	N = 74, Age = 39 y (13.0), 61% female	Digital CBT-I, 6-7 wk	Community	DSM-V and ISI ≥7
Kaldo et al,[55] 2015	N = 73, Age = 47 y (15.2), 81% female	Digital CBT-I, 8 wk	Community	Research diagnostic criteria and ISI >10
Kamen et al,[21] 2019[b]	N = 47, Age = 58.88 y (30–74, for CBT with placebo); 56.26 y (36–73 for CBT-I with armodafinil) 91% female, Comorbidity: cancer	CBT-I, 7 sessions (3 face to face, 4 telephone)	Community and clinic (cancer)	Insomnia ≥3 mo starting/worsening with cancer treatment

(continued on next page)

Table 2
(continued)

Author, Year	Sample	Intervention	Setting	Insomnia Inclusion Criteria
Koffel et al,[53] 2018	N = 18 Age = 48.50 y (14.93) 61% female	CBT-I and CBT-I coach, 5 × 60-min sessions	VA medical center	Receiving CBT-I in a clinic
Lee & Harvey,[23] 2015	N = 17 Age = 39.47 y (13.47) 59% female Comorbidity: bipolar	CBT-I-BP, 8 × 50-min weekly individual sessions	Community	SOL or WASO unrefreshing sleep with daytime impairment for 3 d/wk for at least the last month
Lovato et al,[40] 2013	N = 86 Age = 64.10 y (6.80), 49–85 y (range) 52% female	CBT-I, 4 × 60-min group sessions	Community	WASO>30 min ≥3 nights ≥6 mo, daytime impairment
Ludwin et al,[15] 2018	N = 14 Age = 68.36 y (5.03), 60–83 y (range) 0% female	CBT-I, 6–8 × 75 min group sessions	VA medical center	Self-reported sleep problems
Manber et al,[60] 2011	N = 301, Age = 49.6 y (13.9), 21–88 y (range) 57.5% female	CBT-I, 7 × 90-min group sessions (first weekly, then biweekly for final 2)	Sleep clinic	Complaint of insomnia confirmed by BSM board-certified psychologist or physician
Matthews et al,[11] 2012	N = 34 Age = 53.56 y (7.09), 35–65 y (range) 100% female Comorbidity: cancer	CBT-I, 6 sessions (face to face and telephone)	Cancer centers and referrals	Insomnia that started or was made worse through diagnosis determined by clinical interview
McCrae et al,[41] 2018	N = 32 Age = 67.97 y (5.97) 69% female	Brief behavioral therapy, 4 wk	Community	SOL or WASO >30 min ≥3 nights per week >6 mo, daytime impairment
Miller et al,[49] 2013	N = 9 Age = 46.4 y (34–58 y) 67% female	Sleep restriction therapy, 4 sessions (face to face and telephone)	Community	Research diagnostic criteria

Study	Sample	Intervention	Setting	Inclusion criteria
Miller et al,[45] 2015	N = 75 Age = 45.5 y, 25–60 y (range) 75% female	Sleep restriction therapy	Community	Problems with SOL/WASO or EMA >30 min on ≥3 d/wk for at least 3 mo and daytime impairment
Perlis et al,[51] 2004	N: CBT-I and placebo = 9; CBT-I and modafinil = 10 Age = 47.4 y (1.7, CBT with placebo), 35.0 y (11.7, CBT-I and modafinil) 67% female (CBT and placebo) 80% female (CBT-I and modafinil)	CBT-I (with placebo or modafinil), 8× weekly sessions, 30–90 min	Community and sleep center	ICSD classification of psychophysiologic insomnia and ≥30 min SOL ≥2 awakenings per night ≥15 min and/or WASO 30 min, TST ≤6 h unless SE ≥80%. Problem >4 nights per week with ≥6 mo duration, daytime impairment complaint that had to at least be sleepiness/fatigue
Petrov et al,[32] 2014	N = 53 Age = 18.9 y (1.7), 17–25 y (range) 87% female	Behavioral treatment 1 × 90-min group session	College	ISI ≥8, and ICSD-2 classification, "sometimes" ≥1 out of 11 items of sleep disorders screener
Randall et al,[16] 2019	N = 30 Age = 33.13 y (8.85) 0% female	CBT-I, 1 session	Prison setting	DSM-V criteria (2–3 mo duration) for acute insomnia
Riedel & Lichstein,[36] 2001	N = 22 Age = 67.96 y (7.07), 60–81 y (range) 73% female	Sleep restriction therapy, 6 weekly sessions	Community	SOL or WASO >30 min 3 times a week for ≥6 mo
Savard et al,[12] 2016	N = 161 Age = 52.6 y (8.9) (face-to-face CBT), 55.3 y (8.7) (video-based CBT-I) 100% female Comorbidity: cancer	CBT-I (face to face or digital) 6 wk of 50-min sessions or 6 booklets with 5–20-min video	Cancer centers	ISI ≥8 or use of sleep medication ≥2× in past 2 wk
Seyedi-Chegeni et al,[28] 2018	N = 45 Age = 57.37 y (12.8) 33% female Comorbidity: COPD	Progressive muscle relaxation, 8 wk	Respiratory clinic	PSQI ≥ 21

(continued on next page)

Table 2
(continued)

Author, Year	Sample	Intervention	Setting	Insomnia Inclusion Criteria
Sidani et al,[62] 2015	N = 262 Age = 56 y (16), 21–90 y (range) 60% female	Behavioral therapy 4 group sessions, 2 telephone sessions	NA	SOL or WASO ≥30 min on ≥3 nights per week based on sleep diary and reported problems for ≥3 mo based on ISI
Sidani et al,[37] 2017[a]	N = 213 Age = 56 y (16), 21–90 y (range) 60% female	Behavioral therapy 4 group sessions, 2 telephone sessions	NA	SOL or WASO ≥30 min on ≥3 nights per week for ≥3 mo based on ISI
Smitherman et al,[27] 2016	N = 16 Age = 29.6 y (13.4) 94% female Comorbidity: chronic migraines	Behavioral therapy 3 × 30-min biweekly sessions	Community and neurology clinic	ICSD-3 criteria for insomnia
Tamura & Tanaka,[34] 2017	N = 28 Age = 67.21 y (8.33) 71% female	Behavioral treatment, single 2-h group session	Public health center	SOL or WASO >30 min and >10 points on ISI (Japanese version)
Taylor et al,[63] 2014	N = 17 Age = 19.47 y (1.66), 17–25 y (range) 24% female	CBT-I 6× individual sessions	Student sample	DSM-V insomnia criteria
Tremblay et al,[13] 2009	N = 57 Age = 54.05 y (7.36) 100% female Comorbidity: cancer	CBT-I, 8× weekly 90-min group sessions	Community and referrals	SOL or WASO >30 min, SE <85%, ≥3 nights per week ≥6 mo, daytime impairment
Trockel et al,[66] 2014	N = 696 Age = 52 y (14), 22–85 y (range) 10% female	CBT-I, 5 sessions	Clinic (VA)	DSM-IV insomnia criteria

Study	Sample	Intervention	Setting	Diagnostic criteria
Vincent & Hameed,[65] 2003	N = 50 Age = 51.4 y (11.4) 66% female	CBT-I, 7× weekly 90-min group sessions	Community and referral	DSM-IV-TR and TST <6.5 h SOL >45 or WASO >30 and ≥4 h for ≥6 mo and 2 daytime areas of impairment
Vincent et al,[42] 2008	N = 40 Age = 46.9 y (11.9) 50% female	CBT-I, 6× weekly group sessions	Sleep clinic	SOL or WASO or EMA ≥30 min or nonrestorative sleep ≥3 nights per week ≥6 mo with ≥2 daytime impairment areas
Vincent & Lewycky,[43] 2009	N = 59 68% female	Digital CBT-I, 5 sessions	Community and referrals to sleep clinic	SOL or WASO ≥30 min, 1 daytime impairment and ≥6 mo ≥ nights per week

Abbreviations: CBT-E, CBT-I and environmental changes; COPD, chronic obstructive pulmonary disease; DSM, Diagnostic and Statistical Manual of Mental Disorders; EMA, early morning awakenings; HIV, human immunodeficiency virus; ICSD, International Classification of Sleep Disorders; ISI, insomnia severity index; NA, not available; PSQI, Pittsburgh sleep quality index; SD, standard deviation; SCT, Stimulus Control Therapy; SE, standard error; SOL, sleep onset latency; SRT, Sleep Restriction Therapy; TR; text revision; TST, total sleep time; VA, Veterans' Affairs.

[a] Same trial as Savard et al.[12]

[b] Same trial as Garland et al,[20] summary of direct adherence data.

combined group and telephone sessions.[25,37,39] Mean session duration ranged from 15 minutes (by telephone[25]) to 120 minutes,[50] but most were between 60 and 90 minutes. Most interventions were delivered in 6 to 8 sessions; however, several studies delivered CBT-I in a single dose.[16,32,34,57,58]

Measurement and Magnitude of Adherence

For the purpose of the current review, adherence measures were classified as direct, indirect, and spouse/clinician-reported (see description earlier). **Fig. 2** shows the number of studies included in our review over time (including those reviewed by Matthews and colleagues[9]) and depicted by type of adherence measure.

Direct adherence

Direct adherence included measures where participants were directly asked whether they had been adherent to the treatment recommendations. In instances where adherence was conceptualized as the percentage of participants who were classified as adherent (based on cutoffs using either an arbitrary time frame or a Likert scale), rates ranged from 10%[56] to 100%.[12,52] There was no consistency in the definition of the cutoffs for classifying someone as adherent. Adherence to individual CBT-I components (including stimulus control, sleep restriction, cognitive therapy, sleep hygiene, and relaxation) were measured. With large variability across individual studies, a clear pattern did not emerge. However, self-reported adherence rates to sleep hygiene were at the higher end of the spectrum, varying between 76%[43] and 100%[12,52] of participants adherent. Adherence to relaxation

techniques such as guided imagery and breathing exercises was lower, with most adherence rates less than 70%.[25,41,43,52,56,59] Adherence to sleep restriction, stimulus control, and cognitive therapy was extremely variable, with percentage rates of participants classified as adherent in the 30s and 40s,[33,52,59] in the 60s,[33,43] or in the 80s and 90s.[12,39,52,59]

In studies where the adherence was measured on a scale depicting the degree to which participants followed the recommendation, the adherence rates were high. The authors transposed the average adherence scores from each study as if it had been a 0% to 100% scale, so that we could compare scores across studies. The rates ranged from 56% to 86%.[23,26,27,42,45,49,60] Others reported percentage of time treatment was adhered to (median of 65%[19]) or days per week the participants were adherent to, which was variable (from median 0–1 days[47] to mean 6.23 days[61]). Sidani and colleagues[62] presented data detailing how many days participants used the bed for sleep alone (6.1–6.5 days), got out of bed if unable to sleep (1.3–2 days), and took naps in bed only if necessary (0.4–1 days). Importantly, they also reported days when the techniques were not applicable (eg, participant slept through and therefore did not have to get up if unable to sleep). This aspect of understanding adherence to CBT-I is important, because some components are not always applicable, especially if the patient's sleep starts to improve. Ruiter Petrov and colleagues[32] reported that participants described adhering to 77% of stimulus control instructions and 85% of sleep restriction instructions. Others reported that participants spent on

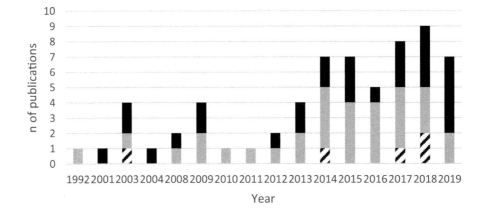

Types of adherence data published

Fig. 2. Types of studies published by year.

Table 3
Direct adherence measures, magnitude, correlation with outcomes and predictors

Author, Year	Adherence Measure	Quality Rating: Description Rating: of Adherence Measure	Quality Rating: Measure of Adherence	Magnitude of Adherence	Correlation Between Adherence and Outcomes	Predictors/ Correlates of Adherence	Nonpredictors/ Correlates of Adherence
Absolon et al,[18] 2016	% of participants who were able to follow treatment recommendation for at least 24/30 d	High	Low	75%	Not associated with any treatment variables	—	Demographic variables
Arem et al,[10] 2019	% of participants who reported home practice as "very often"	Low	Low	71%	—	—	—
Bernatchez et al,[19] 2019	% of time strategies were applied	Low	Low	65% (median)	—	—	—
Blom et al,[22] 2016	How often treatment components were used on a 5-point scale (0 not at all, 4 very much)	Low	Low	—	$r = 0.53$ for correlation between overall CBT-I adherence and improvement in insomnia after treatment	—	—
Buchanan et al,[26] 2018	Self-report (how well did you adhere to treatment on scale 0–7, higher score indicating better adherence)	High	High	5.0 (1.5–7.0) for self-report	—	—	—
Chambers & Alexander,[46] 1992	Self-reported compliance	Low	Low	—	Adherence did not predict treatment outcomes	—	—

(continued on next page)

Table 3
(continued)

Author, Year	Quality Rating: Description Rating: of Adherence Measure	Quality Rating: Measure of Adherence Measure	Magnitude of Adherence	Correlation Between Adherence and Outcomes	Predictors/ Correlates of Adherence	Nonpredictors/ Correlates of Adherence
Ebert et al,[33] 2015	Participants were asked whether they completed exercises at home completely, partly, or not at all	Low	Reported here for % implementing exercise completely: 50.88 for use of recreational activities; 35.09% for stimulus control and sleep restriction, 63% for sleep restriction specifically; 35.09% for strategies overcoming perseverative cognitions	Indirect effects of increased recreational activities that were associated with reduced perseverative cognitions and this with the reduction of sleeping problems (0.11, SE 0.07, 95% CI, 0.41–0.02)	—	—
Edinger et al,[61] 2009	How many days per week implemented each of the 6 core elements of the treatment (standard rise time, avoidance of naps, not worrying in bed, use of the bed only for sleeping, adherence to TIB prescription, getting out of bed when unable to sleep) and adherence to each item was averaged	Low	Mean of 6.23 d/wk adherent	—	—	—

Study	Measure		Results			Correlates	
Epstein et al. (2012)[39]	(1) Self-report (0–4 with higher scores better adherence) and (2) questions about adherence to specific behaviors; eg, did you adhere to the QHR	Low	(1) No means reported for self-reports (2) 89.3% (±9.5%) for SCT, 87.3% (±10.2%) for SRT, and 90.0% (±8.5%) for MCI	Low	—	—	—
Epstein et al,[25] 2013	Self-report questionnaire (how often did you implement components, scale not clear) and % of veterans using audio files	Low	28% indicated very much. Use of audio files: guided imagery 40.7%–79.4% depending on treatment week; breathing awareness 25.9%–58.8%; body scan 22.2%–61.8%	Low	—	—	—
Hebert et al,[59] 2010	% of homework practice for at least 4 nights of the week	High	Clock watching (70.0%), caffeine (60.9%) and alcohol taper (95.6%), avoiding heavy meals before bed (87.0%), sleeping separately from noisy bed partner (87%), exercising (39%), tapering liquids before bed (60.9%), temperature control in bedroom (87%), avoidance of napping (82.6%), regular sleep schedule (82.6%), avoiding reading or TV viewing in bed (82.6%), abdominal breathing (60.0%), progressive muscle relaxation (38.8%), imagery-induced relaxation (38.8%), hypnosis (41.2%), and sleep restriction (44.4%)	Low	—	Perceived behavioral control, support, and higher intention were associated with adherence to sleep hygiene practices. More contemplative individuals were more likely to adhere to exercise and tapering caffeinated beverages	—

(continued on next page)

Table 3
(continued)

Author, Year	Adherence Measure	Quality Rating: Description Rating: of Adherence Measure	Quality Measure of Adherence	Magnitude of Adherence	Correlation Between Adherence and Outcomes	Predictors/ Correlates of Adherence	Nonpredictors/ Correlates of Adherence
Ho et al,[38] 2014	How far they had followed instructions (all, almost all, or more than half)	Low	Low	—	—	—	Support
Holmqvist et al,[52] 2014	Use of homework on >4 nights per week	Low	Low	Telehealth: 75% (clock watching), 73% (relaxation), 72% (sleep restriction and stimulus control), 47.8% (cognitive therapy), 95% (sleep hygiene) Online CBT-I: 65% (clock watching), 72.7% (relaxation), 95% (sleep restriction and stimulus control), 80% (cognitive therapy), 100% (sleep hygiene)	—	Web vs telehealth	—

Study	Measure			Results	Moderators	Type of reminder
Horsch et al,[56] 2017	How often the relaxation exercises were used (in days)	High	Low	Median 0 (IQR 6, for no reminders), median 1 (IQR 3 for self-set reminder), and 1 (IQR 5 for system set reminder)	Reminders vs no reminders, appreciation for the relaxation exercises and ability to use the phone	Type of reminder (self or system set), self-empowerment or opportunity (opportunity to do the relaxation exercises was available), acceptance and use of technology, locus of control, insomnia severity, behavioral intention
Horsch et al,[47] 2017	Number of relaxation exercises performed (also reported % with >35 relaxation exercises)	High	Low	Mean of 49 relaxation exercises completed, (10% of participants adherent for relaxation)	—	—
Kaldo et al,[55] 2015	Hours spent each week using treatment methods	Low	Low	Mean 6.1 h (SD = 4.5)	—	—
Lee & Harvey,[23] 2015	Self-report assessing on a scale of 0–100 to what extent they completed the homework assignment, with higher scores indicating better adherence	High	Low	Mean = 82.08 (SD = 17.02) homework compliance	—	Recall of therapy components, how many therapy components were delivered per session

(continued on next page)

Table 3
(continued)

Author, Year	Adherence Measure	Quality Rating: Description of Adherence Measure	Quality Rating: Measure of Adherence	Magnitude of Adherence	Correlation Between Adherence and Outcomes	Predictors/ Correlates of Adherence	Nonpredictors/ Correlates of Adherence
Manber et al,[60] 2011	Self-report scale from 0–3 for each of the 6 components, with higher scores indicating better adherence	High	Low	Mean of 1.69–2.33 for high depression group and 1.85–2.49 for low depression group	Adherence related to lower posttreatment ISI scores	Lower depression scores, especially for rise time and TIB (no difference for cognitive components	—
McCrae et al,[41] 2018	Self-report logs for sleep hygiene behaviors, stimulus control components, and relaxation practice (supposed to practice twice a day and specify time), and then reported % of items that were adhered to	High	High	Sleep hygiene: 86.19% (SD, 20.13%), stimulus control, 83.01% (SD, 20.21%), and relaxation 68.83% (SD, 30.43%)	—	Adherence higher for sleep hygiene than stimulus control and relaxation	—
Miller et al,[49] 2013	Sleep restriction adherence scale (range 5–30, greater score more adherence	Low	High	Week 1 = 26.1 (3.5), week 2 = 24.0 (3.8), week 3 = 25.1 (1.3), week 4 = 23.1 (6.1)	—	—	—
Miller et al,[45] 2015	Sleep restriction adherence scale (range 5–30, greater score, more adherence)	Low	High	>20 on Sleep Restriction Adherence Scale, "adherence suggested on sleep diary"	—	—	—

Ruiter Petrov et al,[32] 2014	Self-report asking whether they implemented 11 behaviors then average % of behaviors adhered to over the 14-d follow-up period	High	Low	On average, 77% of stimulus control instructions and 85% of sleep hygiene instructions were adhered to	—	Bed partner or pet and higher treatment-related self-efficacy associated with stimulus control adherence. Treatment-related self-efficacy and less alcohol use were associated with better sleep hygiene adherence	Baseline variables not related to sleep hygiene adherence; baseline variables (except bed partner/pet and treatment-related self-efficacy) not related to SCT adherence
Savard et al,[12] 2016	% of participants implementing strategies at least moderately or at least a lot or extremely	Low	Low	Implementing moderately: 100% behavioral, 94% cognitive, and 100% sleep hygiene; implementing a lot or extremely: 97% for behavioral, 65% for cognitive, and 93% for sleep hygiene. For dCBT-I: 96% (behavioural), 81% (cognitive), and 94% (sleep hygiene) reported that they at least "moderately" put into practice the individual components. Reduced to 59% (cognitive), 54% (behavioural) and	—	—	

(continued on next page)

Table 3
(continued)

Author, Year	Adherence Measure	Quality Rating: Description Rating: of Adherence Measure	Quality Rating: Measure of Adherence Measure	Magnitude of Adherence	Correlation Between Adherence and Outcomes	Predictors/ Correlates of Adherence	Nonpredictors/ Correlates of Adherence
				74% (sleep hygiene) if using the 'a lot/ extremely' cut off			
Seyedi-Chegeni et al,[28] 2018	Self-report duration and time of relaxation practice at home (were told to practice 2 times per day for 30 min each)	High	Low	Average exercise time 50 min and 1.8 times per day	—	—	—
Sidani et al,[62] 2015	On diary indicated whether (1) used the bed for sleep only, (2) getting out of bed when unable to fall asleep or fall back to sleep within 15–20 min, and (3) taking a nap in bed only if necessary. Adherence was conceptualized as the number of days within each treatment week that each recommendation was applied and number of days it was not needed Overall rating scale measured overall adherence to	High	Low	(1) Use of bed for sleep only reported in days per week: applied on average (randomized = 6.3–6.5; preference = 6.1–6.4), nonapplicable (randomized = 0.5–0.6; preference = 0.14–0.23) Got out of bed: applied (randomized = 1.6–2; preference = 1.3–1.9), nonapplicable (randomized = 2.3–2.9; preference = 2.3–3.3) Took nap in bed: applied (randomized = 0.7–1; preference = 0.4–0.7),	—	—	Group (allocated based on treatment preference or randomized to treatment)

Source	Adherence measure	Adherence rate	Adherence results	Acceptability measure	Acceptability rate	Acceptability results
Sidani et al,[37] 2017	Self-report on a scale of 0–4 with higher rates indicating better adherence	Low	nonapplicable (randomized = 4.7–5.2; preference = 4.8–5.3) (2) Mean overall compliance score: random group = 3.1, preference group = 2.9	treatment: 5-point scale ranging from not at all (0) to very much (4) — Suitability of the treatment, overall attitude toward and desire for continued treatment use — Utility, therapist competence and interpersonal style, perceived benefits on insomnia/everyday functioning, satisfaction with format and dose of treatment; satisfaction with outcomes and attribution of outcomes to treatment	Low	—
Smitherman et al,[27] 2016	Self-report on a scale of 1–5 with higher scores indicating more frequent implementation (nearly every day)	High	Mean = 4.3 (SD = 0.4)	—	Low	—
Taylor et al,[63] 2014	Self-report to indicate whether they were adherent to various behaviors each day of the week	Low	—	—	High	—

(continued on next page)

Table 3
(continued)

Author, Year	Adherence Measure	Quality Rating: Description of Adherence Measure	Quality Rating: Measure of Adherence of Adherence	Magnitude of Adherence	Correlation Between Adherence and Outcomes	Predictors/ Correlates of Adherence	Nonpredictors/ Correlates of Adherence
Tamura & Tanaka,[34] 2017	Self-reported how often practiced any of the sleep-promoting behaviors with scores from 0 to 23. Also reported % practice individual behaviors	Low	Low	Went from 8.89 (4.84) at baseline to 7.25 (4.29) at posttreatment. The only change in the sleep-promoting behaviors was exposure to sunlight in the morning. % implementing behaviors at posttreatment ranged from 35.7 to 85.7	—	—	—
Vincent et al,[42] 2008	Self-report rating about adherence in general from 1-6 with higher scores (range 5–30) indicating better adherence	Low	High	Mean = 21.4.	—	Barriers (discomfort, annoyance, boredom)	Perceived behavioral control, pretreatment sleepiness, gender, postsecondary education status

							Low	High
Vincent & Lewycky,[43] 2009	Number of participants practicing homework >4 nights per week each week	Low	Low	Clock-watching (73.9%), sleep hygiene (76.8%), stimulus control (64.2%), relaxation training (67.6%), sleep restriction (51.6%), hypnotic tapering (22.6%). Relaxation types: paced breathing exercises 48%, PMR 22%, hypnosis 22%, imagery-induced relaxation 22%	—			

Abbreviation: IQR, interquartile range; QHR, quarter-hour-rule.

average 6 hours each week following the treatment methods (treatment components were not specified).[55] Seyedi Chegeni and colleagues[28] found that participants spent 50 minutes completing relaxation practice, and did this on average 1.8 d/wk (**Table 3**).

Indirect adherence

Indirect measures related to instances where the assessment of adherence behavior was indirect (eg, asking them when they went to bed, and comparing this with the clinician-prescribed bedtime), which is particularly relevant for adherence to SRT. In SRT, the patient's TIB is curtailed to the average total sleep time assessed by sleep diaries (sometimes +15–30 minutes). Adherence to SRT can be derived by comparing the prescribed TIB with the actual TIB reported on the sleep diary or from examining the bedtime and rise time reports. In several studies (n = 9), the percentage of participants within a certain period of their prescribed TIBs (eg, within 15 minutes) was reported. Adherence was conceptualized either as TIB that was identical or within 1 minute,[15] within 15 minutes,[14,36,54,58] or within 30 to 60 minutes of their prescribed TIBs each night.[15,20,21,36,56,58] The proportion of participants who were within 15 minutes of their prescribed TIBs ranged from 36%[36] to 91.7%.[57] Using a more generous cutoff of 30 minutes, the rates increased marginally to 37.5%[21] to 100%.[15] The strictest cutoff for adherence was a TIB that was no more than 1 minute greater than the prescribed TIB,[15] and 57% of participants showed this level of adherence in their sleep diaries. Applying similar criteria (within 15 minutes) for bedtime, Perlis and colleagues[51] reported that 51% of participants were adherent to their prescribed bedtimes; adding modafinil, this increased to 80% of participants. Ruiter Petrov and colleagues[32] reported that 47% of participants were within 30 minutes of their prescribed rise times.

The second most frequently reported measure was days participants were adherent to their prescribed TIBs/bedtimes/rise times (eg, within 15 minutes). The average percentage of days participants' TIBs were within 30 minutes was calculated, and this was between 60% of days[11] and 83.2% of days.[13] Percentage of days participants were with 15 minutes of their bedtimes was high. In 3 studies, the reported percentages were in the high 80s and low 90s.[13,16,48] Matthews and colleagues[11] reported slightly lower rates of 42.8% to 58.5% depending on treatment week. Participants were within 15 minutes of their rise times on 78.4% to 90% of days,[13,16] within

30 minutes on 72.6% to 87.1% of days,[11,48] and within 60 minutes on 72.4% of days.[50]

In two studies, the deviation from prescribed TIB was reported as between 20 and 28 minutes.[36,50] For rise time, the deviation was similar,[50,63] except in Ruiter Petrov and colleagues'[32] study, where the deviation was, on average, 82 minutes. For deviation from bedtime, Taylor and colleagues[63] reported that participants were 8 minutes off their prescribed times.

In several studies it was reported whether the TIB was significantly different from the prescribed TIB as a measure of adherence. No significant differences between average actual and prescribed TIB were reported in 2 studies.[40,41] Some measured adherence as reduction of TIB from pretreatment to posttreatment and they reported reductions of 122[49] and 98[45] minutes. These reductions indicated a significant change from pretreatment values. McCrae and colleagues[41] did not report the mean differences from pretreatment to posttreatment but did report that changes were significant during the treatment phase, but not at follow-up.

In 2001, Riedel and Lichstein[36] published an article in which they conceptualized adherence as the variance of TIB or rise time, and they reported that this variance was a strong predictor of treatment outcome. This finding indicated that it was not the reduction in TIB but the consistency of patients' sleep behaviors that led to improved outcomes. Several studies attempted to replicate their findings and also computed the standard deviation (SD) or the variance of TIB,[15,34,36] bed time,[64,65] or rise time/wake time.[15,34,36,42,64,65] None of the studies clearly state exactly how variance was calculated, but the SD is the square root of the variance. For the rates discussed later, we converted the variance reported in the studies to minutes and then to the SD so the values are more easily interpretable by the reader. Ludwin and colleagues[15] reported a median variance for TIB reduced from 2209 to 1225 after treatment (equivalent to a reduction in the SD from 47 minutes to 35 minutes). Riedel and Lichstein[36] reported slightly higher mean levels of overall variance, but still a reduction after treatment (from 4095 to 1189; this is equivalent to a reduction in the SD from 64 minutes to 34 minutes). When examining rise time variance, Ludwin and colleagues[15] reported a reduction from 1521 to 761 after treatment (this is the equivalent of a reduction in SD from 39 minutes to 28 minutes). These rates were more comparable with those reported by Riedel and Lichstein[36] (1790 to 692 or a change in SD of 42 to 26 minutes).[36] Vincent and colleagues[42] reported variances in wake time of 4277 at baseline to 3249 after treatment (this is equivalent to a reduction in SD from 66 to 57 minutes). Cui and Fiske[64] reported the SDs in wake time as 40.4 minutes and SDs in bedtime as 27 minutes. Tamura and Tanaka[34] reported the coefficient of variance (SD/mean) in bed and rise time. The authors were unable to transform the coefficient of variance into the SD in minutes with the information provided in the article (and we did not receive a response from the investigators after requesting further information), so the coefficient of variance is reported here unchanged. The investigators reported increased consistency in TIB and rise time after treatment compared with baseline (2.6–2.3 for TIB and 8.9–7.3 for rise time).[34]

In some studies, an adherence measure was used that was not common with another study. This include (1) the mean proportion of TIB reduction that was adhered to, and this was reported to be 68.99%[36]; and (2) scores ranging from 0 to 49 depicting adherence to individual components, which was derived from the sleep diary, with scores varying from 42.4 to 45.6 depending on the treatment week.[35] The sleep diary was also used to determine adherence to components of stimulus control (no napping/reducing napping to no later than 3.00–3.15 PM and <60 minutes, and getting out of bed if unable to sleep). Adherence to avoiding naps was reported on a mean of 95.6% of days[13] and 84.3% of days.[48] Adherence to getting out of bed if awake at night was, on average, practiced on 97.73% of days[13] and 64.3% of days[48] (**Table 4**).

Clinician-reported adherence data
Five studies measured adherence using therapist ratings.[44,48,53,65,66] Although in 3 articles therapists were asked to rate adherence to individual intervention components,[53,65,66] the magnitude of therapist-rated adherence was not reported.

In two studies,[53,66] the Patient Adherence Form was used, a validated questionnaire that was created for the Veterans' Affairs CBT-I Training Program.[67] Therapists rated participant adherence to 6 specific behaviors from 1 to 6 (no adherence to complete adherence). This rating was then averaged to create an overall adherence score. In one article,[44] the Treatment Adherence Rating Scale–Therapist Report was used (derived from Lichstein and colleagues,[68] which asked to what extent participants completed practice exercises [0%-100%, with 10% increments]). In two studies,[48,65] original scales were created for therapists to rate the extent to which participants completed their homework. Ratings either ranged from 0 to 100[48] or 1 to 5,[65] with higher values indicating better patient adherence. Dong and colleagues[48] reported the magnitude of therapist-

rated adherence to homework exercises as a mean of 80.99; Vincent and Hameed[65] reported that therapists rated that 48% of participants were at least very much adherent. The same study also measured adherence by asking the spouse about patient adherence to different behaviors. The scores on this questionnaire ranged from 5 to 25, and, on average, spouses rated their partner's adherence as good (mean = 20.58) (**Table 5**).

Relationship Between Adherence and Outcomes

Direct adherence
There were conflicting findings regarding direct adherence measures. Although some found that directly measured[18,46] adherence was not related to treatment outcomes, in 2 studies self-reported frequency of using treatment components was significantly related to lower insomnia severity index (ISI) scores posttreatment, for overall CBT-I use ($r = 0.53$,[22] positive correlation because they used a change in ISI score), and adherence specifically to cognitive ($r = -0.34$[60]) and behavioral components ($r = -0.27$[60]).

Indirect adherence The relationship between indirect adherence and outcome was reported in 8 studies; because there was a large variability in the way adherence was measured, clear patterns did not emerge. Matthews and colleagues[11] reported a significant relationship between adherence to bedtime and reported awakenings at night ($r = -0.35$) and also total sleep time ($r = 0.38$). This finding was not replicated in other studies.[24,48] Similarly, adherence to rise time was not reported to be associated with outcome[48] and neither was adherence to TIB.[15,48]

The first study to operationalize adherence as consistency in TIB/bedtime/rise time was by Riedel and Lichstein.[36] They reported that rise time variance was associated with improvements in sleep quality ($r = -0.60$) and nocturnal awakenings ($r = 0.44$). Variance in TIB was associated with sleep efficiency ($r = -0.51$) and WASO ($r = 0.51$). These associations with outcome were replicated in some studies (consistent wake time was related to more tapering of sleep medication after treatment, $r = -0.49$[65]), but not others.[15,42] However, some of these studies used variance of wake time. The use of wake time as opposed to rise time variance could be challenging, considering that the former is a measure of sleep/wake state and behavior, rather than just behavior.

Adherence to the quarter-hour-rule (getting up at night if unable to sleep) was associated with ISI reduction after treatment (Beta = -0.22), and follow-up (−0.20), as well as with insomnia remission after treatment (odds ratio [OR], 2.63) and follow-up (OR, 2.23).[48] No napping during the day was associated with adherence and objective WASO (Beta = 0.41), TST (0.41), and sleep efficiency (SE) (0.38) in 1 study,[13] but not in another.[48]

Spouse/Clinician-Reported Data Therapist-rated patient adherence rates were significantly related to higher ISI score reduction[48,66] and posttreatment insomnia remission.[48] Therapist ratings of how adherent participants were also related to outcomes including reduction in dysfunctional beliefs, less sleep related impairment, and better sleep quality, although not related to posttreatment SOL or sleep efficiency.[65] Spouse-rated adherence was not related to outcome.[65] Important to note here is that Vincent and Hameed[65] collected therapist ratings at the end of treatment, whereas Dong and colleagues[48] and Trockel and colleagues[66] asked therapists to rate adherence after each session.

Predictors of Adherence

Demographics

In studies using variability in sleep routines as an indirect measure of adherence, younger age was identified as a predictor of wake time variability in one study,[42] but not in another[11]; older age was a predictor of bedtime and rise time variability,[64] although another study did not find a significant relationship between age and adherence.[50] Postsecondary education and employment status was not related to self-reported adherence.[18,42] Having a bed partner or pet was positively related to adherence to stimulus control.[32] Gender was consistently not a predictor of adherence across self-reported[18,42] and indirect[42,50,64] measures.

Baseline insomnia variables Duration of insomnia at baseline was not associated with adherence.[48] Likewise, insomnia severity was unrelated to adherence in several studies,[11,47,64] although one study reported that less severe insomnia was related to rise time adherence.[50] Lower levels of fatigue were significantly related to adherence to rise time[11] and an overall measure of 7 sleep diary behaviors.[48] However, overall daytime impairment was not found to be a significant predictor of behaviors reported in sleep diaries.[48] Lower levels of sleepiness predicted consistency of wake time[42]; however, the use of wake time adherence has limitations, because wake time captures a behavior and a sleep/wake state, and the latter is not under the control of the patient. Dysfunctional beliefs about sleep were negatively related to TIB

and rise time adherence,[50] although another study found that dysfunctional beliefs about sleep and sleep-related safety behaviors were not significant predictors of bedtime, rise time, or getting up at night when unable to sleep.[48] Medication use at baseline was not related to spouse-rated adherence.[65]

Features of the intervention Adherence to relaxation was found to be higher in a telehealth than Web-based intervention, although, in the Web-based treatment, higher adherence to stimulus control, sleep restriction, cognitive therapy, and sleep hygiene was reported.[52] In contrast, treatment modality was not a significant predictor when comparing face-to-face therapy with a mobile application.[53] Relaxation adherence was also positively related to reminders, although the type of reminder (self or system set) had no significant impact.[47] Recall of therapy components and the number of therapy components delivered in a session were not related to self-reported homework adherence.[23] Adherence to prescribed TIB was significantly higher in an individual than group treatment arm.[57] Studies investigating the use of medication to combat sleepiness related to CBT-I (because of changes in sleep routine caused by sleep restriction and stimulus control) found mixed results: modafinil was associated with prescribed bedtime adherence,[51] whereas in another study[20] the use of armodafinil was not associated with adherence (although this study used TIB as its adherence measure).

Health variables Health variables, including perceived health, pain status, health status, and exercise, were not significant predictors of adherence,[32] although less alcohol use was associated with better sleep hygiene adherence.[32] In samples with a cancer comorbidity, the number of health problems,[64] months since cancer diagnosis, and radiation were not significant predictors, although chemotherapy (compared with other treatments) was a predictor of better TIB adherence.[11]

Mental health and sleep-related variables Low levels of depression were related to higher adherence to behavioral components of CBT-I (particularly rise time and reducing TIB)[64,69]; however, psychiatric comorbidities were not identified as significant predictors of bedtime or rise time adherence in other studies.[11,48,65] No significant differences were found between high-depression and low-depression groups in adherence to cognitive components, with the exception of high-depression participants reporting not changing their expectations of sleep as much as the low-depression group.[60] In contrast, another study

Table 4
Indirect adherence measures, magnitude, correlation with outcomes and predictors

Author, year	Adherence Measure	Quality Rating: Description of Adherence Measure	Quality Rating: Measure of Adherence	Magnitude of Adherence	Correlation Between Adherence and Outcomes	Predictors/ Correlates of Adherence	Nonpredictors/ Correlates of Adherence
Birling et al,[54] 2018	TIB difference, calculated by subtracting prescribed TIB from mean TIB reported in the sleep diary	High	High	—	—	—	—
Bouchard et al,[35] 2003	Recorded the presence or absence of 7 behaviors based on a sleep diary, then combined this score for minimum 0 and maximum 49 score (behaviors evaluated included bedtime more than 15 min before prescribed time, get up more than 30 min after prescribed time, does not get out of bed if awake for more than 30 min, naps >60 min and after 3 PM, not following evening routine, used bed for nonsleeping activities)	High	High	Ranged from M = 42.35 (SD = 5.32) in week 2 to M = 45.61 (SD = 3.35) in week 7	—	Self-efficacy	—

(continued on next page)

f-

Table 4
(continued)

Author, year	Adherence Measure	Quality Rating: Description of Adherence Measure	Quality Rating: Measure of Adherence	Magnitude of Adherence	Correlation Between Adherence and Outcomes	Predictors/ Correlates of Adherence	Nonpredictors/ Correlates of Adherence
Boullin et al,[57] 2017	Adherent if TIB on average was 15 min within prescribed TIB	High	High	53.85% (group treatment) 91.67% (individual treatment arm)	—	Individual treatment arm	—
Chakravorty et al,[14] 2019	Adherent if difference between TIB and pTIB in total (for the week) <105 min	High	High	90.9	—	—	—
Cui & Fiske,[64] 2019	SD in bed and rise times (higher SD poorer adherence) based on weekly averages	High	High	27.1 min (SD 29.0) bedtime; 40.4 min (SD 25.9) rise time	—	Higher age, fewer depression symptoms	Gender, ethnicity, education, employment, insurance, marital status, number of health problems, anxiety, baseline PSQI, ISI, or Epworth Sleepiness Scale

| Cvengros et al,[50] 2015 | Difference between TIB/rise time and prescribed TIB/rise time and then calculated % of days/35 when TIB was no more than >30 earlier and rise time was no more than 60 min later | High | High | Mean total TIB = 22 min (SD 38.3) more than prescribed, rise time = 30.5 min (SD 36.4) later than prescribed; participants were adherent with TIB recommendations on 61.6% of days (SD = 27.4, range = 0–96.4%), and rise time recommendations 72.4% of days (SD = 24.8, range = 17.1%– 100%) | — | Fewer dysfunctional beliefs (to TIB and rise time) and less severe insomnia (to rise time) | Age, gender, ethnicity, years of education, duration of insomnia |

(continued on next page)

Table 4
(continued)

Author, year	Adherence Measure	Quality Rating: Description of Adherence Measure	Quality Rating: Measure of Adherence	Magnitude of Adherence	Correlation Between Adherence and Outcomes	Predictors/ Correlates of Adherence	Nonpredictors/ Correlates of Adherence
Dong et al,[48] 2018	(1) Calculated number of adherent days per week for each criterion: bedtime ≤15 min before prescribed bedtime, rise time ≤30 min after the prescribed rise time, 20-min rule in the middle of the night, nap before 3 PM, and ≤60 min, TIB ≤30 min within pTIB	High	High	(1) Bedtime: 6.17 d (SD 0.92); rise time 5.08 d (SD 1.39); naps 5.91 d (SD 1.56); Sleep window 5.05 d (SD 1.41); getting out of bed during night awakenings 4.51 d (SD 2.11)	Beta −0.18 for overall adherence and insomnia improvement. Beta −0.22 for getting out of bed during night and ISI change at posttreatment and at follow-up. Insomnia remission and overall adherence OR 1.99 at posttreatment and OR 1.54 at 6-mo follow-up. Getting out of bed and remission OR 2.63 at posttreatment and OR 2.23 at 6 mo follow-up. Adherence to bedtime, rise time, napping, and sleep window did not significantly predict outcomes	Pretreatment fatigue (for global adherence to behavioral strategies)	Psychiatric comorbidities, daytime impairment, treatment expectation at session 1, duration of insomnia, dysfunctional beliefs about sleep and sleep-related safety behaviors (some of these were reported as significant trends)

Study	Adherence measure						
Edinger et al,[61] 2009	(2) standard deviations in TIB and rise time from baseline to posttreatment from the sleep diary	High	High	Magnitude of TIB/rise time variance not reported	—	—	—
Ellis et al,[58] 2015	% of participants within 15 min of their pTIB and % of participants within 30 min of their prescribed TIB	High	High	60% within 15 min, 65% within 30 min of prescribed TIB	—	—	—
Garland et al,[20] 2016	% of participants within 30 min of their TIB	High	High	67.6 (CBT + A) 54.78 (CBT + P)	—	—	Not whether assigned to placebo or armodafinil
Heenan et al,[24] 2019	Average difference between bedtime and prescribed bedtime	Low	High	—	No correlation with sleep diary and questionnaire outcome measures	—	—
Horsch et al,[56] 2017	Difference between TIB and prescribed TIB (also reported % with difference <60 min)	High	High	M difference to prescribed TIB of 59.2 min (SD 46.4) (68% adherent to sleep restriction)	—	—	—
Kamen et al,[21] 2019	Difference in time of bed and prescribed TIB >30 min, then dichotomous yes/no for adherent vs not adherent	High	High	37.5 wk 1, then ranged 60%–75.7% (depending on week of treatment)	—	Social support	—
Lovato et al,[40] 2013	Difference between TIB and pTIB	Low	High	TIB not significantly different from prescribed TIB	—	—	—

(continued on next page)

Table 4
(continued)

Author, year	Adherence Measure	Quality Rating: Description of Adherence Measure	Quality Rating: Measure of Adherence	Magnitude of Adherence	Correlation Between Adherence and Outcomes	Predictors/ Correlates of Adherence	Nonpredictors/ Correlates of Adherence
Ludwin et al,[15] 2018	(1) Difference between TIB and prescribed TIB in the final week, participants considered adherent if difference in score <1 and nonadherent if difference >0; (2) rise time variability during initial and final treatment weeks; and (3) variability of TIB during the initial and final treatment weeks with greater variability indicating poorer adherence	High	High	(1) 57% had a difference in score between TIB and pTIB that was <1. None had a difference in score >30 min; (2) Median rise variability went from 0.42 (0.08–1.05) to 0.21 (0.05–0.56) (3) Median TIB variance went from 0.62 (0.30–1.23) to 0.34 (0.13–0.65)	No correlation with ISI, SE, WASO, SL, TST (although moderate negative relationships of some outcomes with rise time variability)	—	—

Matthews et al,[11] 2012	Number of days that bedtime/rise time were within 15 min of prescribed time, and TIB was within 30 min of prescribed time	High	High	3–4.1 (rise time), 4.2–5.1 (TIB) and 5.4–6.1 d (bedtime)	$r = -0.35$ (for prescribed bedtime and reported awakenings per night. $r = 0.38$ (for prescribed bedtime and TST) and $r = 0.32$ (for prescribed TIB and TST)	Chemotherapy (vs other treatments for bedtime and TIB), motivation (for TIB and rise time), lower fatigue (for rise time)	Age, full-time employment, marital status, radiation, months since diagnosis, insomnia severity, anxiety and depression
McCrae et al,[41] 2018	(1) Difference between TIB and prescribed TIB, and (2) difference in pretreatment and posttreatment TIB	High	High	No difference between TIB and pTIB. There was a reduction in TIB from baseline to late treatment, posttreatment, but not at follow-up	—	—	—
Miller et al,[49] 2013	(2) TIB reduction from pretreatment to posttreatment	Low	High	Significant reduction in TIB from pretreatment to posttreatment (489 vs 367 min)	—	—	—
Miller et al,[45] 2015	TIB reduction from pretreatment to posttreatment	Low	High	Significant reduction in TIB from pretreatment to posttreatment (526 vs 428 min)	—	—	—

(continued on next page)

Table 4
(continued)

Author, year	Adherence Measure	Quality Rating: Description of Adherence Measure	Quality Rating: Measure of Adherence	Magnitude of Adherence	Correlation Between Adherence and Outcomes	Predictors/ Correlates of Adherence	Nonpredictors/ Correlates of Adherence
Perlis et al,[51] 2004	Difference between bedtime and prescribed bedtime. If it was later or the same, then assigned 0, and if all the weekly values (sum) were at least 105 min then deemed nonadherent. (That equates to on average 15 min deviation per day.) Adherence was conceptualized as % of participants considered adherent	High	High	80% CBT with modafinil, 51% CBT with placebo	—	Modafinil	—
Ruiter Petrov et al,[32] 2014	SD in rise time and % of participants who were more than 30 min different	High	High	81.6 min deviation from rise time (SD 96.5, range 0–540.0); 47% of participants were <31 min different from their prescribed rise time	—	—	—

Study	Adherence measure				Results		
Randall et al,[16] 2019	Number of nights that participants were within 15 min of their prescribed bedtime or rise time on their 1-wk posttherapy diary	Low	High	90%	—	—	—
Riedel & Lichstein,[36] 2001	(1) Difference in TIB and prescribed TIB; (2) % of TIB reduction that was adhered to (in %); (3) change in TIB from baseline to posttreatment; (4) TIB variance; (5) rise time variance	High	High	—	(1) 27.89 min (SD 31.72) more TIB, 64% were within 30 min of TIB, and 36% within 15 min of prescribed TIB; (2) adherence of 68.99% (SD 26.31); (3) TIB posttreatment was M = 400.39, SD = 69.90, and this was significantly lower than baseline (M = 467.92, SD = 66.24); (4) variance of TIB at baseline (4095.01) and posttreatment (1189.80); (5) rise time variance 1790.86 at baseline and 692.37 at posttreatment	$r = 0.51$ for WASO and TIB variance; $r = 0.44$ for rise variance and awakenings, $r = -0.51$ for TIB variance and sleep efficiency, and $r = -0.60$ for sleep quality and rise time variance. Adherence to combined score for TIB difference/TIB %, rise variance and TIB variance was associated with reduced WASO and improved sleep quality	—

(continued on next page)

Table 4
(continued)

Author, year	Adherence Measure	Quality Rating: Description of Adherence Measure	Quality Rating: Measure of Adherence	Magnitude of Adherence	Correlation Between Adherence and Outcomes	Predictors/ Correlates of Adherence	Nonpredictors/ Correlates of Adherence
Tamura & Tanaka,[34] 2017	(1) Variance in bedtime and rise time	Low	High	Bedtime variance reduced from 2.61 (2.40) at baseline to 2.35 (1.86) at posttreatment Rise time variance reduced from 8.89 (4.84) at baseline to 7.25 (4.29) at posttreatment	—	—	—
Taylor et al,[63] 2014	Difference between TIB and prescribed TIB, and difference between rise time and prescribed rise time	Low	High	Difference of 7.65 min between actual bedtime and prescribed bedtime; difference of 20.61 min between prescribed rise time and actual rise time	—	—	

Study		Adherence definition		Results		Association	
						—	
Tremblay et al,[13] 2009	High	Dichotomous yes/no for 5 criteria: (1) <15 min within bedtime, after the sixth session that turned to >30 min earlier and then computed the sum of all bedtimes/ number of days; (2) same as (1) but for rise time; (3) getting up within 30 min of awakenings in the night; (4) any naps <60 min and ending before 3.15 PM; (5) TIB<30 min different to prescribed TIB. Then % of days that the participant was adherent was calculated from the days between session 3 and end of CBT-I	High	Overall: 88.83% days (SE 8.48), Bedtime: 89.20% days (SE 11.60), rise time: 78.36% days (SE 15.60), avoidance of napping 95.63% days (SE 6.02), rising during the night if awake 97.73% days (SE 4.33), adherence to TIB 83.20% days (SE 17.20)	High	Association between adherence to not napping and change in objective WASO B(beta) = -0.41, TST (0.41) and sleep efficiency (0.38)	—
Vincent & Hameed,[65] 2003	High	Consistency of bedtime, consistency of wake time (SDs at 14 d pretreatment and posttreatment)	High	—	High	Tapering of sleep medications at posttreatment was related to more consistent wake time r = -.49	Anxiety, dysthymia

(continued on next page)

Table 4
(continued)

Author, year	Adherence Measure	Quality Rating: Description of Adherence Measure	Quality Rating: Measure of Adherence	Magnitude of Adherence	Correlation Between Adherence and Outcomes	Predictors/ Correlates of Adherence	Nonpredictors/ Correlates of Adherence
Vincent et al,[42] 2008	Consistency of wake time	Low	High	Significant improvement in variance of rise time (before 1.2 h, SD 0.68; after 0.91 h, SD 0.58)	No correlation with wake time consistency	Younger age, less sleepiness	Barriers, perceived behavioral control, gender, postsecondary education status

Abbreviations: CBT, cognitive behavior therapy; OR, odds ratio; pTIB, prescribed time in bed.

Table 5
Spouse/clinician-reported adherence measures, magnitude, correlation with outcomes and predictors

Author, Year	Adherence Measure	Quality Rating: Description of Adherence Measure	Quality Rating: Measure of Adherence	Magnitude of Adherence	Correlation Between Adherence and Outcomes	Predictors/Correlates of Adherence	Nonpredictors/Correlates of Adherence
Dolsen et al,[44] 2017	Therapist adherence scale (0–100, "To what extent did your patient complete the practice exercises outside of session this past week?" (0% to 100% with 10% increments")	High	High	—	—	More total wake time after the session (but this was reversed later on in treatment); longer TST (later on in treatment)	—
Dong et al,[48] 2018	Therapist adherence scale (0–100, "To what extent did your patient complete the practice exercises outside of this session?"	High	High	Mean = 80.99, (SD = 17.85)	ISI reduction posttreatment ($b = -0.14$, $P = .045$), remission at posttreatment (OR = 1.84, $P = .008$)	—	Psychiatric comorbidities, daytime fatigue, daytime impairment, treatment expectation at session 1, duration of insomnia, dysfunctional beliefs about sleep, and sleep-related safety behaviors
Koffel et al,[53] 2018	Therapist rated scale for 6 treatment recommendations, scale 1–6 with higher scores indicating better adherence	High	High	—	—	—	CBT-I coach or not

(continued on next page)

Table 5
(continued)

Author, Year	Adherence Measure	Quality Rating: Description of Adherence Measure	Quality Rating: Measure of Adherence	Magnitude of Adherence	Correlation Between Adherence and Outcomes	Predictors/ Correlates of Adherence	Nonpredictors/ Correlates of Adherence
Trockel et al,[66] 2014	Therapist-rated scale for 6 treatment recommendations, scale 1–6 with higher scores indicating better adherence. Then split group into terciles (high med low adherence)	High	High	—	d = 0.95, higher adherence had 4.1 points greater ISI reduction compared with lower group	—	Therapeutic alliance
Vincent & Hameed,[65] 2003	Therapist questionnaire (on a scale of 1–5 with higher scores indicating better adherence for 5 components of CBT-I) and spouse questionnaire with a range of 5–25 with higher scores indicating better adherence. Adherence to multiple behaviors was assessed in the spouse questionnaire (relaxation practice, sleep diary completion, changes to night routine, QHR)	High	High	47% rated at least very much adherent on therapist questionnaire. Average score on spouse questionnaire was 20.58, highest score was for diary completion, then bedtime routine, sleep restriction, and then relaxation training	Therapist-rated adherence was related to reduction in dysfunctional beliefs, less sleep-related impairment, better sleep quality; not related to posttreatment SOL or sleep efficiency. Spouse rating not related to outcomes	No dysthymia related to higher therapist-rated adherence	Anxiety, medication use, depression

ound that depression and anxiety were not related to therapist-rated adherence, although no dysthymia was significantly positively related to adherence.[65] Sleep-related variables, including more total wake time after the session and longer total sleep time, were positively related to adherence.[44]

Other psychological variables Several variables related to perception of treatment (suitability of the treatment, overall attitude toward and desire for continued treatment) were related to higher directly measured adherence.[37] However, treatment expectations at first session,[48] perceived utility, therapist competence and interpersonal style, perceived benefits on insomnia/everyday functioning, satisfaction with format and dose of treatment, satisfaction with outcomes, and attribution of outcomes to treatment[37] were not predictors of adherence.

Perceived barriers were negatively related to direct adherence, but not a predictor of wake time consistency.[42] Perceived behavioral control did not predict direct overall adherence[42]; however, self-efficacy, a similar construct, was related to sleep diary adherence measures relevant to sleep restriction and stimulus control.[35] Motivation[11] and social support[21] were predictors of adherence to prescribed TIB; motivation was also a predictor of rise time adherence.[11] Locus of control, behavioral intention, perceived opportunity, and acceptance and use of technology did not significantly predict adherence to relaxation exercises.[47]

DISCUSSION

Despite the evidence for the efficacy of CBT-I as the first-line treatment of chronic insomnia, understanding of patients' ability to implement individual recommendations is limited. The lack of reliable data regarding adherence to CBT-I limits knowledge of client engagement and the efficacy of specific intervention components. Although the most recent systematic review in this area[11] identified a lack of articles investigating adherence, the current review shows that recognition of the importance of measuring adherence to CBT-I is increasing. However, variation in study characteristics, definitions of adherence, and a lack of standardized adherence measures remain a barrier to synthesis of adherence research, as outlined in this review. Studies measuring CBT-I adherence vary greatly in sample size, modality, dosage, and intervention components. There is a need for more clinical trials to include a measure of adherence, so that clinicians can determine how these differences in study characteristics affect the magnitude of adherence. For example, it is not

known whether components (such as SRT) administered alone or in combination with other CBT-I components make adherence worse or better. Are less restricted sleep windows, as a result of negotiation between the therapist and the patient, associated with better adherence? If the patient opts to delay bedtime, advance rise time, versus cutting off time at both ends, does this have an impact on adherence? If cognitive components are delivered alongside (or even before) the behavioral components, will adherence to the behavioral components be increased? Measurement of adherence to specific CBT-I components has increased since the most recent review,[11] so, with continued focus on improving the way adherence is measured, authors hope that this will result in answers to these questions. **Our first recommendation is that clinical trials with CBT-I need to include a measure of adherence. There needs to be a focus on the individual components and clinicians need to work toward a consensus of what constitutes optimal adherence to CBT-I.**

Several studies since Matthew and colleagues'[11] review have focused on assessing behavior indirectly through the sleep diary (referred to here as indirect) and have moved away from simply asking patients whether they were adherent or not. This approach is beneficial because these types of measures are less likely to be influenced by social desirability. The drawback of this development is the huge variability in the way adherence is measured, varying from number of participants meeting specific cutoffs (within 15, 30, or 60 minutes of rise time/ bedtime/TIB), number of days participants meet a specific cutoff, and number of raw minutes deviation from bed time/rise time/TIB. This heterogeneity moves clinicians further and further away from a sound understanding of the magnitude of nonadherence in CBT-I trials and makes it difficult to interpret the relationship between adherence and outcome. Therefore, recommendations for optimal cutoffs cannot be made to guide clinicians in monitoring adherence to CBT-I. The most common cutoff used to determine adherence to prescribed TIB was 30 minutes' deviation. This cutoff seems sensible, because it would theoretically translate to a 15-minute deviation at bedtime and 15 minutes at rise time, which is also commonly reported. This cutoff is also consistent with the few studies in which raw minute deviation was reported (22–28 minutes more TIB than prescribed).[36,50] The cutoff for bedtime was typically 15 minutes, but for rise time some used 15 minutes and some 30 minutes. A more generous cutoff for rise time is defendable under the consideration that it might be more difficult for individuals to rise in the morning, because they are going from a state of sleep to wake, which could be influenced by sleepiness/sleep inertia. These are effects that have not been considered as an influence on adherence to treatments for sleep disorders. Non-adherence is always considered as intentional, but sleepiness is powerful and can override the motivation to adhere to the recommendation. A patient might be completely motivated to adhere to the get-up time in the morning but then, when the behavior is to be implemented (after a rapid transition from sleep to wake after the alarm goes off), the patient is driven by extreme sleepiness and is more likely to stay in bed, falls back asleep, and therefore does not comply with the treatment recommendations. It could be said that the patient is adherent (is willing and motivated and has prepared for it by setting the alarm) but is not compliant (does not engage in the behavior). Likewise, the individual might be prepared to adhere to stimulus control when discussing this recommendation with the therapist or the spouse during the day, but then, when the patient is awake in the middle of the night, alone with the partner sleeping, and with impaired decision making (because the areas of the brain involved in decision making are less active than the emotional areas of the brain during sleep), the patient might be less likely to get up. The state in which the patient makes the decision to adhere (during the day) is different to the state in which the behavior has to be implemented. These kinds of issues have yet to be explored (for a detailed discussion of this issue see Ref.[70] and Angela L. D'Rozario and colleagues' article, "Summary and Update on Behavioural Interventions for Improving Adherence with Positive Airway Pressure Treatment in Adults," in this issue). **Our second recommendation is to work toward a consensus on how to measure adherence to SRT, which should be done by reporting (1) raw minute deviations from TIB, bedtime, and rise time; (2) number of days participants were within 15 minutes of bedtime, 15 minutes within their TIBs, and 30 minutes within their rise times; and (3) number of participants who, on average, were within 15 minutes of bedtime, 15 minutes within their TIBs, and 30 minutes within their rise times. If possible, the authors encourage investigators to report adherence to other cutoffs in supplementary material (eg, 30 and 60 minutes of TIB), so that the optimal dose of adherence can be established**.

Since the publication by Riedel and Lichstein[36] in 2001, the variance in TIB/bedtime/rise time was reported frequently. However, the heterogeneity in measures made it difficult to draw conclusions about the magnitude of variance in behavior. Furthermore, many of the studies using this measure did not adequately describe the ways in which variance was calculated. **Our third recommendation is to report variance of bedtime, TIB and rise time in minutes, including clear descriptions of how variance is calculated.**

The proportion of studies using spouse/clinician-reported measures of adherence has increased since Matthews' review[11]; and none of the studies examined adherence using objective measures such as actigraphy (despite this method being tested in healthy patients more than 15 years ago[71]), mattress sensors, or camera technology. The lack of such objective measurements is likely a consequence of adherence mainly being a secondary outcome measure in most clinical trials. **Our fourth recommendation is to explore other objective measurements of adherence in clinical trials of CBT-I and to establish a gold-standard that is (most) unaffected by bias.**

The heterogeneity across studies also meant that drawing conclusions about the relationship between adherence and outcome was challenging. This difficulty was further complicated by different definitions of outcomes used. One important aspect to consider here is the importance of a temporal difference between measuring adherence and outcome in order to establish true causal relationships. It is also imperative to develop unbiased indirect or objective measures of adherence as described earlier. Therapists might rate their patients as more adherent if they are improving. Overall, only a few studies reported the relationship between adherence and outcome. It is important to establish this link, because, if it emerges that adherence is not related to outcome, it will be necessary to understand which aspects of treatment are mechanisms of change. **Our fifth recommendation is to measure the relationship between adherence and outcome.** Usually, the treatment is only as good as when it is correctly implemented; however, this remains an assumption for CBT-I. Importantly, there needs to be a temporal difference between measuring adherence and treatment outcome, in order to establish causality. There was also heterogeneity in the type of predictors linked to adherence; however, some of the psychological variables seemed slightly more consistently associated with adherence compared with nonmodifiable factors (eg, demographics). This finding is similar to the adherence literature in other sleep disorders (eg, continuous positive airway pressure [CPAP] treatment of obstructive sleep apnoea[72]). Studies examining adherence should also test for predictors (particularly those that are modifiable).

One last observation to be made here is that very few studies with digital CBT-I measure adherence that goes beyond attrition, diary completion, or viewed/completed sessions. Twenty studies (50% of all studies) that were excluded because they did not include a measure of adherence were for digital CBT-I. This finding is interesting because adherence should be easy to measure through electronic sleep diaries. Studies that include digital CBT-I should include measures of adherence.

SUMMARY

The current review shows that awareness of adherence and research into adherence to CBT-I has become more prevalent over the past decade. However, these studies show wide variation across sample sizes, comorbidities, treatment dosage, and importantly across adherence measures. The authors hope that researchers can adopt our recommendations, so that a consensus around the optimal measurement and magnitude of adherence can be reached in order to determine the association with treatment outcome and predictors. This approach could guide future adherence intervention studies as well as individual clinicians.

CLINICS CARE POINTS

- Some studies indicate that there is a small to moderate relationship between adherence to CBT-I and outcome (although this is contradicted by others). Because there is some evidence of a relationship, the authors advise clinicians to monitor adherence and explore avenues to improve adherence.
- Adherence to CBT-I is complex, and patients who do not adhere often do so intentionally. However, there is also room to consider patients' unintentional nonadherence, particularly if their behavior is influenced by sleepiness or sleep inertia (eg, not being able to get up at their prescribed rise times because they are too sleepy).
- Patients might be selective when adhering to individual CBT-I components. Clinicians are thus advised to examine nonadherence to one component in the context of adherence to another component.

ACKNOWLEDGMENTS

The authors would like to thank Sarah Kevill, librarian at the University of Strathclyde, for her support during the literature searches.

DISCLOSURE

The authors have nothing to disclose.

REFERENCES

1. Roth T. Insomnia: definition, prevalence, etiology, and consequences. J Clin Sleep Med 2007;3(5): S7–10.
2. Riemann D, Baglioni C, Bassetti C, et al. European guideline for the diagnosis and treatment of insomnia. J Sleep Res 2017;26(6):675–700.
3. Qaseem A, Kansagara D, Forciea MA, et al. Clinical Guidelines Committee of the American College of Physicians. Management of chronic insomnia disorder in adults: a clinical practice guideline from the american college of physicians. Ann Intern Med 2016;165(2):125–33.
4. van Straten A, van der Zweerde T, Kleiboer A, et al. Cognitive and behavioral therapies in the treatment of insomnia: a meta-analysis. Sleep Med Rev 2017; 38:3–16.
5. Trauer JM, Qian MY, Doyle JS, et al. Cognitive behavioral therapy for chronic insomnia: a systematic review and meta-analysis. Ann Intern Med 2015;163(3):191–204.
6. Spielman AJ, Saskin P, Thorpy MJ. Treatment of chronic insomnia by restriction of time in bed. Sleep 1987;10(1):45–56.
7. Kyle SD, Morgan K, Spiegelhalder K, et al. No pain, no gain: an exploratory within-subjects mixed-methods evaluation of the patient experience of sleep restriction therapy (SRT) for insomnia. Sleep Med 2011;12(8):735–47.
8. Chakrabarti S. What's in a name? compliance, adherence and concordance in chronic psychiatric disorders. World J Psychiatry 2014;4(2):30–6.
9. Matthews EE, Arnedt JT, McCarthy MS, et al. Adherence to cognitive behavioral therapy for insomnia: a systematic review. Sleep Med Rev 2013;17(6): 453–64.
10. Arem H, Lewin D, Cifu G, et al. A feasibility study of group-delivered behavioral interventions for insomnia among breast cancer survivors: comparing cognitive behavioral therapy for insomnia and a mind-body intervention. J Altern Complement Med 2019;25(8):840–4.
11. Matthews EE, Schmiege SJ, Cook PF, et al. Adherence to cognitive behavioral therapy for insomnia (CBTI) among women following primary breast cancer treatment: a pilot study. Behav Sleep Med 2012; 10(3):217–29.
12. Savard J, Ivers H, Savard MH, et al. Long-term effects of two formats of cognitive behavioral therapy for insomnia comorbid with breast cancer. Sleep 2016;39(4):813–23.

13. Tremblay V, Savard J, Ivers H. Predictors of the effect of cognitive behavioral therapy for chronic insomnia comorbid with breast cancer. J Consult Clin Psychol 2009;77(4):742–50.

14. Chakravorty S, Morales KH, Arnedt JT, et al. Cognitive behavioral therapy for insomnia in alcohol-dependent veterans: a randomized, controlled pilot study. Alcohol Clin Exp Res 2019;43(6):1244–53.

15. Ludwin BM, Bamonti P, Mulligan EA. Program evaluation of group-based cognitive behavioral therapy for insomnia: a focus on treatment adherence and outcomes in older adults with co-morbidities. Clin Gerontol 2018;41(5):487–97.

16. Randall C, Nowakowski S, Ellis JG. Managing acute insomnia in prison: evaluation of a "one-shot" cognitive behavioral therapy for insomnia (CBT-I) intervention. Behav Sleep Med 2019;17(6):827–36.

17. Zhang B, Wing YK. Sex differences in insomnia: a meta-analysis. Sleep 2006;29(1):85–93.

18. Absolon NA, Balneaves L, Truant TL, et al. A self-administered sleep intervention for patients with cancer experiencing insomnia. Clin J Oncol Nurs 2016;20(3):289–97.

19. Bernatchez MS, Savard J, Savard MH, et al. Feasibility of a cognitive-behavioral and environmental intervention for sleep-wake difficulties in community-dwelling cancer patients receiving palliative care. Cancer Nurs 2019;42(5):396–409.

20. Garland SN, Roscoe JA, Heckler CE, et al. Effects of armodafinil and cognitive behavior therapy for insomnia on sleep continuity and daytime sleepiness in cancer survivors. Sleep Med 2016;20:18–24.

21. Kamen C, Garland SN, Heckler CE, et al. Social support, insomnia, and adherence to cognitive behavioral therapy for insomnia after cancer treatment. Behav Sleep Med 2019;17(1):70–80.

22. Blom K, Jernelov S, Lindefors N, et al. Facilitating and hindering factors in internet-delivered treatment for insomnia and depression. Internet Interv 2016;4:51–60.

23. Lee JY, Harvey AG. Memory for therapy in bipolar disorder and comorbid insomnia. J Consult Clin Psychol 2015;83(1):92–102.

24. Heenan A, Pipe A, Lemay K, et al. Cognitive-behavioral therapy for insomnia tailored to patients with cardiovascular disease: a pre-post study. Behav Sleep Med 2020;18(3):372–85.

25. Epstein DR, Babcock-Parziale JL, Herb CA, et al. Feasibility test of preference-based insomnia treatment for Iraq and Afghanistan war veterans. Rehabil Nurs 2013;38(3):120–32.

26. Buchanan DT, McCurry SM, Eilers K, et al. Brief behavioral treatment for insomnia in persons living with HIV. Behav Sleep Med 2018;16(3):244–58.

27. Smitherman TA, Walters AB, Davis RE, et al. Randomized controlled pilot trial of behavioral insomnia treatment for chronic migraine with comorbid insomnia. Headache 2016;56(2):276–91.

28. Seyedi Chegeni P, Gholami M, Azargoon A, et al. The effect of progressive muscle relaxation on the management of fatigue and quality of sleep in patients with chronic obstructive pulmonary disease: a randomized controlled clinical trial. Complement Ther Clin Pract 2018;31:64–70.

29. American Psychiatric Association. Diagnostic and statistical manual of mental disorders. 5th edition. Washington, DC: American Psychiatric Association; 2013.

30. American Academy of Sleep Medicine. International classification of sleep disorders. 3rd edition. Darien (IL): American Academy of Sleep Medicine; 2014.

31. Edinger JD, Bonnet MH, Bootzin RR, et al. Derivation of research diagnostic criteria for insomnia: report of an american academy of sleep medicine work group. Sleep 2004;27(8):1567–96.

32. Ruiter Petrov ME, Lichstein KL, Huisingh CE, et al. Predictors of adherence to a brief behavioral insomnia intervention: daily process analysis. Behav Ther 2014;45(3):430–42.

33. Ebert DD, Berking M, Thiart H, et al. Restoring depleted resources: efficacy and mechanisms of change of an internet-based unguided recovery training for better sleep and psychological detachment from work. Health Psychol 2015;34S:1240–51.

34. Tamura N, Tanaka H. Effects of sleep management with self-help treatment for the Japanese elderly with chronic insomnia: a quasi-experimental study. J Behav Med 2017;40(4):659–68.

35. Bouchard S, Bastien C, Morin CM. Self-efficacy and adherence to cognitive-behavioral treatment of insomnia. Behav Sleep Med 2003;1(4):187–99.

36. Riedel BW, Lichstein KL. Strategies for evaluating adherence to sleep restriction treatment for insomnia. Behav Res Ther 2001;39(2):201–12.

37. Sidani S, Epstein DR, Fox M. Psychometric evaluation of a multi-dimensional measure of satisfaction with behavioral interventions. Res Nurs Health 2017;40(5):459–69.

38. Ho FY, Chung KF, Yeung WF, et al. Weekly brief phone support in self-help cognitive behavioral therapy for insomnia disorder: relevance to adherence and efficacy. Behav Res Ther 2014;63:147–56.

39. Epstein DR, Sidani S, Bootzin RR, et al. Dismantling multicomponent behavioral treatment for insomnia in older adults: a randomized controlled trial. Sleep 2012;35(6):797–805.

40. Lovato N, Lack L, Wright H, et al. Predictors of improvement in subjective sleep quality reported by older adults following group-based cognitive behavior therapy for sleep maintenance and early morning awakening insomnia. Sleep Med 2013;14(9):888–93.

41. McCrae CS, Curtis AF, Williams JM, et al. Efficacy of brief behavioral treatment for insomnia in older adults: examination of sleep, mood, and cognitive outcomes. Sleep Med 2018;51:153–66.

42. Vincent N, Lewycky S, Finnegan H. Barriers to engagement in sleep restriction and stimulus control in chronic insomnia. J Consult Clin Psychol 2008; 76(5):820–8.

43. Vincent N, Lewycky S. Logging on for better sleep: RCT of the effectiveness of online treatment for insomnia. Sleep 2009;32(6):807–15.

44. Dolsen MR, Soehner AM, Morin CM, et al. Sleep the night before and after a treatment session: a critical ingredient for treatment adherence? J Consult Clin Psychol 2017;85(6):647–52.

45. Miller CB, Kyle SD, Gordon CJ, et al. Physiological markers of arousal change with psychological treatment for insomnia: a preliminary investigation. PLoS One 2015;10(12):e0145317.

46. Chambers MJ, Alexander SD. Assessment and prediction of outcome for a brief behavioral insomnia treatment program. J Behav Ther Exp Psychiatry 1992;23(4):289–97.

47. Horsch C, Spruit S, Lancee J, et al. Reminders make people adhere better to a self-help sleep intervention. Health Technol (Berl) 2017;7(2):173–88.

48. Dong L, Soehner AM, Belanger L, et al. Treatment agreement, adherence, and outcome in cognitive behavioral treatments for insomnia. J Consult Clin Psychol 2018;86(3):294–9.

49. Miller CB, Kyle SD, Marshall NS, et al. Ecological momentary assessment of daytime symptoms during sleep restriction therapy for insomnia. J Sleep Res 2013;22(3):266–72.

50. Cvengros JA, Crawford MR, Manber R, et al. The relationship between beliefs about sleep and adherence to behavioral treatment combined with meditation for insomnia. Behav Sleep Med 2013;13(1):52–63.

51. Perlis ML, Smith MT, Orff H, et al. The effects of modafinil and cognitive behavior therapy on sleep continuity in patients with primary insomnia. Sleep 2004; 27(4):715–25.

52. Holmqvist M, Vincent N, Walsh K. Web- vs. telehealth-based delivery of cognitive behavioral therapy for insomnia: a randomized controlled trial. Sleep Med 2014;15(2):187–95.

53. Koffel E, Kuhn E, Petsoulis N, et al. A randomized controlled pilot study of CBT-I coach: feasibility, acceptability, and potential impact of a mobile phone application for patients in cognitive behavioral therapy for insomnia. Health Inform J 2018; 24(1):3–13.

54. Birling Y, Wang J, Li G, et al. Culturally adapted CBTI for Chinese insomnia patients: a one-arm pilot trial. Int J Behav Med 2018;25(3):331–40.

55. Kaldo V, Jernelov S, Blom K, et al. Guided internet cognitive behavioral therapy for insomnia compared to a control treatment - a randomized trial. Behav Res Ther 2015;71:90–100.

56. Horsch CH, Lancee J, Griffioen-Both F, et al. Mobile phone-delivered cognitive behavioral therapy for insomnia: a randomized waitlist controlled trial. J Med Internet Res 2017;19(4):e70.

57. Boullin P, Ellwood C, Ellis JG. Group vs. individual treatment for acute insomnia: a pilot study evaluating a "one-shot" treatment strategy. Brain Sci 2016;7(1). https://doi.org/10.3390/brainsci 7010001.

58. Ellis JG, Cushing T, Germain A. Treating acute insomnia: a randomized controlled trial of a "single-shot" of cognitive behavioral therapy for insomnia. Sleep 2015;38(6):971–8.

59. Hebert EA, Vincent N, Lewycky S, et al. Attrition and adherence in the online treatment of chronic insomnia. Behav Sleep Med 2010;8(3):141–50.

60. Manber R, Bernert RA, Suh S, et al. CBT for insomnia in patients with high and low depressive symptom severity: adherence and clinical outcomes. J Clin Sleep Med 2011;7(6):645–52.

61. Edinger JD, Olsen MK, Stechuchak KM, et al. Cognitive behavioral therapy for patients with primary insomnia or insomnia associated predominantly with mixed psychiatric disorders: a randomized clinical trial. Sleep 2009;32(4):499–510.

62. Sidani S, Bootzin RR, Epstein DR, et al. Method of treatment allocation: does it affect adherence to behavioural therapy for insomnia? Can J Nurs Res 2015;47(1):35–52.

63. Taylor DJ, Zimmerman MR, Gardner CE, et al. A pilot randomized controlled trial of the effects of cognitive-behavioral therapy for insomnia on sleep and daytime functioning in college students. Behav Ther 2014;45(3):376–89.

64. Cui R, Fiske A. Predictors of treatment attendance and adherence to treatment recommendations among individuals receiving cognitive behavioral therapy for insomnia. Cogn Behav Ther 2020;49(2):113–9.

65. Vincent NK, Hameed H. Relation between adherence and outcome in the group treatment of insomnia. Behav Sleep Med 2003;1(3):125–39.

66. Trockel M, Karlin BE, Taylor CB, et al. Cognitive behavioral therapy for insomnia with veterans: evaluation of effectiveness and correlates of treatment outcomes. Behav Res Ther 2014;53:41–6.

67. Manber R, Carney C, Edinger J, et al. Dissemination of CBTI to the non-sleep specialist: protocol development and training issues. J Clin Sleep Med 2012;8(2):209–18.

68. Lichstein KL, Riedel BW, Grieve R. Fair tests of clinical trials: a treatment implementation model. Adv Behav Res Ther 1994;16(1):1–29.

69. Manber R, Edinger JD, Gress JL, et al. Cognitive behavioral therapy for insomnia enhances depression outcome in patients with comorbid major

depressive disorder and insomnia. Sleep 2008; 31(4):489–95.

70. Crawford MR, Vallières A. The dark side of adherence-a commentary on palm et al.(2018) factors influencing adherence to continuous positive airway pressure treatment in obstructive sleep apnea and mortality associated with treatment failure- A national registry-based cohort study. Sleep Med 2019;51(85):91.

71. Carney CE, Lajos LE, Waters WF. Wrist actigraph versus self-report in normal sleepers: sleep schedule adherence and self-report validity. Behav Sleep Med 2004;2(3):134–43 [discussion: 144–7].

72. Crawford MR, Espie CA, Bartlett DJ, et al. Integrating psychology and medicine in CPAP adherence- new concepts? Sleep Med Rev 2014;18(2): 123–39.

Considering the Role of Adherence in New and Emerging Sleep Treatments

Simon A. Joosten, MBBS, BMedSc, PhD[a,b,c,*], Shane A. Landry, PhD[d,e],
Ai-Ming Wong, MBBS, BMedSc, PhD[a,b], Bradley A. Edwards, PhD[d,e]

KEYWORDS

- Obstructive sleep apnea • Sleep medicine • Positive airway pressure

KEY POINTS

- There are several novel and emerging treatments for obstructive sleep apnea (OSA), including new devices and pharmacotherapies.
- For the most part, long-term efficacy and adherence data for these interventions in the sleep context are lacking.
- Future studies exploring the long-term adherence and efficacy in novel and emerging treatments of OSA are required to fully understand the place of these treatments in treatment hierarchies.
- Such research also should aim to evaluate the use of these novel therapies in real-world clinical settings, because many of the studies performed to date have been done under closely monitored research populations and relatively small sample sizes.

INTRODUCTION

Adherence can be broadly defined as the extent to which a patient's actions agree or correlate with medical or health advice.

In the field of sleep medicine, considerable time and effort have been spent acknowledging the need for patients to adhere to recommended treatments in order to maintain or receive the putative benefits. Not only do patients need to administer treatments on a nightly basis (eg, Did they use the treatment?) but also they are required to achieve certain time goals on treatment (eg, How much treatment did they get while they were asleep?) with the idea being that the more sleep time the treatment is in place the better the outcome. Many studies of continuous positive airway pressure (CPAP) therapy have adopted this approach, including the biggest randomized controlled trials (RCTs) of treatment efficacy.[1]

The additional dimension to consider in adherence is the interaction between the perceived severity of the illness being treated and the apparent side effects of the treatment being used. In the sleep context, this paradigm often takes the form of sleepiness and snoring as the main symptoms being treated and sleep interruption as the main side effect of the treatment. This is a relatively unique balance because sleep-related treatments have the potential side effect of worsening the presenting complaint. Further to this, aspects of the illness being treated can have an impact on adherence. For example, depression is a common comorbidity of

---

[a] Monash Lung and Sleep, Monash Medical Centre, 246 Clayton Road, Clayton 3168, Victoria, Australia;
[b] School of Clinical Sciences, Monash University, Melbourne, Victoria, Australia; [c] Monash Partners – Epworth, Clayton, Victoria, Australia; [d] Department of Physiology, School of Biomedical Sciences and Biomedicine Discovery Institute, Monash University, 264 Ferntreegully Road, Notting Hill 3168, Melbourne, Victoria, Australia;
[e] Turner Institute for Brain and Mental Health, Monash University, Melbourne, Victoria, Australia

* Corresponding author. Sleep and Circadian Medicine Laboratory, Monash University BASE Facility, Ground Floor, 264 Ferntree Gully Road, Notting Hill, Victoria 3168, Australia,
E-mail address: simon.joosten@monash.edu

Sleep Med Clin 16 (2021) 203–211
https://doi.org/10.1016/j.jsmc.2020.12.001

obstructive sleep apnea (OSA) and depression itself can have an impact on adherence.[2]

By way of comparison, the World Health Organization reports that up to 50% of patients living in developed countries who are diagnosed with chronic disease do not adhere to the recommended treatment.[3] These rates are similar to the rates of treatment discontinuation for CPAP at 6 months.[4] It may be more reasonable, however, to compare sleep-based treatments to other time-based treatment strategies, for example, peritoneal dialysis, a treatment that requires patients to commit to actually doing the treatment and to commit the time to allow for the treatment to be effective. In a systematic review of peritoneal dialysis adherence, Griva and colleagues'[5] nonadherence rates for peritoneal dialysis exchanges range from 2.6% to 53%. Again, these are comparable to figures for patients able to achieve adequate time on CPAP (defined in the aforementioned CPAP study as 3 or more hours per night).

Continuous CPAP is the current gold standard and first-line treatment of OSA. It works by delivering a positive pressure through a nasal/face mask interface that works to pneumatically splint the upper airway open. In addition to resolving OSA, CPAP therapy also improves daytime sleepiness, reduces hypertension, improves quality of life, and is associated with a reduction in the risk of fatal and nonfatal cardiovascular events. The chief limitation of CPAP is that it provides therapeutic benefit only when it is used, and evidence from RCTs show that CPAP adherence is consistently low (approximately 3.5 hours use per night). It is estimated that between 29% and 83% of patients are nonadherent to their CPAP therapy, when nonadherence is defined as a mean of less than or equal to 4 hours of use per night.[6,7]

Although there are several alternative treatment options available (ie, mandibular advancement devices, lateral positioning, and weight loss), many of them have a variable effect on improving OSA and its deleterious consequences. The variable efficacy of these therapies is likely attributable to a combination of (1) how good each treatment is at reducing/abolishing OSA severity and (2) how compliant the patient is with the therapy. For example, CPAP and oral appliances have been suggested as having similar effectiveness in treating OSA but the ways they achieve this are different. CPAP is excellent at abolishing OSA but many people do not sleep with the machine for all of the night. By contrast, oral appliances may not be able to reduce the apnea and hypopnea index (AHI) as well as CPAP, but they have better adherence resulting in a similar efficacy. The optimal therapy, therefore, is one that is highly effective at reducing OSA severity and one that patients use regularly for the entire time they are sleeping.

As such, there has been an intense research focus on developing new/novel therapies for the treatment of this disorder that are both highly effective and easy for patients to adhere to. The focus of this review is on patient adherence to emerging and novel treatments for OSA.

HYPOGLOSSAL NERVE STIMULATION

Hypoglossal nerve stimulation (HNS) treats OSA via neurostimulation of the genioglossus muscle, which in turn decreases upper airway collapsibility. It typically is employed as a second-line therapy for patients who either are nonadherent or do not tolerate CPAP. There are 3 main types of devices: unilateral HNS,[8,9] bilateral HNS,[10] and targeted HNS by stimulating the hypoglossal nerve with 6 electrodes at a more proximal location, catching branches to all lingual muscles, including the tongue.[11] Collectively, these studies have shown HNS to be highly efficacious in improving OSA severity (using the AHI) and improving quality of life.

With regard to patient adherence, selective unilateral HNSs are able to objectively record and store patient utilization data. Overall, there was relatively good usage of the device. Kezirian and colleagues[9] monitored 31 participants over 12 months and demonstrated that their participants used the HNS for an average of 5.4 hours ± 1.4 hours per night, and therapy was used for a mean of 86% ± 16% of nights. Kent and colleagues[12] recruited 20 participants following implantation of a unilateral HNS and reported a mean adherence monitoring via device interrogation of 7.0 hours ± 2.2 hours per night, although participants were reviewed between 2 months and 6 months post-HNS implantation. Similarly, Steffen and colleagues[13] reported an average use of 39.1 hours ± 14.9 hours per week among all 60 participants who received unilateral HNS device after 12 month. Among these participants, 89% used HNS for greater than or equal to 20 hours per week.

Two newer studies have also assessed patients' adherence to HNS via a series of questionnaires. Eastwood and colleagues[10] administered a usability questionnaire to participants at 6 months, detailing the number of hours used per night and the number of nights used per week. At 6 months post–bilateral HNS implantation, 91% of participants reported using bilateral HNS greater than 5 days per week and 77% reported an average nightly use of greater than 5 hours. Hofauer and colleagues[14] explored the participants' attitude toward the unilateral HNS treatment toward their OSA and quality of life and collected HNS adherence data. The questionnaires also evaluated (1) the use of different functions of the HNS and (2) the subjective sensation of the stimulation. After 1 month of implantation of the HNS, participants used HNS for an average of 40 hours ± 14.2 hours per week, which is equivalent to an average of 5.7 hours ± 2.0 hours per day. The duration of objective use correlated with the subjective patient reporting of using HNS for an average of 6.8 days ± 0.9 days per week and for between 5 hours and 7 hours per day. Furthermore, 74.5% of participants used HNS for greater than or equal to 4 hours per night. Although up to 13.7% of participants were sometimes awoken by HNS at night, none of the reported sensations influenced the objective nightly usage. The AHI or daytime sleepiness did not have any obvious influence on adherence.

Several adverse events are relatively common among patients, with a meta-analysis investigating the outcomes of HNS in the management of OSA[15] reporting 6.2% of patients experiencing some form of pain; 11% of patients experiencing tongue abrasion with or without lesions; and 3.0% and 5.8% of patients experiencing internal and external device malfunction, respectively. This study, however, did not review patient compliance with the HNS device and whether these adverse effects affected patients' adherence.

Therefore, HNS for treatment of OSA appears to be reasonably tolerated by a majority of participants, with reasonable adherence reported both objectively and subjectively. Future studies reviewing whether patient adherence is affected by HNS adverse events may help provide further insight on whether these complications impact on patient adherence and should form part of counseling when starting patients on HNS.

PHARMACOTHERAPY FOR OBSTRUCTIVE SLEEP APNEA

Given that OSA now is recognized to be a multifactorial disorder caused by a combination of anatomic and nonanatomic causes or endotypes, this has opened up the field to identify pharmacologic agents that might be able to specifically target the abnormal factors. More specifically, the drugs that have been trialed to date all have been focused on improving/correcting the nonanatomic causes of OSA, which contribute its development in a majority of patients. These include (1) ineffective upper airway dilator muscles, (2) a low respiratory arousal threshold, and (3) a hypersensitive ventilatory control system (ie, high loop gain).

Sedatives/Hypnotics Targeting a Low Arousal Threshold

The arousal threshold is the level of ventilatory drive at which a patient arouses (awakens) from sleep. The lower the arousal threshold, the more readily increases in ventilatory drive can cause arousal from sleep. The presence of a low arousal threshold (which occurs in approximately 30%–50% of individuals with OSA) can destabilize breathing (and sleep) and impede the ability for compensatory muscles responses to effectively dilate the airway while maintaining sleep. Several studies have trailed sedatives/hypnotics in an attempt to raise the arousal threshold and treat OSA.[16] The effects of these studies vary dramatically, however, in the degree to which they alter the arousal threshold and/or OSA severity.[17–21] Most of the trials in OSA patients typically give the medication only for 1 night, with no adherence data available for longer-term use in this context. The longest duration trial specifically in OSA patients is that of Carter and colleagues,[22] who performed a randomized double-blind parallel trial of zopiclone for 1 month. Although adherence (assessed as pill count at day 30 of the trial) was reported to be high for both the zopiclone and placebo groups (93.7% ± 9.7% and 93.4% ± 11.0%, respectively), only approximately a third of participants said that they would continue with the study medication if available.

Although long-term studies in OSA patients currently are lacking, there are more data available regarding the longer-term use of sedatives for the treatment of chronic insomnia. In a 6-month double-blind trial of eszopiclone (vs placebo) in 830 patients with chronic insomnia, Krystal and colleagues[23] demonstrated that although the discontinuation rates were not different, they were approximately 40%, a rate that has been reported by another study of similar duration.[24] In the trial by Krystal and colleagues,23, adherence to the treatment regimen was calculated using the number of doses taken (determined by tablets counts) divided by the number of doses to be taken (calculated as the number of days on study), multiplied by 100. The mean adherence rates were 94.4% and 90.6% for eszopiclone and placebo, respectively. The investigators also performed an open-label extension in a subset of these patents for a further 6 months (total 12 months) and showed that discontinuation rates were at approximately 20% and adherence during this phase was quite high, at 96%.[25]

Serotonergic, Noradrenergic, and Antimuscarinic Medications Targeting the Ineffective Upper Airway Dilator Muscles

In order for the upper airway dilator muscles to hold open the small pharyngeal airway present in OSA and protect against collapse, the airway dilator muscles have to be responsive to collapsing forces and the increased muscle activity has to be effective at reopening the upper airway. Unfortunately, a proportion of patients with OSA display poor pharyngeal dilator muscle effectiveness or responsiveness, which describes the amount of additional ventilation or muscle activity, respectively, that can be achieved by compensatory activation of the pharyngeal dilator muscles of the upper airway in response to increases in ventilatory drive. Several medications with varying serotonergic, noradrenergic, and antimuscarinic activities have been trialed in patients with OSA, with varying degrees of efficacy, in order to improve dilator muscle activity.[26] Most of the studies exploring the effects of drug treatments on upper airway dilator muscle function involve very small numbers of patients, studied for a single night (often delivered only a single dose of medication). Perhaps the most promising drug combination is that of atomoxetine and oxybutynin. In a single-night study of 20 participants, Taranto-Montemurro and colleagues[27] demonstrated an improvement in genioglossus responsiveness, with subsequent improvement in AHI of 63%.

Because centrally acting medications can have varying effects on a range of neurotransmitter receptors, drawing broad conclusions about groups of side effect profiles and adherence issues is difficult. Atomoxetine is a stimulant with predominantly noradrenergic effects that is prescribed primarily for attention-deficit/hyperactivity disorder (ADHD) in children. In 1 study of 32,937 adult patients receiving stimulants for ADHD, of whom 4113 received atomoxetine, it was demonstrated that adherence to atomoxetine administration is lower than for other stimulants.[28] The study utilized a method of proportion of days covered to measure treatment adherence. It is calculated as the number of days covered by the prescribed drug divided by the days in the study period (which was 12 months). Adults naïve to stimulants who were prescribed atomoxetine had a proportion of days covered of only 0.31 ± 0.28, the worst adherence rate of all stimulants studied in this article. It is not clear how this poor adherence rate would translate to a sleep population.

Oxybutynin is an antimuscarinic agent typically prescribed in adults with detrusor hyperactivity or hyperhidrosis. In a large study of prescription database of general practitioners in the United Kingdom involving 6189 patients prescribed antimuscarinics for overactive bladder over 12 months, oxybutynin was the most poorly adhered to medication, with a median number of days on therapy of 86.5 days to 116.4 days over the 12 months. Over the 12-month period, only 13.3% to 24.4% of patients received antimuscarinics for more than 80% of the time.

Currently, small-number physiology studies demonstrating pharmacotherapy efficacy at improving dilator muscle effectiveness and AHI in OSA patients have utilized medicines with poor adherence rates within their class and indication strata. No data exist to date on the adherence to these medicines in the sleep medicine context.

Acetazolamide Targeting High Loop Gain

There is growing evidence indicating that a hypersensitive ventilatory control system (high loop gain) is a key factor contributing to the pathogenesis of OSA in many individuals. In OSA physiology, loop gain represents the inherent stability of the negative feedback loop that controls breathing. A high loop gain constitutes an unstable system, where a small disturbance in breathing (ie, a hypopnea) can lead to a large corrective overshoot, resulting in cyclical fluctuations in breathing/ventilatory drive, perpetuating subsequent obstructive events. As such, acetazolamide (ACZ) has been trialed for treatment of OSA, largely due to its ability to lower loop gain and stabilize respiratory control.

ACZ is a carbonic anhydrase inhibitor that has been used in therapeutically for a variety of conditions, such as glaucoma,[29] idiopathic intracranial hypertension,[30] acute mountain sickness,[31] obstructive,[32] and central sleep apnea (CSA).[33] ACZ commonly is taken orally; however, dosage amount and regime can vary considerably between conditions and studies. Key side effects of ACZ include paresthesias, dysgeusia (ie, taste alteration), polyuria, and fatigue. A meta-analysis of 53 studies reporting ACZ's side effects demonstrates that they are experienced commonly by participants, in particular, paresthesias, which had an odds ratio of 12.3.[34] Paresthesia and dysgeusia demonstrated clear dose-dependent relationships that did not appear to plateau at any particular dose.

With regard to ACZ's ability to treat OSA, a recent meta-analysis of 28 studies by Schmickl and colleagues[35] demonstrated that ACZ significantly reduced the AHI by 37.7% (approximately 13.8/h) and improved the oxygen saturation as measured by pulse oximetry nadir by 4.4%. This effect was similarly strong for both CSA and OSA. Furthermore, meta-regression demonstrated a dose-response relationship, indicating greater therapeutic benefits, occurred at higher dosage levels. This effect plateaued, however, at 500 mg/d, with reduced benefit observed at higher dosage. Together, these recent meta-analyses indicate that an ideal effective dose for the treatment of OSA/CSA may be between 125 mg/d and 500 mg/d.

Despite a large and diverse series of RCTs and case series evidence examining the efficacy and side-effect profile of ACZ, there are limited published data on adherence. This is not surprising given that a majority of published trials have involved short periods of use, typically greater than or equal to 7 days (mean = 17 days).[34,35] Furthermore, doses have tended to be high, particularly in short trials focused on demonstrating efficacy (OSA/CSA studies mean dose 556 mg/d[35]). Despite the high doses used in this study, discontinue/dropout rates tend to be low, with several trials reporting all participants completing the trial.[36–41]

Several longer-term trials provide more relevant information with regard to tolerance. Vahedi and colleagues[42] performed a parallel-group (n = 26/25) RCT using 500 mg/d for 90 days for migraine prophylaxis. Twelve (46%) participants in the ACZ group discontinued the trial compared with 6 in the placebo group. Although noncompliance was approximately equal (ACZ = 3 and placebo = 4), discontinuation due to side effects (mainly paresthesia, 81%, and fatigue, 58%) was the predominate cause in the ACZ group. Two parallel-group RCTs using 250-mg/d doses of ACZ in patients with chronic mountain sickness showed numerically higher number of participants lost to follow-up in ACZ arms compared with placebo: 7/22 (31%) over 42 days[43] and 6/40 (15%) over 90 days.[44] ten Hove and colleagues[30] performed a 6-month RCT in patients with idiopathic intracranial hypertension. Patients started at a 250-mg/d dose and increased by 250 mg per week in an attempt to achieve a maximum dose of 4000 mg/d. Only 9.5% (9/95) participants randomized to the ACZ group discontinued. Of the 86 who completed the trial, 38 (44.2%) were able to tolerate the maximum dose (4 g/d), with a further 39 (45.3%) tolerating a dose 1000 mg/d to 3750 mg/d, and 9 (10.5%) tolerating a dose between 125 mg and 750 mg.

Only a few studies report conducting pill counts[30,33,39,45,46] or any other means of direct adherence monitoring, but, to the authors' knowledge, only 1 study has reported these data in publication. Basnyat and colleagues[46] performed a 2-day to 3-day RCT exploring a 250-mg/d dose of ACZ for prophylaxis of acute mountain sickness. Participants were trekkers who were recruited during their assent to Everest Base Camp. Although participants lost to follow-up were consistent between the ACZ (22/96 [23%]) and the placebo arms (20/101 [19.8%]), 20% of participants in the ACZ had missed doses versus 3.7% in the placebo group. Participants missing doses also were more likely to have experienced paresthesias.

Compliance with therapy often has been monitored by blood tests analyzed for markers of metabolic acidosis, in particular, reduced serum pH and bicarbonate. Although individual data for these variables rarely has been reported, the group differences typically are of large effect size, which may indicate high adherence in most short trials. ACZ has a relatively short plasma half-life (approximately 4 h); however, metabolic acidosis often takes 2 days to 3 days of dosing to accumulate. At present, it is relatively unknown how intermittent/missed dosing affects day-to-day bicarbonate/pH data or treatment efficacy. Individual data reflecting changes in metabolic acidosis have been presented in only a few studies. Eskandari and colleagues[45] demonstrated a linear relationship between reduction in bicarbonate and AHI.[45] These data indicate that all participants (treated with mean dose of 658 mg/d) experienced a reduction in bicarbonate of at least 5 mmol/L. Conversely, 2 studies[44,47] show a subset of participants with relatively small or unchanged bicarbonate levels on ACZ, which may be indicative of poor adherence in these individuals. In a 12-week 500 mg/d trial, Vahedi and colleagues[42] examined bicarbonate levels every 4 weeks, and there appears an acute reduction in bicarbonate in the first 4 weeks of ACZ followed by a small and gradually increase over subsequent weeks. This may indicate reduced adherence over time or a reduced acidosis. Consistent with these data, White and colleagues[48] reported good tolerance of 1000-mg/d ACZ at a 1-year follow-up in 2 participants, 1 of whom no longer demonstrated evidence of metabolic acidosis (normal pH and bicarbonate) at follow-up.

NASAL DILATORS

Nasal dilators are devices that dilate the nasal passages either externally (usually worn on the skin of the nose) or internally (usually placed inside the opening of the nose). Although these devices have been reported on in medical literature since approximately 1993, they usually are not considered an established OSA treatment, although they have been tested in OSA populations with mixed efficacy results on OSA metrics in various studies. The most common reported reasons for discontinuation of use include skin irritation, nasal discomfort, poor fit (ie, device falls out/off), and perceived lack of efficacy compared with other treatments.

Although several single-night studies have reported on the use of external nasal dilators,[49–52] few studies report medium-term use and no studies report on long-term use of external nasal dilators. In a 1-week run in as part of single-night crossover trial of external nasal dilators Djupesland and colleagues[53] found the dilator was "well tolerated" without reporting actual figures. Over a 3-month period in a randomized crossover study of external nasal dilators in patients with acromegaly in Brazil, Amaro and colleagues[54] found a compliance rate of 98%, using a pill count method (ie, patients given just the right amount of dilator strips to account for the number of days in the study and any left over strips counted and recorded), although this method of compliance testing does not account for nights when the device was fitted but fell off during the night. In an RCT conducted by Redline and colleagues,[55] external nasal dilator treatment was applied to 46 patients for a period of 8 weeks to 12 weeks, with reported compliance 82% ± 26% of nights. This arm of treatment was a conservative treatment arm of a larger study of effectiveness of CPAP for mild OSA. At the end of the study, the investigators asked participants if they were interested in continuing therapy and 72% answered affirmatively (although use of external nasal dilator strips was combined with use of nasal spray in addition to dilators). In summary, data regarding the long-term efficacy of external nasal dilators are lacking. Short-term and medium-term data suggest compliance above 80% in small numbers of patients.

For comparison, the use of internal nasal dilators is documented in several small studies of short-term, medium-term, and long-term usage. Most of these studies report some degree of participant dropout, presumably due to device discomfort or lack of efficacy. In a 1-month run in of an internal nasal dilator prospective study, Schonhofer and colleagues[56] reported a dropout rate of 5/26 patients. Of the 21 patients who completed the study, 16 participants found that the device was lost several times a night (ie, fell out). Furthermore, over 6-month period of use as part of an observational trial, Loth and colleagues[57] reported that 5/42 patients dropped out in the first month, 15/42 dropped out in 6 months, and, when followed-up 5 years later, 9/42 were still using the device.[58]

EXPIRATORY RESISTANCE VALVES

Nasal resistance valves restrict nasal exhalation creating a backlog of pressure (ie, positive end-expiratory pressure) that splints the airway open. They typically are 1-time use, disposable devices worn nightly and consist of a small valve held in place just inside each nostril by a hypoallergenic adhesive. Efficacy for treating snoring and OSA has been reported to be variable (reductions in the AHI ranging between 43% and 59%), with most studies trialing these devices in those with mild to moderate OSA and some studies reporting a better response in those that do not have existing nasal obstruction. The most common reported reasons for discontinuation of devices are skin irritation and lack of efficacy.

There are both medium-term and longer-term adherence data reported on small numbers of individuals. In an RCT of nasal resistance valves of 127 patients with mild to moderate OSA randomized to receive the device, 119 patients completed the trial with dropout due to a combination of noncompliance, adverse effects, and lost to follow-up.[59] In the 119 patients who received 3 months of treatment, the device was worn the entire night for median 88.2% (67.5, 96.4) of nights and experienced a 43% reduction in the AHI. Similarly, in a study by Walsh and colleagues,[60] a dropout rate of 11/59 patients was reported. Of the 24 participants randomized to receive treatment device, use of 92% to 97% of sleep time was reported over a 5-week period as well as experiencing a 45% reduction in their AHI. Friedman and colleagues[61] reported a similar adherence of 86.4% in 38/59 patients who completed a 30-day trial of nasal expiratory valve device. In a longer-term follow-up of a nasal expiratory valve device, Kryger and colleagues[62] found that 34/51 patients continued to use the nasal valve device after 12 months and that they reported wearing the device for the entire night 89% of the time.

In summary, most studies report an initial noncompliance/dropout rate of approximately 20% with nasal expiratory valve devices. Medium-term compliance appears to be approximately 90% and longer-term rates in smaller number studies are approximately 70%.

SUCTION DEVICES

Oral suction devices are designed to apply negative pressure to structures of the oropharynx in order to anteriorize soft tissue structures and create space at the back of the throat. Efficacy is variable.

Reasons for discontinuing this treatment usually hinge on oral discomfort and mouthpiece fitting/poor vacuum seal.

There is little in the way of long-term compliance data on these devices. In a multicenter RCT of device, Colrain and colleagues[63] demonstrated over a 4-week period that 57 subjects used the device for 6.0 hours $\pm$ 1.4 hours per night and 84% of patients use exceeded a median of 4 hours. Furthermore, Farid-Moayer and colleagues observed that 19/54 subjects reported oral tissue discomfort of the palate and throat with this device and 12% reported oral abrasion or erythema.[64]

In summary, many patients experience some level of oral discomfort with these devices in the short/medium term, and long-term adherence data are lacking.

SUMMARY

There are several novel and emerging treatments for OSA, including new devices and pharmacotherapies. For the most part, long-term efficacy and adherence data for these interventions in the sleep context are lacking. In some cases, however, it is possible to infer possible adherence rates from treatments of other conditions in cases of pharmacotherapies.

Adherence to device treatments entails an extra dimension in the sleep context. Not only are patients required to apply the device treatment, they often are required to reapply or adjust during the course of the night to ensure the device is in situ for the duration of sleep. Device treatment of OSA is a unique situation in which the device itself has the potential to worsen sleepiness, often one of the cardinal symptoms of a sleep disorder.

Future studies exploring the long-term adherence and efficacy in novel and emerging treatments for OSA are required to fully understand the place of these treatments in treatment hierarchies. Such research also should aim to evaluate the use of these novel therapies in real-world clinical settings, because many of the studies performed to date have been done under closely monitored research populations and relatively small sample sizes.

CLINICS CARE POINTS

- New and emerging treatments for OSA by definition lack long term efficacy and adherence data.
- When considering emerging treatments for OSA, understanding the barriers to adherence is important and these barriers can very

depending on the treatment and its relevant side effects.
- Adherence to sleep therapies not only encompasses the binary consideration of if the treatment was taken but also how much of the sleep period the treatment was being used and if the treatment itself became a barrier to treatment.

DISCLOSURE

S.A. Joosten have received equipment to support research from ResMed, Philips Respironics, and Air Liquide Healthcare. B.A. Edwards has received funding from Apnimed. B.A. Edwards is supported by a Heart Foundation of Australia Future Leader Fellowship (101167). S.A. Joosten is supported by an NHMRC early career fellowship (1139745).

REFERENCES

1. McEvoy RD, Antic NA, Heeley E, et al. CPAP for preventions of cardiovascular events in obstructive sleep apnea. N Engl J Med 2016;375:919–31.
2. Phillips KD, Moneyham L, Murdaugh C, et al. Sleep disturbance and depression as barriers to adherence. Clin Nurs Res 2005;14:273–93.
3. Sabat. Adherence to long-term therapies: evidence for action. Geneva (Switzerland): World Health Organization; 2003.
4. Kribbs NB, Pack AI, Kline LR, et al. Objective measurement of patterns of nasal CPAP use by patients with obstructive sleep apnea. Am Rev Respir Dis 1993;147:887–95.
5. Griva K, Lai AY, Lim HA, et al. Non-adherence in patients on peritoneal dialysis: a systematic review. PLoS One 2014;9:e89001.
6. Sawyer AM, Gooneratne NS, Marcus CL, et al. A systematic review of CPAP adherence across age groups: clinical and empiric insights for developing CPAP adherence interventions. Sleep Med Rev 2011;15:343–56.
7. Weaver TE, Grunstein RR. Adherence to continuous positive airway pressure therapy: the challenge to effective treatment. Proc Am Thorac Soc 2008;5:173–8.
8. Strollo PJ Jr, Soose RJ, Maurer JT, et al. Upper-airway stimulation for obstructive sleep apnea. N Engl J Med 2014;370:139–49.
9. Kezirian EJ, Goding GS Jr, Malhotra A, et al. Hypoglossal nerve stimulation improves obstructive sleep apnea: 12-month outcomes. J Sleep Res 2014;23:77–83.
10. Eastwood PR, Barnes M, MacKay SG, et al. Bilateral hypoglossal nerve stimulation for treatment of adult obstructive sleep apnoea. Eur Respir J 2020;55.

11. Friedman M, Jacobowitz O, Hwang MS, et al. Targeted hypoglossal nerve stimulation for the treatment of obstructive sleep apnea: six-month results. Laryngoscope 2016;126:2618–23.

12. Kent DT, Lee JJ, Strollo PJ Jr, et al. Upper airway stimulation for OSA: early adherence and outcome results of one center. Otolaryngol Head Neck Surg 2016;155:188–93.

13. Steffen A, Sommer JU, Hofauer B, et al. Outcome after one year of upper airway stimulation for obstructive sleep apnea in a multicenter German post-market study. Laryngoscope 2018;128:509–15.

14. Hofauer B, Steffen A, Knopf A, et al. Patient experience with upper airway stimulation in the treatment of obstructive sleep apnea. Sleep Breath 2019;23: 235–41.

15. Kompelli AR, Ni JS, Nguyen SA, et al. The outcomes of hypoglossal nerve stimulation in the management of OSA: a systematic review and meta-analysis. World J Otorhinolaryngol Head Neck Surg 2019;5: 41–8.

16. Jordan AS, O'Donoghue FJ, Cori JM, et al. Physiology of arousal in obstructive sleep apnea and potential impacts for sedative treatment. Am J Respir Crit Care Med 2017;196:814–21.

17. Heinzer RC, White DP, Jordan AS, et al. Trazodone increases arousal threshold in obstructive sleep apnoea. Eur Respir J 2008;31:1308–12.

18. Eckert DJ, Owens RL, Kehlmann GB, et al. Eszopiclone increases the respiratory arousal threshold and lowers the apnoea/hypopnoea index in obstructive sleep apnoea patients with a low arousal threshold. Clin Sci (Lond) 2011;120:505–14.

19. Smales ET, Edwards BA, Deyoung PN, et al. Trazodone effects on obstructive sleep apnea and non-REM arousal threshold. Ann Am Thorac Soc 2015; 12:758–64.

20. Carberry JC, Fisher LP, Grunstein RR, et al. Role of common hypnotics on the phenotypic causes of obstructive sleep apnoea: paradoxical effects of zolpidem. Eur Respir J 2017;50.

21. Carberry JC, Grunstein RR, Eckert DJ. The effects of zolpidem in obstructive sleep apnea - an open-label pilot study. J Sleep Res 2019;28:e12853.

22. Carter SG, Carberry JC, Cho G, et al. Effect of 1 month of zopiclone on obstructive sleep apnoea severity and symptoms: a randomised controlled trial. Eur Respir J 2018;52.

23. Krystal AD, Walsh JK, Laska E, et al. Sustained efficacy of eszopiclone over 6 months of nightly treatment: results of a randomized, double-blind, placebo-controlled study in adults with chronic insomnia. Sleep 2003;26:793–9.

24. Walsh JK, Krystal AD, Amato DA, et al. Nightly treatment of primary insomnia with eszopiclone for six months: effect on sleep, quality of life, and work limitations. Sleep 2007;30:959–68.

25. Roth T, Walsh JK, Krystal A, et al. An evaluation of the efficacy and safety of eszopiclone over 12 months in patients with chronic primary insomnia. Sleep Med 2005;6:487–95.

26. Taranto-Montemurro L, Messineo L, Wellman A. Targeting endotypic traits with medications for the pharmacological treatment of obstructive sleep apnea. a review of the current literature. J Clin Med 2019;8.

27. Taranto-Montemurro L, Messineo L, Sands SA, et al. The combination of atomoxetine and oxybutynin greatly reduces obstructive sleep apnea severity. A randomized, placebo-controlled, double-blind crossover trial. Am J Respir Crit Care Med 2019; 199:1267–76.

28. Setyawan J, Hodgkins P, Guerin A, et al. Comparing treatment adherence of lisdexamfetamine and other medications for the treatment of attention deficit/hyperactivity disorder: a retrospective analysis. J Med Econ 2013;16:962–75.

29. Lusthaus J, Goldberg I. Current management of glaucoma. Med J Aust 2019;210:180–7.

30. ten Hove MW, Friedman DI, Patel AD, et al. Safety and tolerability of acetazolamide in the idiopathic intracranial hypertension treatment trial. J Neuroophthalmol 2016;36:13–9.

31. Low EV, Avery AJ, Gupta V, et al. Identifying the lowest effective dose of acetazolamide for the prophylaxis of acute mountain sickness: systematic review and meta-analysis. BMJ 2012;345:e6779.

32. Edwards BA, Sands SA, Eckert DJ, et al. Acetazolamide improves loop gain but not the other physiological traits causing obstructive sleep apnoea. J Physiol 2012;590:1199–211.

33. Javaheri S. Acetazolamide improves central sleep apnea in heart failure: a double-blind, prospective study. Am J Respir Crit Care Med 2006; 173:234–7.

34. Schmickl CN, Owens RL, Orr JE, et al. Side effects of acetazolamide: a systematic review and meta-analysis assessing overall risk and dose dependence. BMJ open Respir Res 2020;7:e000557.

35. Schmickl CN, Landry SA, Orr JE, et al. Acetazolamide for OSA and central sleep apnea: a comprehensive systematic review and meta-analysis. Chest 2020;158(6):2632–45.

36. DeBacker WA, Verbraecken J, Willemen M, et al. Central apnea index decreases after prolonged treatment with acetazolamide. Am J Respir Crit Care Med 1995;151:87–91.

37. Sakamoto T, Nakazawa Y, Hashizume Y, et al. Effects of acetazolamide on the sleep apnea syndrome and its therapeutic mechanism. Psychiatry Clin Neurosci 1995;49:59–64.

38. Latshang TD, Nussbaumer-Ochsner Y, Henn RM, et al. Effect of acetazolamide and AutoCPAP therapy on breathing disturbances among patients with obstructive sleep apnea syndrome who travel to

altitude: a randomized controlled trial. JAMA 2012; 308:2390–8.

39. Ulrich S, Keusch S, Hildenbrand FF, et al. Effect of nocturnal oxygen and acetazolamide on exercise performance in patients with pre-capillary pulmonary hypertension and sleep-disturbed breathing: randomized, double-blind, cross-over trial. Eur Heart J 2015;36:615–23.

40. Tojima H, Kunitomo F, Kimura H, et al. Effects of acetazolamide in patients with the sleep apnoea syndrome. Thorax 1988;43:113–9.

41. Sutton JR, Houston CS, Mansell AL, et al. Effect of acetazolamide on hypoxemia during sleep at high altitude. N Engl J Med 1979;301:1329–31.

42. Vahedi K, Taupin P, Djomby R, et al. Efficacy and tolerability of acetazolamide in migraine prophylaxis: a randomised placebo-controlled trial. J Neurol 2002;249:206–11.

43. Sharma S, Gralla J, Ordonez JG, et al. Acetazolamide and N-acetylcysteine in the treatment of chronic mountain sickness (Monge's disease). Respir Physiol Neurobiol 2017;246:1–8.

44. Richalet J-P, Rivera-Ch M, Maignan M, et al. Acetazolamide for monge's disease. Am J Respir Crit Care Med 2008;177:1370–6.

45. Eskandari D, Zou D, Grote L, et al. Acetazolamide reduces blood pressure and sleep-disordered breathing in patients with hypertension and obstructive sleep apnea: a randomized controlled trial. J Clin Sleep Med 2018;14:309–17.

46. Basnyat B, Gertsch JH, Johnson EW, et al. Efficacy of low-dose acetazolamide (125 mg BID) for the prophylaxis of acute mountain sickness: a prospective, double-blind, randomized, placebo-controlled trial. High Alt Med Biol 2003;4:45–52.

47. Fontana M, Emdin M, Giannoni A, et al. Effect of acetazolamide on chemosensitivity, cheyne-Stokes respiration, and response to effort in patients with heart failure. Am J Cardiol 2011;107:1675–80.

48. White DP, Zwillich CW, Pickett CK, et al. Central sleep apnea: improvement with acetazolamide therapy. Arch Intern Med 1982;142:1816–9.

49. Bahammam AS, Tate R, Manfreda J, et al. Upper airway resistance syndrome: effect of nasal dilation, sleep stage, and sleep position. Sleep 1999;22: 592–8.

50. Gosepath J, Amedee RG, Romantschuck S, et al. Breathe Right nasal strips and the respiratory disturbance index in sleep related breathing disorders. Am J Rhinol 1999;13:385–9.

51. Hoffstein V, Mateika S, Metes A. Effect of nasal dilation on snoring and apneas during different stages of sleep. Sleep 1993;16:360–5.

52. Pevernagie D, Hamans E, Van Cauwenberge P, et al. External nasal dilation reduces snoring in chronic rhinitis patients: a randomized controlled trial. Eur Respir J 2000;15:996–1000.

53. Djupesland PG, Skatvedt O, Borgersen AK. Dichotomous physiological effects of nocturnal external nasal dilation in heavy snorers: the answer to a rhinologic controversy? Am J Rhinol 2001;15:95–103.

54. Amaro AC, Duarte FH, Jallad RS, et al. The use of nasal dilator strips as a placebo for trials evaluating continuous positive airway pressure. Clinics (Sao Paulo) 2012;67:469–74.

55. Redline S, Adams N, Strauss ME, et al. Improvement of mild sleep-disordered breathing with CPAP compared with conservative therapy. Am J Respir Crit Care Med 1998;157:858–65.

56. Schonhofer B, Franklin KA, Brunig H, et al. Effect of nasal-valve dilation on obstructive sleep apnea. Chest 2000;118:587–90.

57. Loth S, Petruson B. Improved nasal breathing reduces snoring and morning tiredness. A 6-month follow-up study. Arch Otolaryngol Head Neck Surg 1996;122:1337–40.

58. Petruson B, Loth S. Five-year compliance with a nostril dilator. Arch Otolaryngol Head Neck Surg 2000; 126:1168–9.

59. Berry RB, Kryger MH, Massie CA. A novel nasal expiratory positive airway pressure (EPAP) device for the treatment of obstructive sleep apnea: a randomized controlled trial. Sleep 2011;34:479–85.

60. Walsh JK, Griffin KS, Forst EH, et al. A convenient expiratory positive airway pressure nasal device for the treatment of sleep apnea in patients nonadherent with continuous positive airway pressure. Sleep Med 2011;12:147–52.

61. Friedman M, Hwang MS, Yalamanchali S, et al. Provent therapy for obstructive sleep apnea: impact of nasal obstruction. Laryngoscope 2016; 126:254–9.

62. Kryger MH, Berry RB, Massie CA. Long-term use of a nasal expiratory positive airway pressure (EPAP) device as a treatment for obstructive sleep apnea (OSA). J Clin Sleep Med 2011;7:449-53B.

63. Colrain IM, Black J, Siegel LC, et al. A multicenter evaluation of oral pressure therapy for the treatment of obstructive sleep apnea. Sleep Med 2013;14: 830–7.

64. Farid-Moayer M, Siegel LC, Black J. A feasibility evaluation of oral pressure therapy for the treatment of obstructive sleep apnea. Ther Adv Respir Dis 2013;7:3–12.

Can Smartphone Apps Assist People with Serious Mental Illness in Taking Medications as Prescribed?

Cynthia L. Bianco, MS[a], Amanda L. Myers, BS[b,1], Stephen Smagula, PhD[c], Karen L. Fortuna, PhD, LICSW[d,*]

KEYWORDS

• Serious mental illness • Smartphone apps • Medication • Treatment

KEY POINTS

• Individuals with serious mental illness (SMI) have high rates of not taking medication as prescribed.
• Smartphone applications (apps) designed for people with SMI have been found feasible and acceptable among this population—yet, developing technologies that promote adherence among vulnerable populations presents unique challenges to adherence.
• Smartphone apps may serve to promote taking medications as prescribed.

INTRODUCTION

Medication nonadherence is common among adults with serious mental illness (SMI), with rates of nonadherence estimated to be at least 40% to 50%.[1–3] SMI is defined by a psychiatric diagnosis of schizophrenia spectrum disorders, bipolar disorder, or persistent major depressive disorder. In an effort to promote recovery language consistent with the mental health movement that originated as a medical model and now focuses on a recovery model of mental health, medication adherence henceforth is referred to as taking medication as prescribed. Not taking medication as prescribed is associated with increased risks of hospitalizations and relapse and increased severity of symptoms among people with SMI.[4–6] Reasons for not taking medication as prescribed vary and commonly include forgetting to take medications, poor insight into illness and the need to take medications, negative attitudes toward medications, and negative side effects from medications.[6–8]

Advances in technology, specifically mobile technology, provide a unique and potentially advantageous avenue for promoting taking medications as prescribed among vulnerable populations, including people with SMI. It is estimated that approximately 77% of US adults own a smartphone.[9] Although national rates of smartphone ownership among adults with SMI currently is not known, some reports suggest rates of ownership between 66% and 72%.[10,11] Previously, researchers expressed concern over the disparities in smartphone ownership among the SMI population due to socioeconomic factors and high rates of unemployment; however, a recent meta-analysis indicates an increasing trend in smartphone ownership among this population.[11] Developing and implementing mental health smartphone applications (apps) may serve to increase taking medication as prescribed as well as monitoring symptoms and functioning. This article reviews some of the smartphone

[a] Department of Psychiatry Research, Dartmouth-Hitchcock, 2 Pillsbury Street, Suite 401, Concord, NH 03301, USA; [b] Department of Public Health, Rivier University, Nashua, NH, USA; [c] Department of Psychiatry, University of Pittsburgh School of Medicine, 3811 O'Hara Street, Room E-1120, Pittsburgh, PA 15213, USA; [d] Department of Psychiatry, Dartmouth College, 2 Pillsbury Street, Suite 401, Concord, NH 03301, USA
[1] Present address: 2 Pillsbury Street, Suite 401, Concord, NH 03301.
* Corresponding author.
E-mail address: klfortuna@gmail.com

Sleep Med Clin 16 (2021) 213–222
https://doi.org/10.1016/j.jsmc.2020.10.010
1556-407X/21/© 2020 Elsevier Inc. All rights reserved.

apps designed for people with SMI that have functionality pertaining to taking medication as prescribed and compares with and contrasts against those available for sleep apnea.

SMARTPHONE APPLICATIONS

Few smartphone apps were designed to specifically address taking medication as prescribed among adults with SMI.[12–14] Most apps commonly included monitoring of medication adherence as a secondary feature[15–22] or utilized psychosocial interventions to provide information and strategies to enhance taking medication as prescribed while not measuring adherence directly.[23–25]

Smartphone Applications with Medication Adherence as Primary Feature

Wenze and colleagues[12,26] developed the smartphone app MyTreatment (MyT) to improve taking medication as prescribed among adults with bipolar disorder. MyT incorporates psychoeducation components and cognitive behavior therapy (CBT) elements. MyT alerts users twice daily to enter the app and complete the available surveys. During the morning, users are asked which medications they need to take that day and if they have any appointments. During the evening, users are asked if their medication was taken and if they attended their appointments. Both sessions assess for symptoms and potential risk factors for not taking medication as prescribed (eg, concern over medication side effects and need to engage in treatment). A small pilot study (N = 8) over 3 months deemed MyT feasible and found a decrease in missed medication doses by 22% and a decrease in missed appointments by 71%.[12] Additional research is needed to examine the full efficacy of the app on taking medication as prescribed.

MedActive is a smartphone app designed specifically to increase taking antipsychotic medication as prescribed among adults with schizophrenia.[13] Users designate a scheduled time in which they typically take their medications. Five minutes prior to the scheduled dose, MedActive notifies users with a personalized auditory and visual alert. Five minutes after the scheduled dose, MedActive asks people whether or not they took their medication. If medication is reported as not taken, participants are asked why. Additionally, if medication is not taken due to side effects, people are given the option to send an automated message to their psychiatrist. In a 2-week open trial,[13] MedActive was deemed feasible and acceptable. Participants (N = 7) reported taking their medication 100% of the time and a majority agreed that MedActive

made it easier to talk to their psychiatrists about their medication. Due to the short time frame of the study, however, the results are limited and future research is needed to examine outcomes during a longer duration of MedActive use.

MedLink was designed to improve taking antidepressant medications as prescribed among adults with major depressive disorder.[14] MedLink utilizes Wisepill, an electronic pill dispenser that sends wireless signals to the MedLink app, indicating that the pill bottle has been opened. MedLink users enter their daily scheduled time for medication; if a signal from Wisepill is not received within 10 minutes of that time, MedLink sends a smartphone alert asking users if they have taken their medication. This alert stays on the smartphone screen until the user responds or actively declines. If users state that the medication has not been taken, MedLink follows-up, asking users if they are planning on taking their medication. In addition to daily reminders, MedLink provides weekly brief lessons on antidepressants, strategies for taking medication as prescribed, and general self-management techniques. In a small pilot study (N = 11),[14] users experienced some technical difficulties, in particular connectivity problems, between Wisepill and MedLink. Despite this, users generally favored MedLink, and taking medication as prescribed was shown to be 82%, although it is not known how this compares to not using the app.

Smartphone Apps with Medication Adherence as Secondary Feature

MONARCA (I and II), developed by Faurholt-Jepsen and colleagues,[15,16] is a smartphone-based self-monitoring (SM) system designed for people with bipolar disorder. Participants receive smartphone notifications at a self-chosen time of day to evaluate mood and emotional states, functioning, behaviors, activity levels, individualized early warning signs, and use of medications. In 2 randomized controlled trials of MONARCA I (N = 78) and MONARCA II (N = 129), using a single-blind, parallel-group design, participants randomized to use MONARCA did not show significantly different levels of taking medication as prescribed at follow-up compared with control groups (lithium: $P = .49$, n = 64; lamotrigine: $P = .21$, n = 56; and quetiapine: $P = .16$, n = 48) or at 6 months' follow-up (lithium: $P = .22$, n = 29; lamotrigine: $P = .43$, n = 26; and quetiapine: $P = .99$, n = 17).[15,16]

Ginger.io is a smartphone app designed for adolescents and young adults with recent-onset psychosis.[19] Users received daily prompts to assess mood, medication use, and social interactions. Additionally, users completed weekly surveys on symptoms, sleep, and taking medication as prescribed. Daily surveys could be completed any time between 5:00 PM and 11:55 PM, while weekly surveys were available from Sundays at 10:00 AM to Mondays at 11:55 PM. In a longitudinal feasibility study using a within-person design (N = 76), a majority of participants in a feasibility study of Ginger.io felt that the app helped remind them to take their medication[19]; medication adherence rates were not reported.

App4Independence (A4i) was designed for individuals with schizophrenia to enhance self-management.[20] Twice-daily notifications prompt users to complete surveys assessing mental health and goal progress. Users also can custom set medication and appointment reminders. Additionally, A4i consists of information promoting engagement in recovery. Results from a feasibility study using a pre–post design (N = 38) report significant improvements in medication adherence; however, the investigators caution the interpretation of results.[20] Despite this caution, participants felt A4i significantly helped them remember to take their medications. Furthermore, measures of psychiatric symptoms significantly improved postintervention.

Two European information technology companies designed apps for SM of mood, activity levels, sleep, and medication adherence for people with bipolar disorder.[27] The 2 apps, Pulso and Trilogis-Monsenso, were compared with feasibility and usability in 3 European countries (Italy, Spain, and Denmark). Pulso allows users to evaluate their mood, activity levels, social media activity, and medication intake daily. Participants were not prompted to complete these assessments, however. Trilogis-Monsenso sent users daily prompts to evaluate mood, activity levels, sleep, and medication intake. Medication adherence rates for the 2 apps were not reported. Both apps were found acceptable and feasible for this population.[27]

Kumar and colleagues[21] assessed the usability and feasibility of the LifeData system, containing the smartphone app RealLife Exp, among individuals with early psychosis. RealLife Exp sends daily notifications to prompt users to complete surveys on mood, medication use, socialization, and conflict. Approximately 49% of users felt RealLife Exp helped them remember to take their medications. A majority of users felt the app was easy to use and 37% felt the app was useful overall.

SIMPLe was designed for people with bipolar disorder to monitor psychiatric symptoms and provide psychoeducation.[17] The app administered daily prompts for individuals to answer questions pertaining to mood, energy, sleep, medication adherence, and irritability. In addition to daily questions, weekly "yes" or "no" questions were included, based on *Diagnostic and Statistical Manual of Mental Disorders* (Fifth Edition)[28] criteria for manic and depressive episodes, as well as questions pertaining to suicidal ideation. In a 3-month feasibility study, 86% of participants found use of the app satisfactory and 82% found the app useful. Active use of the app decreased, however, from 94% within the first month to 74% during the third month.[17] This is not surprising because active app use generally drops off after 2 weeks of use among people with mental health conditions.[29]

Heal Your Mind (HYM) was designed to provide real-time case management and self-directed CBT for people with early psychosis.[22] This app includes 6 modules, giving users a space to record their thoughts and emotions, rate their psychiatric symptoms, and record daily activities, such as social activities and medication regimens. Additionally, the app provides a space where users can communicate with case managers in real time as well the as the ability for users to share their self-directed CBT and self-rated psychiatric symptoms.[22] In a feasibility study,[22] a majority of participants used the HYM app once or twice a week. Overall, participants found the app easy to use and were satisfied with using the app. Additionally, 71% of participants reported receiving psychiatric help through use of the app.

CBT2go is an app designed for individuals with bipolar disorder or schizophrenia.[30] Participants receive a single session of in-person CBT that is augmented through use of CBT2go.[30] The app prompts users 3 times daily. During the morning, the app asked participants questions pertaining to mood or presence of auditory hallucinations. In the afternoon, participations were asked questions regarding their socialization. In the evening, participants were asked about their medication routine. Depp and colleagues[30] conducted a randomized controlled trial to explore the impact of CBT2go on global psychiatric symptoms and overall functioning, as measured by the Brief Psychiatric Rating Scale (BPRS) and Specific Levels of Function (SLOF) scale, respectively. Participants (n = 255) were randomized to CBT2go, to SM (similar to CBT2go without CBT elements), or to receive treatment as usual (TAU). Modest improvements were found in BPRS scores in both the CBT2go and SM groups compared with TAU; CBT2go and SM scores were not significantly different from each other. The CBT2go group showed significant improvements in SLOF scores, whereas the SM group did not.

The PeerTECH app is an adaptation of Integrated Illness Management and Recovery (I-IMR).[18] The app provides users with personalized self-management support, intervention components relevant to the user's needs and goals, medication reminders, and a Health Insurance Portability and Accountability Act–compliant chat feature. A small pilot study (N = 8) explored the feasibility and acceptability of PeerTECH among older adults with SMI.[18] In addition to access to the app, participants met weekly with a certified peer specialist to review modules adapted from I-IMR using a tablet. A certified peer specialist is a person with a lived experience of a mental health condition. This lived experience is used to promote recovery, instill hope, enhance engagement with treatment and services, and help strength social support. Over the 12-week study duration, 4 participants used the medication adherence feature and reported that they took their medication daily. Within the field of mental health and the recovery movement, taking medications is a personal choice. As such, participants were not required to use the medication adherence feature.

Psychiatric self-management skills improved significantly among all participants. Additionally, participants reported increased levels of hope, social support, and empowerment.

FOCUS is a smartphone system consisting of 3 apps and designed specifically for people with schizophrenia to promote self-management skills.[23] Users are prompted daily to check in with FOCUS; once in the app, users can complete interventions pertaining to taking medication as prescribed, mood regulation, sleep, and social functioning.[23] In a feasibility trial, approximately 90% of participants found the app acceptable and useable.[24] When compared with a peer-led, group-based, self-management intervention, participants were more likely to use FOCUS than attend group sessions.[31] Additionally, FOCUS was found to significantly reduce depressive symptoms among individuals with schizophrenia spectrum disorders, bipolar disorder, and major depressive disorder (**Table 1**).[25]

TECHNOLOGY FEATURES THAT FACILITATE MEDICATION ADHERENCE

In a study of an online psychosocial intervention for psychosis, participants were more likely to be engaged if they received weekly e-mail support in which online coaches provided participants with encouragement to engage in the intervention.[32] Reciprocal accountability[33] and supportive accountability[34] both are frameworks that suggest

incorporating human factors in digital interventions may increase engagement, because users are held accountable through the use of a clinician (supportive accountability[34]) or a peer support specialist (reciprocal accountability[33]) (ie, synchronous or asynchronous communication with another person via e-mail or other digital avenues, such as text messaging or in-app chat features). Accountability also may be enhanced by making users aware of what is expected from them, allowing users to set pertinent and relevant goals, and including some form of performance monitoring. Incorporating elements of the reciprocal accountability,[33] supportive accountability,[34] and object relations[35] within smartphone apps for people with SMI may increase rates of adherence and engagement among users. A recent systematic review examined features of apps and their impact on engagement.[36] Researchers found that live (not automatic or artificial) peer support had the highest engagement (17%) compared with other features (ie, trackers = 6.3%; mindfulness/mediation = 4.1%; breathing exercises = 1.6%; and psychoeducation = 3%).[36] As such, utilizing peer support specialists as the social presence element may increase engagement further, which, in turn, may increase taking medication as prescribed.[37] Peer support specialists are individuals with a lived experience of mental illness who use their experience to promote recovery, instill hope, promote treatment engagement, and strengthen social supports.

Functional factors of smartphone apps, such as efficiency and ease of use, also may play a role in user engagement. Community-engaged research and user-centered design can facilitate the development, implementation, and acceptance of digital interventions by partnering with the target population to better understand their needs and desired outcomes of the intervention.[37] Several of the apps, described previously, were designed in this manner.[13,16–18,20,23]

PARALLELS TO TREATMENT OF SLEEP APNEA

The use of positive airway pressure (PAP) is a well-established, efficacious way to alleviate moderate-to-severe obstructive sleep apnea (OSA) symptoms and improve overall quality of life.[38] Unfortunately, rates of using PAP as prescribed is relatively low.[39] The rates of adherence may be associated with education level, socioeconomic status, disease severity, perception of control over one's illness, social support, and marital status or the presence of a bed partner.[40] Given the success in other disease states, a smartphone app may help improve PAP usage

Table 1
Summary of application adherence, feasibility, and acceptability

Smartphone Application for Serious Mental Illness	Adherence (Primary vs Secondary Feature)	How Were Factors Measured (Objectively vs Self-report)?	Adherence Results	Feasibility	Acceptability
A4i	Secondary	—	Not significant	Users reported improvements in medication adherence, focus, thoughts, and mental health.	Some users reported ease of use; others reported the app to feel "old school" and that it could function more smoothly.
CBT2go	Secondary	Self-report	—		
Focus	Secondary	—	—	—	90% of participants found the application acceptable and useable.
Ginger.io	Secondary	—	—	A majority of users reported the application helped them remember their medication doses.	—
HYM	Secondary	Self-report	—	83% of users reported the application was easy to learn and use.	Approximately 80% of users were satisfied with the application.
MedActive	Primary	Self-report	100%	Only 14% (n = 1) of participants reported technical difficulties.	80% of users responded to ecological momentary assessments.
MedLink	Primary	Objective	82%	Users gave the application a 6.6 for learnability on a 7-point Likert scale.	Users gave the application a 5.6 for likability on a 7-point Likert scale.
Monarca (I and II)	Secondary	Self-report	Not significant compared with control		

(continued on next page)

Table 1
(continued)

Smartphone Application for Serious Mental Illness	Adherence (Primary vs Secondary Feature)	How Were Factors Measured (Objectively vs Self-report)?	Adherence Results	Feasibility	Acceptability
MyT	Primary	Self-report	Decreased missed doses by 22%		
PeerTECH	Secondary	Self-report	Of those who used the medication adherence feature (n = 4), 100%	Feasibility was established by users' capacity to use the smartphone application. Users completed 42% of self-management tasks.	
Pulso	Secondary	—	—	On a scale of 1 = strongly agree to 7 = strongly disagree, the mean score for usefulness was 3.8.	On a scale of 1 = strongly agree to 7 = strongly disagree, the mean score for application satisfaction was 3.8.
RealLife Exp	Secondary	Self-report	49% reported it helped them remember medication doses.	A majority of users found the application easy to use.	37% of users felt the application was useful overall.
SIMPLe	Secondary	Self-report	—	82% of users found the application useful.	86% agreed the application was acceptable and satisfactory.
Trilogis-Monseno	Secondary	—	—	On a scale of 1 = strongly agree to 7 = strongly disagree, the mean score for usefulness was 4.2.	On a scale of 1 = strongly agree to 7 = strongly disagree, the mean score for application satisfaction was 4.5.

as prescribed; however, current use of mobile technology in this manner is limited.

The smartphone app, APPnea,[41] sends daily prompts for users to answer 2 yes-or-no questions pertaining to PAP use, physical activity, and dietary habits. A 6-week pilot study found the app feasible and acceptable.[41] Overall, participants had high levels of PAP use; however, pre–post use or use over time was not analyzed. Thus, associations between APPnea and PAP adherence are not yet known.

Appnea-Q was designed to deliver SM tools to individuals with OSA in an effort to increase using therapy as prescribed.[42] The app is divided into 3 sections: follow-up questionnaire, frequent problems, and recommendations. The follow-up questionnaire consists of 10 questions pertaining to PAP use and effectiveness, common side effects, exercise and diet, and weight. The frequent problems section contains a library of information addressing common side effects and issues that PAP users experience. If users do not find the information they are looking for, they are provided with a phone number for a consultation with a sleep unit nurse. The final section contains general information about PAP use, sleep hygiene, and diet. A pilot study found the app feasible and acceptable; however, the app's effect on taking medication as prescribed has yet to be ascertained.[42]

Smartphone apps integrated with elements of CBT may serve to improve PAP adherence. In-person CBT has been shown to increase PAP adherence.[43] As described previously, MyT is an app designed to improve taking medication as prescribed among individuals with bipolar disorder. MyT incorporated elements of CBT and a small pilot study found an increase taking medication as prescribed.[12] Furthermore, educational elements may add additional benefits to taking medication or using therapy as prescribed. Increasing an individual's understanding and awareness of their illness may increase the likelihood of utilizing treatments. Similar to SMI, poor perception of control over illness may adversely affect taking medication as prescribed among individuals with OSA.

DISCUSSION

Medication nonadherence or not taking medication as prescribed is common among adults with SMI and is associated with increased risks of hospitalizations and relapse as well as increased severity of symptoms. Digital interventions, or smartphone apps, may serve to increase taking medication as prescribed among this population.

Currently, there are several smartphone apps designed specifically for individuals with SMI.[12–24,31] A majority of these apps focus on symptom management and psychoeducation, with taking medication as prescribed as a secondary feature. The apps that focus specifically on medication adherence[12–14,26] include small nonrandomized samples and are at risk for bias associated with self-report. Only 1 study relied on objective tracking of medication usage (via the smart pill bottle).[14] In comparison to the sleep field, all modern PAP machines track adherence objectively. Due to the history of people with SMI and their potential traumatic experience with monitoring within institutionalized settings, people with SMI may not find objective monitoring of medication adherence acceptable. For example, the Abilify MyCite is an ingestible sensor on an antipsychotic medication for people with schizophrenia, bipolar disorder, or depression and after ingestion sends a message from the pill's sensor to a smartphone app. In 2019, Abilify MyCite has lost many investors due to the "treatment never gained material traction with patients."[44] In developing technologies for people with SMI, consideration of acceptability is a major issue that may be the culprit in the some of the lowest levels of engagement in digital technologies,[45] thus, subsequently having an impact on adherence.

To address adherence issues with technology, the field is calling for user-centered design in smartphone technology development.[46,47] User-centered design has developed out of the field of engineering and incorporates end users' perspectives in the development of technology through methodologies, such as verbal probing or think aloud,[48] empathy mapping,[49] and/or field usability studies.[50] Promising evidence indicates a combination of user-centered design and community-engaged research.[51] By doing so, end users work as equal partners through the software development lifecycle and have complete decision-making authority.[37] The result has been more acceptable technologies for populations of interest, as evidenced by high engagement rates. For example, a recent systematic review found that a combination of these approaches resulted in the highest levels of engagement by people with SMI.[51]

Poor insight into illness is among the many reasons that contribute to not taking medication as prescribed.[7] Poor insight into illness includes denying, failing to acknowledge, or lack of awareness of psychiatric disorder or psychiatric symptoms. Thus, simple prompts to take medications may not be enough to increase taking medication as prescribed among this population. Participants might not feel as though they need medication or may lack awareness of benefits associated with taking medications.[7] Psychoeducation may help reduce or eliminate poor illness insight. In-person psychoeducation has been found to improve rates of taking medication as prescribed among adults with SMI[36,52]; incorporating these elements within a smartphone app may serve to improve taking medication as prescribed further. Current smartphone apps containing psychoeducation components, such as SIMPLe[17] and PeerTECH,[18] have been found feasible and acceptable among this population; however, associations between use and taking medication as prescribed have not yet been ascertained.

Smartphone apps, including elements pertaining to self-management skills, psychiatric symptom monitoring, and CBT, also may serve to improve rates of taking medication as prescribed. A majority of studies on the apps that included these elements did not report results on rates of medication adherence over time.[19,21,27] The 1 study that did report significant improvements in taking medication as prescribed cautioned views on the interpretation of the result.[20] Lastly, incorporating elements of the supportive accountability model[34] and utilizing peer support specialists may increase rates of taking medication as prescribed further.

Currently, research on smartphone interventions to assist with taking medications as prescribed among adults with SMI still is in its infancy. Future studies not only should explore changes in medication usage after utilization of the app but also examine which intervention components may be associated with improvements in taking medication as prescribed. Additionally, barriers and predictors of engagement and taking medication as prescribed need to be explored further. Adherence research commonly happens in a silo, focused on a particular disease state or type of therapy. Yet, learning from outside disciplines can bring new insights and ideas to challenges. Developing technologies that promote adherence among vulnerable populations, such as people with SMI, presents unique challenges to adherence related to history of people with SMI and potentially their experiences with the mental health system.

DISCLOSURE

The authors have no relevant financial disclosures to report. Dr K.L. Fortuna was funded by a K01 award from the National Institute of Mental Health (K01MH117496).

REFERENCES

1. Lacro JP, Dunn LB, Dolder CR, et al. Prevalence of and risk factors for medication nonadherence in patients with schizophrenia: a comprehensive review of recent literature. J Clin Psychiatry 2002;63(10):892–909.
2. Sajatovic M, Valenstein M, Blow FC, et al. Treatment adherence with antipsychotic medications in bipolar disorder. Bipolar Disord 2006;8(3):232–41.
3. Sansone RA, Sansone LA. Antidepressant adherence: are patients taking their medications? Innov Clin Neurosci 2012;9(5–6):41–6.
4. Phan SV. Medication adherence in patients with schizophrenia. Int J Psychiatry Med 2016;51(2):211–9.
5. Levin JB, Krivenko A, Howland M, et al. Medication adherence in patients with bipolar disorder: a comprehensive review. CNS Drugs 2016;30(9):819–35.
6. Ho SC, Chong HY, Chaiyakunapruk N, et al. Clinical and economic impact of non-adherence to antidepressants in major depressive disorder: a systematic review. J Affect Disord 2016;193:1–10.
7. Velligan DI, Sajatovic M, Hatch A, et al. Why do psychiatric patients stop antipsychotic medication? A systematic review of reasons for nonadherence to medication in patients with serious mental illness. Patient Prefer Adherence 2017;11:449–68.
8. Garcia S, Martinez-Cengotitabengoa M, Lopez-Zurbano S, et al. Adherence to antipsychotic medication in bipolar disorder and schizophrenic patients: a systematic review. J Clin Psychopharmacol 2016;36(4):355–71.
9. Center PR. Mobile fact sheet. 2019. Available at: https://www.pewinternet.org/fact-sheet/mobile/. Accessed February 17, 2020.
10. Ben-Zeev D, Davis KE, Kaiser S, et al. Mobile technologies among people with serious mental illness: opportunities for future services. Adm Policy Ment Health 2013;40(4):340–3.
11. Firth J, Cotter J, Torous J, et al. Mobile phone ownership and endorsement of "mHealth" among people with psychosis: a meta-analysis of cross-sectional studies. Schizophr Bull 2016;42(2):448–55.
12. Wenze SJ, Armey MF, Weinstock LM, et al. An open trial of a smartphone-assisted, adjunctive intervention to improve treatment adherence in bipolar disorder. J Psychiatr Pract 2016;22(6):492–504.
13. Kreyenbuhl J, Record EJ, Himelhoch S, et al. Development and feasibility testing of a smartphone intervention to improve adherence to antipsychotic medications. Clin Schizophr Relat Psychoses 2019;12(4):152–67.
14. Corden ME, Koucky EM, Brenner C, et al. MedLink: a mobile intervention to improve medication

adherence and processes of care for treatment of depression in general medicine. Digit Health 2016; 2. 22055207616663069.

15. Faurholt-Jepsen M, Frost M, Ritz C, et al. Daily electronic self-monitoring in bipolar disorder using smartphones - the MONARCA I trial: a randomized, placebo-controlled, single-blind, parallel group trial. Psychol Med 2015;45(13):2691–704.

16. Faurholt-Jepsen M, Frost M, Christensen EM, et al. The effect of smartphone-based monitoring on illness activity in bipolar disorder: the MONARCA II randomized controlled single-blinded trial. Psychol Med 2020;50(5):838–48.

17. Hidalgo-Mazzei D, Mateu A, Reinares M, et al. Psychoeducation in bipolar disorder with a SIMPLe smartphone application: feasibility, acceptability and satisfaction. J Affect Disord 2016;200:58–66.

18. Fortuna KL, DiMilia PR, Lohman MC, et al. Feasibility, acceptability, and preliminary effectiveness of a peer-delivered and technology supported self-management intervention for older adults with serious mental illness. Psychiatr Q 2018;89(2): 293–305.

19. Niendam TA, Tully LM, Iosif AM, et al. Enhancing early psychosis treatment using smartphone technology: a longitudinal feasibility and validity study. J Psychiatr Res 2018;96:239–46.

20. Kidd SA, Feldcamp L, Adler A, et al. Feasibility and outcomes of a multi-function mobile health approach for the schizophrenia spectrum: app4Independence (A4i). PLoS One 2019;14(7):e0219491.

21. Kumar D, Tully LM, Iosif AM, et al. A mobile health platform for clinical monitoring in early psychosis: implementation in community-based outpatient early psychosis care. JMIR Ment Health 2018;5(1): e15.

22. Kim SW, Lee GY, Yu HY, et al. Development and feasibility of smartphone application for cognitive-behavioural case management of individuals with early psychosis. Early Interv Psychiatry 2018;12(6): 1087–93.

23. Ben-Zeev D, Kaiser SM, Brenner CJ, et al. Development and usability testing of FOCUS: a smartphone system for self-management of schizophrenia. Psychiatr Rehabil J 2013;36(4):289–96.

24. Ben-Zeev D, Brenner CJ, Begale M, et al. Feasibility, acceptability, and preliminary efficacy of a smartphone intervention for schizophrenia. Schizophr Bull 2014;40(6):1244–53.

25. Ben-Zeev D, Buck B, Chu PV, et al. Transdiagnostic mobile health: smartphone intervention reduces depressive symptoms in people with mood and psychotic disorders. JMIR Ment Health 2019;6(4):e13202.

26. Wenze SJ, Armey MF, Miller IW. Feasibility and acceptability of a mobile intervention to improve treatment adherence in bipolar disorder: a pilot study. Behav Modif 2014;38(4):497–515.

27. Faurholt-Jepsen M, Torri E, Cobo J, et al. Smartphone-based self-monitoring in bipolar disorder: evaluation of usability and feasibility of two systems. Int J Bipolar Disord 2019;7(1):1.

28. Association AP. Diagnostic and statistical manual of mental disorders (DSM-5®). Washington, DC: American Psychiatric Pub; 2013.

29. Arean P, Hallgren K, Jordan J, et al. The use and effectiveness of mobile apps for depression: results from a fully remote clinical trial. J Med Internet Res 2016;18(12):e330.

30. Depp CA, Perivoliotis D, Holden J, et al. Single-session mobile-augmented intervention in serious mental illness: a three-arm randomized controlled trial. Schizophr Bull 2019;45(4):752–62.

31. Ben-Zeev D, Brian RM, Jonathan G, et al. Mobile health (mHealth) versus clinic-based group intervention for people with serious mental illness: a randomized controlled trial. Psychiatr Serv 2018;69(9): 978–85.

32. Arnold C, Villagonzalo KA, Meyer D, et al. Predicting engagement with an online psychosocial intervention for psychosis: exploring individual- and intervention-level predictors. Internet Interv 2019; 18:100266.

33. Fortuna KL, Brooks JM, Umucu E, et al. Peer support: a human factor to enhance engagement in digital health behavior change interventions. Journal of Technology in Behavioral Science 2019;4(2):152–61.

34. Mohr DC, Cuijpers P, Lehman K. Supportive accountability: a model for providing human support to enhance adherence to eHealth interventions. J Med Internet Res 2011;13(1):e30.

35. Cohen J, Torous J. The potential of object-relations theory for improving engagement with health apps. JAMA 2019.

36. Bauml J, Pitschel-Walz G, Volz A, et al. Psychoeducation improves compliance and outcome in schizophrenia without an increase of adverse side effects: a 7-year follow-up of the Munich PIP-Study. Schizophr Bull 2016;42(Suppl 1):S62–70.

37. Fortuna K, Barr P, Goldstein C, et al. Application of community-engaged research to inform the development and implementation of a peer-delivered mobile health intervention for adults with serious mental illness. J Particip Med 2019; 11(1):e12380.

38. Giles TL, Lasserson TJ, Smith BJ, et al. Continuous positive airways pressure for obstructive sleep apnoea in adults. Cochrane Database Syst Rev 2006;(1):CD001106.

39. Rotenberg BW, Murariu D, Pang KP. Trends in CPAP adherence over twenty years of data collection: a flattened curve. J Otolaryngol Head Neck Surg 2016;45(1):43.

40. Mehrtash M, Bakker JP, Ayas N. Predictors of continuous positive airway pressure adherence in patients

with obstructive sleep apnea. Lung 2019;197(2):
115–21.

41. Isetta V, Torres M, Gonzalez K, et al. A New mHealth
application to support treatment of sleep apnoea
patients. J Telemed Telecare 2017;23(1):14–8.

42. Suarez-Giron M, Garmendia O, Lugo V, et al. Mobile
health application to support CPAP therapy in
obstructive sleep apnoea: design, feasibility and
perspectives. ERJ Open Res 2020;6(1):
00220–2019.

43. Weaver TE. Novel Aspects of CPAP treatment and
interventions to improve CPAP adherence. J Clin
Med 2019;8(12):2220.

44. Farr C. Digital health start-up once worth $1.5 billion is
racing to keep lights on as investors flee. 2019. Available at: https://www.cnbc.com/2019/12/08/proteus-
digital-struggles-to-raise-cash-after-1point5-billion-
valuation.html. Accessed May 20, 2020.

45. Yeager C, Benight C. If we build it, will they come?
Issues of engagement with digital health interventions for trauma recovery. mHealth 2018;4:37.

46. Torous J, Andersson G, Bertagnoli A, et al. Towards
a consensus around standards for smartphone apps
and digital mental health. World Psychiatry 2019;
18(1):97–8.

47. Rosso P, St-Cyr O, Purdy B, et al. Hype, harmony
and human factors: applying user-centered design
to achieve sustainable telehealth program adoption
and growth. Stud Health Technol Inform 2015;209:
121–7.

48. Priede C, Farrall S. Comparing results from different
styles of cognitive interviewing: 'verbal probing' vs.
'thinking aloud.' International Journal of Social
Research Methodology 2011;14(4):271–87.

49. Neubauer D, Paepcke-Hjeltness V, Evans P, et al.
Experiencing technology enabled empathy mapping. The Design Journal 2017;20(1):4683–9.

50. Duh H, Tan G, Chen V. Usability evaluation for mobile device: a comparison of laboratory and field
tests. Paper presented at: 8th conference on
human-computer interaction with mobile devices
and services. Helsinki, September, 2006.

51. Fortuna K, Naslund J, LaCroix J, et al. Digital peer
support mental health interventions for people with
a lived experience of a serious mental illness: systematic review. JMIR Ment Health 2020;7(4):e16460.

52. Rahmani F, Ebrahimi H, Ranjbar F, et al. The effect of
group psychoeducation program on medication
adherence in patients with bipolar mood disorders:
a randomized controlled trial. J Caring Sci 2016;
5(4):287–97.